Health
Boosters
for Seniors

PREVENTION SENIOR **HEALTH LIBRARY**

Health Boosters for Seniors

300 Ways to Improve Your Health after 50

By the editors of
PREVENTION Health Books™

Rodale Press, Inc.
Emmaus, Pennsylvania

Printed in the United States of America on acid-free ∞, recycled paper ♻

Cover and Book Designer: Diane Ness Shaw

The chart on pages 100–102 was reprinted by permission of *The M-Fit Grocery Shopping Guide: Your Guide to Healthier Choices* by Nelda Mercer, R.D.; Lori Mosca, M.D.; and Melvyn Rubenfire, M.D. Copyright © 1995 by Regents of the University of Michigan.

The recipes by Constance Pittman Linder on pages 144–45 are reprinted by permission of the *Tufts University Diet and Nutrition Letter.*

The sidebar on pages 272–73 is adapted from *Thin Tastes Better* by Stephen P. Gullo, Ph.D. Copyright © 1995 by Stephen Gullo Food Control Center. Reprinted by permission of Crown Publishers Inc.

ISBN 1-57954-220-4 paperback

2 4 6 8 10 9 7 5 3 1   paperback

Notice

This book is intended as a reference volume only, not as a medical manual. The information given here is designed to help you make informed decisions about your health. It is not intended as a substitute for any treatment that may have been prescribed by your doctor. If you suspect that you have a medical problem, we urge you to seek competent medical help.

Contents

Part 3: A Lifestyle of Longevity

Part 4: Defeating Disease

Part 5: Answers for a Longer Life

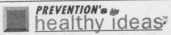

PREVENTION's
healthy ideas

For the best interactive guide to healthy active
living, visit our Web site at **www.healthyideas.com**

Introduction

By virtually every measure we are living longer, healthier, and more productive lives than any generation in history. More people are reaching their eighties, nineties, *and* one-hundreds than ever before. And life expectancy—the average for all people regardless of health—is now more than 72 years for men and roughly 78 years for women.

But getting older would be even better if we could banish heart disease, stroke, cancer, and other dangerous diseases from our lives. In fact, if all major forms of heart disease could be eliminated, average Americans could add nearly a decade to their life expectancy, according to the American Heart Association. And if all forms of cancer were eradicated, the gain would be three years—years you could use to give hundreds more hugs to your grandchildren and marvel at a thousand more sunrises.

The unfortunate truth is that these and other preventable diseases disable thousands of people each year. But as you'll discover in this book, many dreaded diseases don't have to happen to you.

Even if you've been a little lax about exercise and diet in the past, even if high stress and too little sleep have been part of your work ethic for years, it's never too late to turn over a new leaf. You can improve your health and greatly reduce your chances of getting a life-threatening disease by making lifestyle changes now. Some of them are so simple that you may not notice the difference. (See the chart starting on page 100 for some proof.) And if you should develop a serious disorder, lifestyle changes may help you slow or reverse its progress.

If you assume a lower-risk lifestyle—eat less fat and more fruits and vegetables, exercise, and quit smoking—this will put you on the track to good health at any age, say leading doctors. In fact, it is entirely possible to die healthy at an old age.

Our wish is that you find a new vision of healthy aging in the words on these pages. We hope you will be inspired to make changes that will oust the threat of killer diseases from your life.

PART 1

Live Long and Prosper

Why We Die

It's a Small World After All

People in white lab coats have been pondering the "why" behind our imminent mortality since before there was such a thing as white lab coats. And it turns out that the answer, anticlimactically enough, is our reproductive capacity. "The price we pay for sex is death," says S. Jay Olshansky, Ph.D., associate professor, biodemographer, and scientist in the department of medicine at the University of Chicago, Division of Biological Sciences, Pritzker School of Medicine.

In other words, precisely because humans are a sexually reproducing species, all humans will die. That's because once we've passed on our genes, we as individuals are disposable, from a species-wide perspective. That's true, by the way, whether you as an individual reproduce or not. So a life of abstinence won't help you live longer.

Bad as it is for dreams of immortality, this system benefits humankind in the long haul. And, says Dr. Olshansky, it does in a sense provide for a true measure of immortality, since our genetic material is passed on through sex from generation to generation. "Our immortality lies in our genes," he says.

Talkin' about Evolution

The current life-death cycle leaves room for variety in the species, giving our genes the chance to adapt to an ever-changing environment, explains Dr. Olshansky.

3

Each generation can adapt as the world changes and then can pass those adapted genes on to the next generation, he says.

There is a careful orchestration of all our living and dying. "The life spans of most species are linked to their reproductive periods," Dr. Olshansky says. "Mice and insects have short reproductive periods and very short lives. Humans, elephants, and turtles have long reproductive periods and, consequently, long life spans."

The connection is so strong that some researchers are even investigating how pushing back the reproductive period can extend life. "We've already done it with fruit flies," says Leonard Guarente, Ph.D., professor of biology at the Massachusetts Institute of Technology in Cambridge. "If you force them to mate late, over a few generations, you end up with flies that like mating late and that live longer."

But alas, they still age and die. And so do we, despite our best attempts to foil Mother Nature, says George Webster, Ph.D., researcher in molecular biology and aging in Satellite Beach, Florida, and author of *Hello, Methuselah!: Living to 100 and Beyond.* Biologists have determined that each cell in an organism will divide only so many times before it shuts down and becomes inactive, Dr. Webster says. What they haven't figured out yet is how cells decide when they're going to shut down.

The wear and tear of living also pushes this process along, says Siegfried Hekimi, Ph.D., professor of biology at McGill University in Montreal. "You accumulate defects from being alive," he says. "Cells get damaged. Cells wear out. You can slow this down, but there's no way to completely avoid it."

Beating the Clock

Okay, so death is inevitable. But dying before your time is not. Granted, lots of people do make a hasty exit from the human race long before they're ready to pass the baton, but that's not because they're built that way. Often, they simply do things to accelerate the process. The saying "live fast, die young" applies here, says Dr. Webster.

For example, people smoke. They eat fatty foods. They watch television. They sit around and don't exercise. "They do all these wrong things, then they end up with real trouble, like heart disease or cancer, and act like it's a sudden occurrence," Dr. Webster says. "Those diseases aren't a consequence of aging; they're a consequence of living poorly. Start laying plaque in your arteries, and you'll end up with heart disease. Injure your cells with toxins from cigarette smoke, and you'll get cancer."

And even if you somehow escape disease from the damage you've done, you may still accelerate the aging process, so you won't live as well or as long as you should have, adds Dr. Hekimi.

You can affect how long your cells continue to reproduce healthily by taking care of yourself, Dr. Hekimi says. "It's not like your clock is going tick, tock, tick, tock—bang!—you're dead." Your environment, especially your lifestyle, influences the ticking of that clock, he says.

Indeed, there's evidence that controlled, healthy environments such as zoos increase life expectancy in animals. "The animals we take care of in captivity generally live longer in the habitats here than they do in the wild because we make sure that they have a good diet and are tended to when they're sick," says Victor Goldie, of the Docent Council at the Philadelphia Zoo.

"And animals in the zoo are not subject to predation." For example, an elephant's life expectancy in the wild is 35 years, but that could double to 70 in captivity.

If people lived in similar situations—where all our needs were seen to and we were kept from any dangerous environment—we, too, could live years longer, says James Enstrom, Ph.D., associate research professor in the School of Public Health at the University of California, Los Angeles. It wouldn't double, mind you, but an extra decade is a possibility. That assumes a conservative lifestyle, dietary moderation, strong family and spiritual ties, a commitment to education, being health-conscious, no tobacco, no alcohol, no caffeine, no illegal drugs and no sexual promiscuity. (It does sounds like life in captivity, doesn't it?)

But you don't have to check yourself into a human zoo to help your health environment. "You know what to do to live as long as you're supposed to," Dr. Hekimi says. "Don't smoke. Drink in moderation. Be active, but don't overdo it. Don't work too hard. Don't eat garbage."

What it all comes down to, then, is that living to your maximum life span is mostly in your own hands. Experts can help you know what to do. But then you have to do it.

How Long Should We Live?

Testing the Limits

Reaching 100 years of age used to be such an extraordinary accomplishment that NBC weatherman Willard Scott would regularly devote a few seconds of the *Today* show to congratulating any such long-lived "pretty lady" or "fine gentleman." Nowadays, *Today* could dedicate half its airtime to wishing 100-year-olds well.

Just in the 10 years between 1980 and 1990, the population of people older than 85 years increased by 40 percent. By 1990, there were about 30,000 people who lived past the 100-year mark. If we stay this course, researchers predict that by the time 2080 rolls around, there could be as many as 10 million centenarians. With such a growing legion of triple-digit Americans, it's likely that the record for maximum life span—currently set at 122 years—will be broken.

How high can the record go? It depends on whom you ask, because the study of longevity is split into two camps that differ sharply over the limits of the human life span.

One holds that medical technology promises to churn out a future of modern-day Methuselahs. Those who belong to this camp contend that life expectancy, which is the estimated number of years that a person is expected to live on average, will reach 100 in the next generation. And soon, they say, living to 200, 300, or more will not be out of the question.

Researchers in the other camp believe that all species have a genetic program for growth, development, and reproduction that inadvertently leads to a biological limit to life. As far as life expectancy goes, they say, we've just about reached the practical limit.

Pushing the Envelope . . .

Through a combination of curing chronic disease and controlling biological aging factors, the day will come when we live in an "ageless society," says biomedical researcher Ronald Klatz, D.O., M.D., president of the American Academy of Anti-Aging Medicine in Chicago and one of the folks who believes that we've just begun to climb the ladder of longevity. "We won't suffer from degenerative diseases like heart disease and cancer that plague us today," Dr. Klatz says. "We'll just die of total organ shutdown when our cells are no longer able to repair and reproduce. That's at least around age 160."

Unthinkable? Well, splitting an atom was unthinkable in 1928—but by 1938 it was a done deed. Similarly, medical technology will advance in ways we can't begin to imagine, says George Webster, Ph.D., researcher in molecular biology and aging in Satellite Beach, Florida, and author of *Hello, Methuselah!: Living to 100 and Beyond*. "Each year, the National Library of Medicine receives about 1,700 reports on findings in biomedical research," Dr. Webster says. "Who ever imagined that we'd be able to clone a sheep? Yet it didn't take scientists long to figure that out."

Scientists already understand how hormones de-

Life Span versus Life Expectancy

Contrary to what you might think, life expectancy charts don't tell you much about how long you, specifically, have to live. They only predict an average age that you, your next-door neighbor, the president, Larry Bird, Liza Minnelli, and millions of other men and women are expected to live—72.4 years for men, about six years longer for women.

Your life *span*, on the other hand, is how long you actually do live. And if you're in much better physical shape than the average Jane or Joe your age, chances are that your life span will be higher than the life expectancy. "The life span of an individual may turn out to be very different from the life expectancy," says David Smith, M.D., professor in the department of pathology and the Buehler Center on Aging at Northwestern University Medical School in Chicago. "You may die tomorrow, or you could live to be more than 100 years old." In fact, Dr. Smith says, life expectancies aren't very good predictors. "Life expectancies are a prediction of what is to occur in the distant future yet are based on data from people who have recently died," he says. "So they are not very relevant to people living or being born today."

In other words, life expectancy charts are statistical tools, not long-range death sentences. Just because the chart says 72, don't schedule yourself to die then.

cline over time. They have a handle on how our DNA gets damaged over the years. They've studied ways to slow metabolism to prolong life. And they've discovered genes that contribute to aging. Now, says Dr.

Webster, it's just a matter of putting it all together. "We've been able to more than quadruple the life spans of worms by altering certain genes," he says. "Once we understand how these genes work, we can start producing substances that stop their action."

All of which is a good incentive to start living healthfully, Dr. Webster says. Whatever your age is now, if you can make it another 25 years, you'll be able to reap the benefit of the coming anti-aging technology. "If medical technology grows during the next 50 years at the pace it has grown during the past 50 years," Dr. Webster says, "we could push life expectancy into the hundreds.

. . . Or Hitting the Ceiling?

In Genesis 6:3, man's living days are numbered at "one hundred and twenty years." Skeptical scientists don't agree with this. It's not that they doubt that hundreds of thousands of people will be celebrating their 100th birthdays in the years to come. But the buck pretty much stops there, they say.

"It's true that we're living about 30 years longer than we did at the beginning of the century," says S. Jay Olshansky, Ph.D., associate professor, biodemographer and scientist in the department of medicine at the University of Chicago, Division of Biological Sciences, Pritzker School of Medicine. "But if you look at the data, those advances are due to how much we've been able to lower infant and child mortality. Now that we're trying to extend life expectancy on the back end of life, those improvements have slowed dramatically."

In 1993, there was actually a small dip in life expectancy, followed by a stagnant period in 1994. Since then, we've made some gains, and the U.S. Census Bureau expects the numbers to pick up some steam again. So more and more of us will be reaching the century mark, but it doesn't follow that many will go much beyond that mark.

"Though people like to talk about how much we understand the aging process, that doesn't mean that we'll be able to do anything about it," says Siegfried Hekimi, Ph.D., professor of biology at McGill University in Montreal. "We can mutate certain genes in worms so that they live five times longer, but that's by slowing them down metabolically so that they live five times slower. You have to stop living to stop aging, and I doubt that people want to do that."

Quality versus Quantity

Living Life to the Max

T he only way to keep your health is to eat what you don't want, drink what you don't like, and do what you'd druther not."

There are times, to be sure, when it feels like Mark Twain hit the nail right on the head when he wrote that. But with all due respect to the great American author, that's Pudd'nheaded thinking. For the record, you don't have to give up everything that makes life worth living in order to live a long life.

In fact, the whole idea of healthy living is to be able to live life to its fullest in your fifties, sixties, and beyond. For example, you've surely known folks who like to say "I don't want to live forever anyway" as they smoke their cigarettes and eat their fatty foods. "But when they reach an age they used to consider old, they're not any more ready to die than they were before," says Royda Crose, Ph.D., associate professor and associate director of the Fisher Institute for Wellness at Ball State University in Muncie, Indiana, and author of *Why Women Live Longer Than Men*. "And they sure don't say, 'Gee, I'm glad I smoked all those cigarettes and ate all those burgers because now I have emphysema and arteriosclerosis.'"

When it comes to life, the choice is not quantity versus quality, says Ken Goldberg, M.D., founder and director of the Male Health Institute in Dallas and author of *How Men Can Live as Long as Women*. You can have it both ways. The idea is not to extend life for the sake of living longer but to be able to have sex, participate in sports, travel, and enjoy life right up to the very end, he says. "If you're willing to make some changes, that can be for a very long time," Dr. Goldberg says.

You don't have to make New Year's resolutions like "I'll never eat a cheese steak again."

"Small changes, like taking the stairs instead of the elevator and getting enough sleep, can make big differences for the average person," says James Enstrom, Ph.D., associate research professor in the School of Public Health at the University of California, Los Angeles. Aside from the lifestyle changes you hear about all the time, there are loads of honestly enjoyable ways you can make your life happier, healthier, and longer. Here are a few to try.

Living the Sporting Life

Take up a sport, suggests Dr. Goldberg. Almost any sport will do, he says. Recruit some friends to play with on a regular basis. And chances are good that you'll still be living the sporting life all the way into your seventies, if not beyond.

A team of Swedish researchers studied the effects of regular activity throughout life on the physical ability of 233 men at age 76. The volunteers were asked to describe their involvement in competitive sports, recreational sports, occupational physical work, and household work as well as their means of transportation during five periods of their lives, beginning at age 10. The men who had the highest levels of activity after age 35 were the most mobile at 76. And the best activity for ensuring that you'll still be brisk at three-quarters of a century is playing recreational sports.

Regular physical activity has been linked to lower rates of high blood pressure, diabetes, osteoporosis, colon cancer, anxiety, and depression. That doesn't mean you have to join a coed rugby team to reap the benefits of physical activity. "Even making small changes like walking briskly to the bus stop, mowing the lawn without a riding mower, and climbing the stairs at work can make a difference," says Dr. Goldberg. On the other hand, by choosing absolute inactivity, you can shave almost six years off your life span, according to findings from a study of 27,000 people by researchers in California.

As a nice bonus, studies show what we've known

since the days of the recess bell: Taking time to go out and play can sure take the edge off a stressful day.

Curiouser and Curiouser

Research has uncovered an interesting connection between high levels of curiosity and longer life spans. Not only is curiosity a driving force that keeps your gray matter stoked, but maintained over time, it can also help you find ways to cope with the myriad challenges that life throws your way as you age, says Gary E. Swan, Ph.D., director of the Center for Health Sciences at SRI International (formerly Stanford Research Institute) in Menlo Park, California.

"Older adults should attend as many continuing education classes as possible because they provide the environmental support for you to solve problems creatively, to try new things, and to listen to new ideas," Dr. Swan advises.

Saying "I Do" to Health

Comedians have been getting cheap laughs at the expense of marriage for as long as it's been an institution. After all, they keep joking, who wants to live in an institution? But what's really funny about those eternal vows is that as much as we joke about our spouses, the fact is they actually add years to our lives. Finding a mate and being happily married is at least as good for your health as quitting smoking, maintaining healthy blood pressure, eating a low-fat diet, or exercising more than 60 minutes a day.

Marriage may also be the key to disease survival, say experts. When researchers at the Veterans Administration Medical Center in Miami checked the survival rates of 143,969 men with prostate cancer, they found that those who were married lived almost three years longer than those who either were never married or were separated or divorced.

As it turns out, men may get even more out of marriage than women, research shows. "The findings are pretty consistent that being married has plenty of health benefits for men," says study author Joan Tucker, Ph.D., assistant professor of psychology at Brandeis University in Waltham, Massachusetts. "Women traditionally do things for men that have health benefits—things like improving his diet, reducing his risky behavior, providing stress relief, and helping him remember to take medication are all strong health supports."

But whether you are female or male, marriage is even better for your health if you do it only once. Researchers found that the trauma of divorce can be bad enough to negate the benefits of being remarried.

You Are What You Eat

Remember the tired old "an apple a day" cliché? Well, a 20-some-year study of almost 10,000 people in Finland confirmed it. Those who ate the most flavonoids, which are natural antioxidants found in many fruits and vegetables, had lower risks for all cancers and half the risk for lung cancer than those who ate the least. The clear winner for lowering lung cancer rates? You guessed it: apples.

But apples aren't the only fruit of paradise for your health. Those subjects in a Welsh study who ate the most of *any* kind of fruit had half the risk for all cancers as those who ate the least.

Healthy eating in general has become such an accepted life-improver that even major-league ballpark stadiums are hawking fruits and vegetables next to the weenies and fries these days. Busch Stadium, the Astrodome, Dodger Stadium, Jacobs Field, Oriole Park at Camden Yards, Riverfront Stadium, and Shea Stadium all offer vegetables, garden salads, or fruit and vegetable platters. Others, including Candlestick Park and Wrigley Field, offer garden burgers and other healthful stadium snacks.

Laughing in the Face of Death

Most of us were forced to listen to Bobby McFerrin's little ditty "Don't Worry, Be Happy" a few thousand times more than necessary in the last decade or so, but his advice was scientifically sound. If you can laugh in the face of adversity, you can live better, longer.

A Japanese researcher studying 157 men and women ages 65 and older has found a strong connection between maintaining a general sense of well-being and having low levels of total cholesterol, low levels of artery-blocking low-density lipoprotein (LDL) cholesterol, and high levels of healthful high-density lipoprotein (HDL) cholesterol. Lifting your spirits, he concluded, is important in caring for your heart.

Any moves that you make to relieve your stress and lighten your mood will probably decrease your risk for heart attack, says Ichiro Kawachi, M.D., Ph.D., associate professor of health and social behavior at the Harvard School of Public Health.

Getting the Best from Your Genes

The Lifestyle That Fits

Scientists recently found a bad bit of DNA floating around in the genetic coding of mankind. If you inherit it from one of your parents, this dangerous DNA can increase your risk for having a heart attack by 50 percent. Inherit it from both your mother and your father and your risk doubles.

This is just the latest in a slew of findings from geneticists who are reporting that a person's susceptibility to common killers such as heart disease, high blood pressure, and colon cancer can be passed down at birth, putting you in a high-risk category from the moment the cord is cut. This news has left many wondering how much control we actually have over our own health.

The answer: a lot. Scientists are investigating these genetic connections not to dole out death sentences but, rather, to show people what may lie down the road so that they can take the proper measures to head it off at the pass. The doctors who have been telling us that a healthy lifestyle is key to bypassing most life-threatening conditions were right. And they're still right. Lifestyle changes can have an enormous impact on decreasing your risk for diseases, says Walter M. Bortz II, M.D., clinical associate professor of medicine

17

at Stanford University School of Medicine and author of *Dare to Be 100*.

Researchers at the Southwest Foundation for Biomedical Research and the University of Texas Health Science Center, both in San Antonio, found that among 1,236 Mexican-Americans who were part of 42 extended families studied, genes accounted for only 15 to 30 percent of various risk factors for heart disease. So in most cases, Dr. Bortz says, our risk for the diseases that commonly kill us is determined by how we live.

All in the Family

A lot of hospitals are equipped with Orwellian, high-tech equipment that can read your genetic legacy from a single drop of blood. But the easiest way to know what's in your genes is to look at your family tree, says John J. Mulvihill, M.D., professor of human genetics and founder of the Cancer Genetics program at the University of Pittsburgh. "You can definitely see your prominent risk factors in your family history," Dr. Mulvihill says. "And we're learning more all the time. Ten years ago, we didn't think there was any family linkage to prostate cancer. Then people started talking about it and uncovered a strong family connection."

The problem is, most people don't know their family medical history. And most of those who do know don't give it a second thought. Of the 58 people interviewed for one study, nearly half of those having family members who suffered from heart disease or cancer did not believe that their family history had any bearing on their own risk. And men were even less likely than women to think that having a family member afflicted with cancer was relevant to their own risk for the disease.

Thunder in Your Genes

If one of your early childhood memories is Dad or Mom sawing logs on the La-Z-Boy after a good evening's meal, you are ripe to carry on the tradition whether you care to or not. Like the color of your eyes, snoring can be passed down the gene line.

In one study, researchers from Denmark found family history to be the factor most strongly separating habitual snorers from nonsnorers. It was also a major factor in separating typical, garden-variety snorers from those whose snoring is so serious that they have to be relegated to separate rooms during nonwaking hours.

Edmund Pribitkin, M.D., an otolaryngologist at Thomas Jefferson University Hospital in Philadelphia, advises perpetual snorers to try sleeping on their sides rather than their backs, to steer clear of late-night alcoholic drinks or sleeping pills, and to lose weight and exercise.

Snoring is certainly a nuisance for anyone who shares your bed. But sometimes it's a danger signal. Snoring can be a symptom of sleep apnea, a condition in which breathing actually stops during sleep, causing oxygen deprivation and, over time, leading to high blood pressure and an enlarged heart.

Despite this disbelief, studies show clear connections. In Japan, for instance, researchers comparing 363 people with colorectal cancer with an equal number of people who were cancer-free found that those having one first-degree relative (a parent, sibling, or child) with colorectal cancer had almost twice the risk of developing the disease as those with no family history of colon cancer.

Almost nowhere is family history a stronger link than it is for heart disease. As mentioned earlier, just inheriting one tiny bit of faulty DNA from both Mom and Dad can double your risk for developing heart disease.

In the final analysis, we're all likely to be at genetic risk for something, concludes Reed E. Pyeritz, M.D., Ph.D., professor of human genetics, medicine, and pediatrics at Allegheny University of the Health Sciences in Pittsburgh. "I'm fairly convinced that, to some degree, all disease is genetic. So far, the major common diseases to which we've identified genetic links include Alzheimer's disease; arteriosclerosis and all that comes with it, like heart disease, hypertension, and stroke; diabetes; and, of course, most forms of cancer. There's surely more to come."

But despite this bad news, studies still show that these genetic risk factors can be largely offset by making appropriate lifestyle changes or by seeking early medical help in some cases.

What's in Your Hands

Family history may be a strong indicator of the diseases that loom in your future, but it's far from the last word, Dr. Pyeritz says. "Two people can have the same high-risk gene mutation, and one will get the disease and the other will not," he says. "It's hard to know one way or another when we're talking about one gene among 99,999 other genes that also have some influence."

But the greatest influence is exerted by the lifestyle choices—some small, some large—that you make every day: whether you smoke, how much you drink, what you eat, whether you exercise.

The following are some tips that experts offer for taking your health into your own hands.

Keep a running tab. Knowing that you're at risk does you little good if you don't bother to watch for signs of disease. Ken Goldberg, M.D., founder and director of the Male Health Institute in Dallas and author of *How Men Can Live as Long as Women*, recommends keeping tabs on yourself via monthly self-examinations that should include checking for changes in moles or unusual markings on your skin, a quick review of your glands for swelling, heart-rate monitoring, and a search for lumps around your chest. Men should perform a monthly testicular self-exam.

If you have high blood pressure or have had a high blood-pressure reading, you should also have your blood pressure checked monthly. And if you have a family history of diabetes (or are otherwise at risk for it), you should have your blood glucose measured monthly as well, says Dr. Goldberg. If your blood pressure and blood glucose are normal, you only need to have them checked once a year, he adds.

Recognize your inherited habits. Bad habits often can run as strongly down the family lines as bad genes, says James Enstrom, Ph.D., associate research professor in the School of Public Health at the University of California, Los Angeles.

Take an inventory of your habits, Dr. Enstrom says. Do you smoke? Do you exercise? Do you sleep enough? How much do you drink? Do you eat too much? While these things are important for all of us, they're particularly important for folks who have a history in their family of poor health, he says.

Don't pull that trigger. Once you've tracked down your disease profile, learning the common envi-

A History Lesson

A quick look at the ailments that have been hanging around your family for a generation or two can tell you what diseases you need to be on the alert for, says Reed E. Pyeritz, M.D., Ph.D., professor of human genetics, medicine, and pediatrics at Allegheny University of the Health Sciences in Pittsburgh.

"Your doctor should be especially aware of conditions that are 'special' within your family—meaning any common disorders that occur with high frequency and diseases that occur at particularly young ages," Dr. Pyeritz says.

When it comes to discussing your family medical history with your doctor—or to just knowing it yourself—it helps to have your thoughts organized. The following questions suggested by Ken Goldberg, M.D., founder and director of the Male Health Institute in Dallas and author of *How Men Can Live as Long as Women*, can help you do just that. Note that "family" includes father, mother, grandparents, brothers, sisters, uncles, aunts, and cousins.

1. What have your family members died from, and at what age?
2. What medical problems do or did they have?
3. What medications do or did they take?
4. What habits, good and bad, do or did they have?
5. What kind of surgeries or other hospitalizations have they had?
6. What kind of exposures to toxins have they had at work or elsewhere?

ronmental factors that trigger that disease and avoiding them is your best line of defense, Dr. Mulvihill says.

People who are at high genetic risk for colon cancer may be able to lower their risk for polyps by following a low-fat, high-fiber diet because they're staying away from known triggers, Dr. Mulvihill says.

Likewise, diabetes is often a case of a genetic tendency meeting an environmental trigger, says Dr. Mulvihill. Genes that predispose many people to adult-onset diabetes were probably survival genes for our ancestors to help them store energy during prolonged periods of near-starvation. Today, when these genes are combined with the typical sedentary Western lifestyle and high caloric intake, we end up with obesity, insulin resistance, and adult-onset diabetes. Again the answer, Dr. Mulvihill says, is to control what you can, which is how you live. It's well-known that avoiding high-fat, high-sugar fare is a good way not only to keep off excess pounds but also to avoid adult-onset diabetes.

Clean house. When it comes to beating your odds for heart attack, there's still nothing better than giving your lifestyle a good spring cleaning, says Ichiro Kawachi, M.D., Ph.D., associate professor of health and social behavior at the Harvard School of Public Health. "Things like not smoking cigarettes, eating less fat and junk food, eating more fruits and vegetables, exercising, and relieving stress are a whole lot more important than worrying about your genes," Dr. Kawachi says.

The incidences of heart disease and stroke have decreased markedly during the past 30 years. That's because people have been taking their health into their own hands, says Dr. Pyeritz, genes or no genes.

PART 2

The Age Extenders Arsenal

Alcohol

The Spirit of Good Health

There hasn't been much middle ground when it comes to alcohol and health. Prophets, poets, and medicine men have been extolling its life-enhancing virtues since biblical times. Modern medicine, on the other hand, has been reluctant to give even the slightest nod of approval to drinking alcohol. That's not hard to understand, given alcohol's potentially harmful effects on the liver and other organs and its tremendous contribution to accidents.

But as the evidence mounts in alcohol's favor, even the most stoic medical heads are nodding acknowledgment that in moderate amounts it can actually do a body good. The key word here is "moderate." That means no more than two drinks a day, with one drink equaling 12 ounces of beer, 5 ounces of wine, or 1½ ounces of 80-proof hard liquor.

To Your Heart's Content

It all started with the French. They smoke. They eat cheese and crackers. They practically make butter a food group. Yet somehow they manage to have a death rate from heart disease 2½ times lower than ours. When scientists explored the reason why, they uncorked an answer that surprised everyone—red wine.

Red wine is brimming with chemical compounds sporting $10 names such as quercetin, resveratrol, and catechin. These phenolic compounds, as they're called, give red wine its rich scarlet hue. They also may give you some protection from heart disease. Though we need more research to understand exactly how phenolic compounds work, scientists suspect that they operate against heart disease on two fronts.

First, they work similarly to aspirin, keeping the platelets in your bloodstream from sticking together and forming blood clots. Second, they are antioxidants that help neutralize unstable oxygen molecules called free radicals. According to Andrew L. Waterhouse, Ph.D., wine chemist and assistant professor in the department of viticulture and enology at the University of California, free radicals damage your body's low-density lipoprotein cholesterol and make it more likely to stick to your artery walls, causing them to block and harden. "Besides heart disease, free radicals may also contribute to cancer and even aging," Dr. Waterhouse says.

Though wine was the first "adult beverage" scientists said could actually be good for your heart, they've recently given some good news to Guinness-lovers as well. Dark beer can provide protection similar to red wine, and even lighter beer seems to provide mild protection, according to John D. Folts, Ph.D., head of the coronary thrombosis research laboratory at the University of Wisconsin Medical School in Madison and a renowned researcher of a type of phenolic compounds called flavonoids—natural substances which are supposed to lower heart disease risk. To prove that flavonoids in beer might have some health benefits, Dr. Folts mechanically narrowed the arteries of 16 dogs and gave them drugs to make their blood clot. Then he poured each dog either a Guinness Extra Stout or a light-colored lager made by Heineken.

The 11 lucky dogs who got the Guinness had all their clots cleared. Those given the Heineken had their average number of clots reduced from seven to four. Dr. Folts attributes the benefits to the more numerous flavonoids found in dark beer.

There's even a bit of good cheer for those who prefer vodka, white wine, and other drinks that don't contain many dark-colored flavonoids. Just plain alcohol in small amounts may provide heart protection all its own, says Ichiro Kawachi, M.D., Ph.D., associate professor of health and social behavior at the Harvard School of Public Health. A review of a number of studies on the effects of moderate drinking and heart disease concluded that four found benefits from drinking wine; four found benefits from beer; and four from spirits. "That's because alcohol raises your levels of healthy HDL (high-density lipoprotein) cholesterol," says Dr. Kawachi. The evidence is clear, he says: Moderate drinkers do better than abstainers in decreasing their risks of heart attack.

The Cancer Connection

Though heavy drinkers have higher risks for cancers in areas like the mouth, esophagus, and liver, people who drink less—six or fewer drinks a week—show no increased risk. And those who drink moderately may actually lessen their risk for lung, prostate, and other cancers, scientists say.

Researchers in Chicago found that one particularly potent wine compound, resveratrol, not only fought cancer at several stages but also actually seemed to reverse it. In a similar study, researchers from the University of California, Davis, found that when they fed dehydrated wine solids to mice who had been genetically altered to develop cancer, those who ate the wine feed took approximately 40 percent longer to develop tumors than the mice who didn't eat the wine solids. "The antioxidant properties of the phenolic compounds like catechin and quercetin may play a major role in this cancer prevention," says researcher Susan E. Ebeler, Ph.D., of the University of California, Davis. "But we need more research to know for sure."

Living Longer, Living Better

Alcohol doesn't just help against the big life-threatening ailments such as heart disease and cancer. There's plenty of research to show that moderate drinking can ward off other common health problems—the kind that can make life miserable sometimes. Here's a catalog of the conditions you can raise a glass to.

Beating the runs: Diarrhea may not be particularly life-threatening to you, but there's no doubt that it diminishes your quality of life, especially if it threatens to turn your dream vacation into a grand tour of international restroom facilities. Believe it or not, wine may help here, too.

Around the world, wine has long been used as a digestive aid. Now researchers know why. When scientists were experimenting with ways to kill some of our most vicious intestinal foes, including *Escherichia coli* and salmonella, they tried dousing them in test tubes with wine, tequila, ethanol, and bismuth salicylate—better known as Pepto-Bismol. Though the bismuth salicylate did okay, wine was the overall winner—killing more than six times as many bacteria as the pink stuff. (The tequila and the ethanol had no effect on the bugs.) And it seems that just six ounces may be enough to do the trick.

30

Getting unstoned: Kidney stones may not be lethal, but passing one is painful enough to make you wish it were. You'll be happy to know that a couple of beers a day can keep the kidney stones away, according to Harvard researchers. In a large-scale survey over a six-year period, the researchers found that the subjects who drank two or more beers a day were four times less likely to develop kidney stones than those who didn't drink. Wine was not quite as effective, but it still cut the kidney stone risk in half.

Keeping your wits: Maybe you already know about alcohol's ability to remove all memory of your behavior when under its influence. What you may not be aware of is that in smaller, more responsible amounts, alcohol may actually boost your memory capacity. Again, more research is needed, but studies are pointing in that direction.

For example, a study in the Netherlands showed that folks who have a drink or two a day seem to be half as likely to have poor thinking ability as teetotalers. And French researchers found that among 2,273 people older than 65, those who drank 8 to 16 ounces of wine a day were much less likely to develop dementia, which may be an early stage of Alzheimer's disease, than people who drank less or no wine.

Living longer in general: With the combination of all these benefits, a daily bottle of beer or a glass of wine may actually extend your life. In the land Down Under, Australian researchers whose subjects were all over 60 found that those who drank reasonable amounts of alcohol regularly—anywhere from one to three drinks a day—lived significantly longer than the ones who completely abstained. That study was men-only, but in a 12-year study of more than 13,000 subjects of both sexes, researchers in Denmark found that people who drank a couple of glasses of wine a day lived longer than folks who never touched the stuff, the reason being that the wine-drinkers had lower risks for heart disease and stroke. And an American Cancer Society study of 490,000 women and men ages 35 to 69 concluded that moderate alcohol intake in this age group slightly reduced deaths from all causes.

Rules to the Drinking Game

It's worth another reminder: The benefits of alcohol result from responsible drinking. If you customarily say goodnight after parties from a prone position in the back of a taxi, you likely won't enjoy any of the good things you've just read about. While moderate drinking yields health benefits, problem drinking wrecks lives.

If you have trouble with alcohol, you should not drink at all, according to the National Council on Alcoholism and Drug Dependence. One in 10 people who drink will become an alcoholic. Here are some warning signs that you might be that one out of 10.

Heredity: If your mother or father had a drinking problem, your risk is fourfold.

Overdoing it: The national government and other experts draw the line at two drinks a day. Drink more than that and you put yourself at higher risk for developing a problem.

High tolerance: If you drink excessively without really feeling any ill effects, you also may have a drinking problem.

Secret sipping: If you're sneaking drinks, won't talk about your drinking, feel loss of control, or have blackouts, you need help with your drinking.

If you're lucky enough to be problem-free, you

still have to drink responsibly to get the most out of alcohol. According to guidelines established by the federal government, here's how.

Don't play averages. You can't save up your one or two drinks a day and have 14 on Friday night instead. You should drink no more than two drinks a day. Don't binge.

Wait until the dinner hour. Lunchtime is not Miller time. Even one drink during the workday slows you down mentally and physically. Save it for when you get home.

Go right on red. Though health benefits of moderate alcohol consumption are associated with all types of alcohol, remember that red wine is the way to go for antioxidant phenolic compounds. Researchers from the University of California, Davis, tested 20 California wines and listed the most phenolic-rich types. So next time you're poring over a wine list, try one of the winners: Merlot and Petite Sirah.

Companionship

"Opening Our Hearts" Is Good Medicine

It's been a while now since any of us have had the pleasure of hearing the late Roy Orbison sing his hit "Only the Lonely." But we might be treated to a cover version by the Grim Reaper himself. No less an authority than modern medical science maintains that it might just be his favorite song.

That's because the lonely—that is, the disenfranchised, the disconnected, those who feel their lives have no purpose—are the folks at greatest risk for coming down with a bad case of premature death or life-threatening disease, says Dean Ornish, M.D., president and director of the Preventive Medicine Research Institute in Sausalito, California, and author of *Dr. Dean Ornish's Program for Reversing Heart Disease*.

Studies bear this out, including one directed by psychologist Sheldon Cohen, Ph.D., professor of psychology at Carnegie Mellon University in Pittsburgh, in which people with the most diverse types of social contacts and networks were the least likely to be susceptible to a cold virus intentionally squirted up their noses.

Why does social interaction seem to have a life-lengthening and health-promoting effect? Why does mingling and sharing your feelings with others appear to be healing? "Bottom line: Nobody knows," Dr. Ornish says. Theories abound, however. Dr. Cohen and his researchers at Carnegie Mellon believe that having a wide range of social environments is distracting—in a good way. "For example," Dr. Cohen says, "someone whose only social role is worker will find problems at work more distressing than someone who works, has a family, and belongs to social groups."

The stress factor may be key, Dr.Ornish says. Much of his program for heart attack patients is devoted to helping them learn to reduce stressful responses. "We know that when people are under stress, their immune systems are impaired and their cardiovascular system is more prone to heart attacks or sudden cardiac death," he says.

In Dr. Cohen's study, participants' blood levels of norepinephrine and epinephrine were measured regularly. These two hormones are released when we are under acute stress. Dr. Cohen's researchers squirted the common cold virus up the nostrils of all the test participants. Those who became infected were those who had the highest levels of the stress-indicating hormones and were those with the fewest types of social contact.

So perhaps positive interaction with others strengthens our immune systems by encouraging our brains to order the release of protective chemicals or to emit specific electrical impulses. At this point in the medical research, however, it is too early to make that conclusion, Dr. Ornish says.

That's What Friends Are For

Dr. Ornish and colleagues have implemented and studied the effects of programs that include increasing the sense of connection and community. "We have found that the patients initially think that this is the

35

part of the program that will be least helpful," Dr. Ornish says. "And yet when they have gone through the program, they find that it is the most powerful and meaningful part." That's because the peer interaction encourages people to stick with helpful behaviors, such as healthy diets, ceasing smoking, and other goals the programs set forth for the patients, Dr. Ornish says.

Looked at the other way, disconnected people are more likely to engage in behaviors that increase their risk of premature death or disease, according to Dr. Ornish. "People who feel lonely and isolated are more likely to smoke, abuse other drugs or alcohol, eat too much, work too hard, or watch too much television as ways of numbing, distracting, or killing the emotional pain that they feel," he says. "I think the real epidemic in our society is this emotional or psychological or spiritual heart disease—this sense of loneliness, isolation, and alienation that's so common when people feel that sense of disconnection."

Dr. Ornish emphasizes that there's a difference between being alone and being lonely. What it comes down to is that the quality, not the quantity, of relationships is what matters. "It's not so much the number of social contacts you have but the perception of whether you feel loved and cared for and nurtured by them," he says. "Someone could be alone by choice—in a monastery, for example—and they can also feel that sense of interconnection with something spiritual."

Indeed, the benefits of connectedness may not even require a lot of human contact. "It doesn't necessarily have to be another person," adds Dr. Ornish. "Some studies show that even having a plant to take care of, or a pet, prolongs life. Anything that takes us

Good Marriages = Good Health

Scientific studies have consistently demonstrated that companionship contributes to good health. But also keep in mind that the *quality* of your relationship—whether marriage or cohabitation—also affects your health. So says Xinhua Steve Ren, Ph.D., assistant professor at the Boston University School of Public Health and research health scientist with the Center for Health Quality, Outcome, and Economic Research of the Veterans Affairs Medical Center in Bedford, Massachusetts. Here are some of his other findings.

■ Those in unhappy relationships are at a higher health risk than those who are in happy relationships. In fact, their health risk is even higher than those who are divorced.

■ Being separated is more injurious to health than divorce. The separated are more than twice as likely to consider themselves in poor health than married folks are, while divorced people were only about 1.3 times more likely to think themselves in ill health.

■ Separation and divorce can actually improve health—but only in cases where there were serious ongoing marital problems.

■ Separation and divorce are most detrimental to health when the marriage had no prior serious problems and the crisis arose with the sudden discovery of infidelity.

■ All in all, marriage is best. Compared to married people, the unmarried tend to have higher death rates from all causes, higher stress levels, and higher use of health services.

outside of the belief that we are separate and only separate, I think, is healing."

Feeling Better

So how do you go about getting connected? Step one is to learn how to communicate openly with other humans in ways that let them hear you better. A key, says Dr. Ornish, is to practice expressing feelings rather than thoughts.

He recommends adding the words *I feel* and *I want* to your vocabulary, while ridding your language of such phrases as "You should," "I think," "You ought," "You never," and "You always."

There are lots of reasons why this is good communication strategy at any age. Here are some that Dr. Ornish points out.

♦ Feelings connect. But thoughts isolate, especially if they're judgmental.

♦ A thought ("I think you're wrong") can make your listener feel attacked and in no mood to listen. But a feeling ("I feel sad about what you said") is more likely to encourage a listener to hear you.

♦ Feelings are indisputably true statements. Your listener may feel argumentative about what you think. But no one can argue about how you feel. How you feel is how you feel.

♦ Express feelings and you exhibit a bit of vulnerability that people generally recognize and respond to in kind. This raises the level of the communication.

♦ Feelings—that is, emotions—are more effective than thoughts in influencing people.

◆ You can communicate negative feelings (which is just as important as expressing positive ones) without expressing them as judgments or attacks.

Of course, communication means listening as well as talking. You communicate more intimately when you make an effort to hear what other people are saying. Focus on their feelings and expressions, rather than paying more attention to what you're going to say next. Make it clear that you really listened and understood the meaning, Dr. Ornish says. Try it and you'll see that people warm to you as they feel more understood.

Getting a Connection

Once you've mastered the art of talking and listening more effectively, there are other steps you can take to widen and deepen your social circle, Dr. Ornish says. Here are some actions he recommends.

Practice altruism. A major 12-year study showed that those who never do volunteer work are more likely to die young than those who volunteer at least once weekly. So it's in your own selfish best interest to be altruistic, Dr. Ornish says. Help others in ways that you feel comfortable doing, he advises, and never do it because you feel forced to.

Forgive and forget. Make an effort to feel others' pain and forgive their trespasses, Dr. Ornish advises. Simply put, compassion and forgiveness are healing emotions, he says.

Share secrets. There should be at least one other person in the world with whom you can feel free to be completely yourself. Confide in that person. Find people and groups you can let your hair down with and feel comfortable doing it.

Be a joiner. Belonging to a group encourages you to be self-disclosing. That's healing and helpful, Dr. Ornish says. So check out clubs, churches, study groups, support groups, or any other organization that provides ongoing positive social interaction and an opportunity to develop a sense of community.

Meet your "higher self." Develop your sense of communion and connectedness with God or a higher sense of being, advises Dr. Ornish. "On one level we're all separate, you and I," he says. "On another level, we're part of something larger that connects us. . . . Having that spiritual vision, that double vision, being able to see both the unity and the diversity, is a very powerful healing experience for many people."

Breathing Techniques

Take It All In

At 20,000 or so breaths a day, you probably passed the 400 million mark not much after your 50th birthday. You'd think you'd have it down by now, but the truth is that most of us could use some breathing lessons, says breath researcher and psychologist Gay Hendricks, Ph.D., who has taught breathing techniques to Olympic athletes and thousands of others at his Hendricks Institute in Santa Barbara, California.

Dr. Hendricks' criticism of our breathing skills comes after conducting experiments and reviewing more than 300 scientific studies of "breathwork" while researching his popular book *Conscious Breathing*. That has important health implications for people over 50, since breathing is how we rid most toxins, like carbon dioxide, from our bodies and how we cleanse and oxygenate our blood and every cell. If we aren't breathing right, other purification systems—such as our kidneys—get overworked, Dr. Hendricks says.

So what are we doing wrong? "There is one universal breathing problem: the tendency to hold your belly muscles too tense so that you can't get a deep breath down into the center of your body," Dr. Hendricks says. Instead most of us breathe from the top of our lungs, which is inefficient. "Less than $\frac{1}{10}$ liter of blood per minute flows through the top of the lungs," Dr. Hendricks says. "While $\frac{2}{3}$ liter per minute flows through the middle of the lungs, and more than a liter flows through the bottom."

The chest breather constantly discharges too much carbon dioxide and takes in too little oxygen through short, shallow breaths. The imbalance forces the heart to work unauthorized overtime, and that raises the blood pressure.

Health Benefits

Correct, deep, belly breathing, says Dr. Hendricks, has been shown to:

♦ Melt tension. (It counters the shallow tight breaths produced by the instinctive fight-or-flight response that we find ourselves kicked into frequently.)

♦ Clarify and focus the mind.

♦ Increase energy and endurance.

♦ Clear unpleasant emotions. (Two or three big breaths at the onset of an injurious emotion such as fear, anxiety, or depression are often enough to move it out of the body.)

♦ Help manage pain. (This is why it's taught in natural childbirth classes.

♦ Improve athletic performance.

♦ Significantly lower blood pressure.

Deep breathing and breathing in general help in treating many modern-day maladies. "Breathing exercises are a major emphasis of the yoga classes I teach in Hawaii," says Arthur Brownstein, M.D., medical director of the Princeville Medical Clinic and clinical instructor of medicine at the University of Hawaii John A. Burns School of Medicine in Honolulu. Breathing exercises are also a major component of the highly touted stress-management program for heart patients conducted by the Preventive Medicine Research Institute in Sausalito, California.

Doing It Right

To remind yourself to breathe correctly, associate the term *breathe* with normal everyday activities such as standing, sitting, or turning, suggests Larry J. Feldman, Ph.D., director of the Pain and Stress Rehabilitation Center in New Castle, Delaware. Then, he says, taking healthy, deep breaths at intervals throughout your day will be as natural as, well, breathing.

Following are some more basic breathing tips from Dr. Hendricks and Barbara Lang, who teaches Yogic breathing at the Duke University Center for Living in Durham, North Carolina, in an intensive medically supervised program for people with heart problems and other degenerative diseases.

Get past tense. Tense your abdomen. Relax your abdomen. Tense your abdomen. Relax your abdomen. Do this maybe a dozen times, until you are well aware of how a relaxed abdomen feels.

Give yourself a hand. Put your hand on your abdomen. Breathe slowly, comfortably, deeply enough to make your hand rise with each inhalation and fall with each exhalation.

Go for ribs. Keep breathing slowly, comfortably and into your belly. If you are truly breathing correctly, you will feel your rib cage expand to the side with each inhalation.

Move your spine. "Babies can lie in a crib all day without getting a backache because they move their spines with each breath," says Dr. Hendricks. "We tend to hold ourselves more stiffly as we age." With each in-breath, let your spine move away from the chair back (if you're sitting) or away from the floor (if you're lying on your back). On each out-breath, let it flatten against the chair or floor.

Use your finger. Dr. Hendricks suggests the following tension tamer that (like many breathing exercises taught in the West) comes from Asian spiritual teaching.

Close off one nostril with the index finger of your dominant hand and breathe out and then in through the open nostril, slowly, gently, fully. Then close off the other nostril, still using your dominant index finger, and breathe out and then in through the open nostril. Keep your belly muscles relaxed and breathe comfortably, slowly, in and out of your abdomen. Put your attention on the sensations of the breath as it leaves your nose and as it returns. Alternate like this for two minutes, and then switch to the index finger of your nondominant hand and continue for two minutes. Switch back to your dominant hand for one more minute, and then rest for a minute with your hands in your lap. Just don't try it while you have a runny nose.

Herbs

The World's Oldest Medicines

Weeds, seeds, stems, leaves, roots, flowers—these are the stuff of the kind of medicine that people over 50 are increasingly turning to. And with considerably success. Really.

For example, there's a palm seed that relieves prostate enlargement as well as or better than prescription drugs and with fewer side effects. In your spice rack, there's a seasoning that will lower cholesterol levels, decrease your blood pressure, fight minor bacterial infections, and help guard against cancer. Chewing certain roots makes you feel more vibrant. In short, herbs can help you live longer and live better.

Herbal remedies have been used, in some cases, for thousands of years.

What's more, about a quarter of modern prescription medicines in North America are derived or synthesized from natural plant remedies. These days, though, you can find many of the natural originals at your nearest health food store. A lot of herbal remedies are even available in drugstores and supermarkets. Some may even be growing in your backyard.

None of this should encourage you to self-diagnose and self-treat any potentially life-threatening illness. Far from it. But it does make sense to be aware of your options, including the availability of natural healing compounds that often are effective in guarding against ailments that commonly strike people over 50.

The Healing Herbs

Just what are herbs good for? Here's just a partial list of the things healing plants can do for you.

Reduce cholesterol, fight infections. Good ol' garlic does double-duty here. Garlic kills many bacteria, including those that cause ear infections. It also reduces cholesterol and keeps blood from clumping and sticking to artery walls, thus avoiding the deadly narrowing of the arteries that can lead to high blood pressure and heart attacks.

Eating about a clove per day ought to do it, says Varro E. Tyler, Ph.D., dean emeritus of Purdue University School of Pharmacy Sciences in West Lafayette, Indiana, and distinguished professor emeritus of pharmacognosy

Be Careful Playing Doctor

There are those who might think that herbs, being "natural," are therefore safe. But not always, warns Varro E. Tyler, Ph.D., dean emeritus of Purdue University School of Pharmacy Sciences in West Lafayette, Indiana. For example, hemlock is an herb, but it's also a deadly poison, as Socrates found out the hard way.

Even more often-used herbs have their dangers. Ephedra, also known as ma huang, is popular but can cause heart problems. Comfrey, borage, and coltsfoot, all in common use until recently, can cause severe liver problems.

So be careful using herbs. Dr. Tyler offers the following six guidelines for safe, effective herb use.

1. Let your doctor know what you're doing.

2. Consult scientific literature to determine whether an herb is good for a particular condition. Dr. Tyler often credits German studies, reported by the German government's Commission E, as reliable herbal information, in addition to referring people to his own book, *The Honest Herbal*, third edition.

3. When possible, buy products that guarantee standardized potencies on the label. And buy from reputable, reliable companies.

4. Read the label carefully. Make sure that the ingredients you want are in the herbal medication and in the dosage you need.

5. Buy in stores that sell a lot of each product because you want fresh herbs. Many lose their potency as they age—whether in your cabinet or on a store shelf.

6. If you experience side effects or unusual reactions like rashes, stop taking the herb immediately.

(natural pharmaceuticals). But if you're eating it raw, you have to chew it, Dr. Tyler says. That's because garlic gets its power from a natural antimicrobial ingredient called allicin (pronounced like Allison), which is formed when the garlic is chewed or crushed. An odorless alternative that Dr. Tyler recommends is a coated tablet or capsule. Make sure that the label indicates allicin content or allicin potential.

Reverse liver damage. Prescription medication, alcohol, pollutants—all of these things gets processed by your liver. Taking in too much of all that stuff over the years is likely to damage or wear out that vital organ. To the rescue comes an herb known as milk thistle, which Dr. Tyler says seems to guard the liver and even help reverse some damage. The active ingredient here is silymarin. An effective formulation of milk thistle herb should state on the label that it contains 80 to 85 percent silymarin, says Dr. Tyler. Follow the dosage instructions on the label.

In Europe, doctors have been able to counter often deadly mushroom poisoning by injecting a standardized form of silymarin into patients. But that doesn't mean you can use milk thistle as some kind of poisoning preventive. Don't down a handful of capsules just because you know you'll be having some drinks later in the day, Dr. Tyler warns. Taken as an herb, milk thistle is a gentle liver healer, not a short-term liver protector.

Inhibit aging. Sometimes it seems like everybody's *anti* this or *anti* that. Well, that holds true for some herbal remedies, too. Grape seed, for example, is *anti*oxidant. Oxidation is basically the body's equivalent of rust, at the cellular level. It tears down, weakens, and ultimately kills cells that make up our skin and tissues—a process associated with aging and degenerative diseases. Antioxidants, which are found mainly in fruits and vegetables, help counter the cellular wear and tear. How much grape seed should you use? Follow the instructions on the label, says Dr. Tyler.

End constipation, guard against colon cancer. All you have to do is drink slime. That's right. Nice, slimy psyllium in water. Take it flavored or unflavored. Take it as raw husks (which you'll find at the health food store) or as ground-up seeds like those contained in the commercial preparation called Metamucil (which you'll find in the supermarket, along with less-expensive generic versions). Use psyllium daily, says Dr. Tyler, with water and other liquids. *Lots* of liquid—that's key.

This bulking fiber, used daily or more often, gently pushes wastes through the intestinal tract. "It acts like a giant sponge going through the gut, swabbing it out," Dr. Tyler says. "And it tends to remove carcinogens before they can have much effect." As a bonus, psyllium can cut cholesterol, too. For regularity, though, you have to use it, um, regularly. Follow the instructions on the label.

Boost your vitality. Studies show that taking ginseng along with a multivitamin lifts your spirits and makes you feel better, Dr. Tyler says. The active ingredients in this tonic root are called ginsenosides. Since the concentration of ginsenosides varies widely among the many ginseng products on the market, Dr. Tyler recommends that you buy a standardized extract that contains 4 percent ginsenosides. Follow the dosage on the label, he says.

Another herb called Siberian ginseng, which really is not a member of the true ginseng family, works similarly, says Terry Willard, Ph.D., herbalist and director of the Wild Rose School of Natural Healing in Calgary, Alberta, Canada. Dr. Willard suggests taking

A Boost from Nature

Couples in their fifties and sixties deserve a rich and fulfilling sex life. And there's certainly no reason not to accept a little help from your natural friends. Certain herbs, taken as teas or in capsules, have gained a rather sexy reputation over the centuries. James A. Duke, Ph.D., herbalist and ethnobotanist in Fulton, Maryland, offers the following rundown from his book *The Green Pharmacy* of herbs that just might help rekindle the matrimonial fires.

Anise. Its estrogen-like substances reportedly increase libido.

Cardamom. Does this common spice's stimulation of the central nervous system have any sexual effect? Arab tradition holds that it does. It can't hurt to sprinkle a little into your tea or coffee.

Ginger. Arab folk medicine says this common kitchen spice can help men rise to the occasion.

Wild oats. It works for stallions, and some studies say that men also get friskier on a wild oats diet. So if ennui has set in on the male side of the bed, look for products containing *Avena sativa*, the botanical name for wild oats.

Yohimbine. According to controlled scientific studies, one-third of men with erectile problems taking yohimbine get the desired result. But the side effects are dangerous—including anxiety, increased heart rate, elevated blood pressure, and hallucinations. So ask your doctor for the prescription version, yohimbine hydrochloride, which contains only the active ingredient and seems to have far fewer side effects than the herb.

from 500 to 1,000 milligrams of Siberian ginseng twice daily.

Faster thinking. *Ginkgo biloba* may be something of a godsend for folks over 50, because it addresses a problem that often increases with age—memory. By increasing blood flow without affecting blood pressure, ginkgo improves cognition (thinking ability) and has been shown to help with memory problems, concentration difficulties, depression, and dizziness. It is one of the most frequently prescribed medicines in Germany and France, says Adriane Fugh-Berman, M.D., former head of field investigations for the Office of Alternative Medicine at the National Institutes of Health in Bethesda, Maryland, and author of *Alternative Medicine*.

For best results, take ginkgo in a 50-to-1 extract, says Dr. Willard. That means the label should say that it contains 24 percent flavonoid glycosides—the active ingredient that increases blood flow. It's best not to exceed 240 milligrams daily, warns James A. Duke, Ph.D., herbalist and ethnobotanist of Fulton, Maryland, in his book *The Green Pharmacy*. Higher doses can cause diarrhea and irritability.

Shrink an enlarged prostate. Saw palmetto helps, Dr. Tyler says. However, he warns that men should not self-diagnose prostate problems. Let the doctor do that, then discuss alternative treatments, he advises. If the problem *is* an enlarged prostate, then consider the herb. In Germany, doctors prescribe saw palmetto and other herbal remedies nearly 90 percent of the time to relieve enlarged prostates.

Read saw palmetto labels carefully, Dr. Tyler advises, and purchase a brand that contains 85 to 95 percent fatty acids and sterols. The fatty acids and sterols contain the plant medicine that benefits prostate tissue, so you want to be sure that you're getting a potent percentage of that. A usual dose is 80 to 160 milligrams twice daily, Dr. Tyler says.

Cope with depression. Several active principles in the herb St.-John's-wort are proving to be effective antidepressants for mild to moderate depression. It doesn't work instantly, though. The antidepressant effect should be evident within six weeks.

Although St.-John's-wort can be taken as a tea, it is best consumed in capsule or tablet form, Dr. Tyler says. He recommends products standardized to hypericin, an ingredient used as a marker, though not necessarily the active component. Follow label dosage directions carefully.

Solve upset stomachs. Ginger, the cooking spice and the flavor in real ginger ale, is a great stomach-soother and a pleasant motion-sickness preventive, says Dr. Tyler. This root can stop nausea quickly. You can make a cup of tea with ½ to 1 teaspoon grated fresh ginger, or with 1 teaspoon ground ginger. Be forewarned that ginger does have a pepperlike bite. So if you prefer, you can eat some crystallized ginger candy. Or drink real ginger ale (not "artificially flavored"). For motion-sickness prevention, take the cure 20 to 25 minutes before you take off.

Ease sleep. Valerian is a mild tranquilizer that has been shown to help people fall asleep. And it doesn't leave you with the morning hangover associated with sleeping pills, Dr. Tyler says. Valerian smells terrible, so it's better taken in capsule form than as a tea. Follow the instructions on the label, advises Dr. Tyler.

Laughter

Humor as Healer

It sounds funny, but it's true: Laughter is good medicine.

Ever since the late *Saturday Review* editor Norman Cousins published *Anatomy of an Illness*, documenting how he used laughter in combination with his therapy to overcome a potentially fatal connective tissue disease, the medical profession has taken a serious look at the therapeutic power of humor. In one study the production of disease-fighting white blood cells increased by 39 percent in people who watched a 60-minute comedy video, while their levels of a stress-triggering hormone dropped by 46 percent. In another study in 1996, one of the leading humor and health researchers found that blood samples from subjects who viewed a humorous video contained increased levels of a chemical that fights viruses and strengthens the immune system.

But that researcher, Lee Berk, M.D., Ph.D., clinical preventive care clinician and assistant research professor of pathology and laboratory medicine at Loma Linda University School of Medicine in Loma Linda, California, does not take credit for first recognizing the health of humor. He points to a much earlier document, the Bible. "A merry heart doeth good like a medicine, but a broken spirit drieth the bones," we are told in Proverbs 17:22.

Anatomy of a Mirther

Someone tells a joke. The corners of your mouth curl up. Your face crinkles. Depending on the virtue of the humor, you emit a chuckle, a giggle, a chortle, a heh-heh, or a deep-bellied riotous guffaw. That laughter is the behavioral response to a perceptual process known as humor, explains Patty Wooten, R.N., of Santa Cruz, California, who performs as a professional clown for hospital patients and is the author of *Compassionate Laughter*.

Wooten breaks down the physical action into two stages similar to exercise: the arousal phase, when you're the most physiologically active; and the resolution phase, when that guffaw simmers down and you return to a normal resting rate. During vigorous sustained laughter, your heart rate can rise as high as 120 beats per minute, with faster and deeper breaths sending more oxygen into your blood. A variety of muscle groups become active: diaphragm, abdominal, facial—even legs, arms, and back muscles when it's a real knee-slapper. This increases the flow of blood throughout the body. All in all, laughter gives you a good physical workout. In fact, researchers have found that 100 laughs are the aerobic equivalent of 10 minutes on a rowing machine. And, as we all know by now, aerobic exercise is one of the best ways to keep our hearts hardy and assure us years more of laughter.

As for the mind, Wooten says a good yuk "helps us change our perspective on our problems and enables us to develop an attitude of detachment, a sense of self-protection, and control over our environment and other nasty negative influences."

He Who Laughs Last . . .

But in addition to the boon to body, mind, and soul, does humor have long-term benefits? This was the question that tickled Richard Haude, Ph.D., professor emeritus of psychology at the University of Akron in Ohio. Based on the short-term pluses, he and his colleagues speculated that "an ongoing appreciation of humor" just might help people live longer.

To test their hypothesis, Dr. Haude and his colleagues asked 33 older adults with a mean age of 72.3 to rate themselves and a deceased sibling (mean age at death was 64.6) on a scale that evaluates one's sense of humor. The results showed that the surviving siblings had a better sense of humor than their dead relatives. The data are still limited, Dr. Haude says, but the indications are clear.

Now this is all well and good for natural-born comedians, but what about the rest of us? Is there hope for the humor-impaired? Michelle Gayle Newman, Ph.D., assistant professor of psychology at Pennsylvania State University in University Park, thinks so. She found that two groups of people—one that tended to use humor to cope with stress and another that didn't—both benefited from using humor during exposure to a stressful film. All the study participants, even those who didn't have a sense of humor, demonstrated fewer stress reactions to the film when they used humor coping than participants who did not use humor coping. As a result of her study, Dr. Newman now believes that "humor can be learned."

So keep practicing those punch lines. You may never make it to the open mike night at your local comedy club, but you could still be standing to hear the next generation of stand-up comedians.

Medical Testing

Taking Your Health Inventory

When it comes to monitoring health, women do a lot better than men. Because of that, when he treats men Ken Goldberg, M.D., often feels like a mechanic trying to salvage cars after they've been run into the ground. "I see these men who have neglected themselves for years," groans the founder and director of the Male Health Institute in Dallas and author of *How Men Can Live As Long As Women*. "Now they come to me with tons of damage and want to be repaired. Maybe if men had inspection stickers on themselves, they'd take as good care of their own bodies as they do their cars and trucks."

But while men are traditionally more doctor-shy than women, it's equally important for both sexes to have themselves tested medically on a regular basis. That's more true than ever after the age of 50. While you should talk to your doctor about tailoring a medical test schedule that specifically fits your medical needs, there are some general guidelines for the more important tests. Here we'll present a quick overview of these critical tests. Elsewhere in the book you'll find more detailed explanations.

Upping the Ante

Remember how invincible you were in your twenties? Or so you thought. Sure, there was less chance then of serious health problems than there is now, but if you started regular testing early, you're ahead of the game now. Congratulations. But whatever you did in your younger years, it's now time for regular (and more frequent) testing in the following areas.

The Seven Signs

No matter what your age, it's important for women and men to keep an eye out for the seven warning signs of cancer, says Ken Goldberg, M.D., founder and director of the Male Health Institute in Dallas and author of *How Men Can Live as Long as Women*. If you notice one of these signs or symptoms, make an appointment with your doctor right away. The sooner you catch cancer, the better your chance for successful treatment. Here they are.

1. Any change in bowel or bladder habits, such as a thinner stool, a change in color of urine or stool, or a change in frequency

2. A sore that doesn't heal

3. Unusual bleeding or discharge in your stool or your urine (or, for men, in your ejaculate) or coughing up blood

4. A lump or thickening anywhere on your body, particularly under your arm or in or around the chest area

5. Prolonged indigestion or difficulty swallowing

6. An obvious change in a wart or mole

7. A nagging cough or hoarseness

History and physical: It's here that your physician learns, among other things, all about you and your family history: health problems dating back to childhood; any current medical conditions such as allergies, diseases, or medications; lifestyle factors, such as whether you drink or smoke; and any other pertinent information. After age 50, Dr. Goldberg says, this history and physical should be an annual event.

Blood pressure: From age 40 on, you should have your blood pressure checked every two years, says John Coulehan, M.D., professor of medicine and preventive medicine at the State University of New York at Stony Brook School of Medicine. "This might be one of the most important screenings you can have done," Dr. Coulehan says. "There are absolutely no symptoms to high blood pressure. Untreated, it can lead to heart attack, stroke, kidney failure, and many other problems."

Blood count: This test measures the quality of your blood and the levels of three types of blood cells needed for optimum health: red cells, which carry oxygen; white cells, which fight infection; and platelets, which help with blood clotting. Low levels of red blood cells can be a sign of anemia, a major cause of fatigue. Women and men over the age of 50 should have their blood count done every two years, says Dr. Coulehan.

Urinalysis: Fill that cup with a small urine sample and the resulting tests can tell you how well your kidneys function, whether you're drinking enough water, whether you have any kidney stones or urinary tract infections, and even if you have diabetes or some cancers. From age 40 on up, this should be done every two years, says Dr. Goldberg.

Tuberculosis test: Tuberculosis has gone from the history books to the newspaper headlines. And today's strains are harder to fight with traditional medications, making early detection essential. So have a tuberculin skin test every three to five years throughout your life, Dr. Goldberg suggests. You are particularly vulnerable if you live in crowded conditions or work in the teaching or health-care professions.

Cholesterol screening: Those over 50 should have their cholesterol—or lipid profile—screened every two years, Dr. Goldberg says.

Eye exam: After age 40, have your eyes checked every two years to be sure that you're seeing as clearly as possible, says Dr. Coulehan. This should include glaucoma testing, he adds.

Electrocardiogram: You should get a baseline electrocardiogram done at every decade throughout your life, says Dr. Goldberg. This test uses electrodes on your wrists and ankles and chest to determine the electrical activity of your heart.

Any abnormalities that the electrocardiogram shows will alert your doctor that there may be some form of heart disease in progress and that there should be further tests.

Pap test: Reaching menopause is no reason for women to stop monitoring for cervical cancer, says Joseph Aisner, M.D., director of clinical science at the Cancer Institute of New Jersey in New Brunswick.

But after three consecutive yearly Pap tests that show normal, you shouldn't need another for three more years, says Ruth Peters, Sc.D., professor of preventive medicine at the University of Southern California School of Medicine in Los Angeles.

Do It Yourself

Thanks to modern technology, there are plenty of medical tests you can do in the comfort of your own home. Here are some that experts recommend.

Inspect your skin. To guard against non-melanoma skin cancer, do a monthly inventory of your skin for any persistent sores, new molelike growths, or changes in existing moles.

Watch your sugar. If you have diabetes, your doctor may suggest that you monitor your blood sugar levels. You can buy a home monitoring system from most drugstores.

Check your chest. Joseph Aisner, M.D., director of clinical science at the Cancer Institute of New Jersey in New Brunswick, recommends that women ask their doctors to show them how to perform monthly self-exams for breast cancer.

Men should do this too, says Ken Goldberg, M.D., founder and director of the Male Health Institute in Dallas and author of *How Men Can Live as Long as Women*. "Check the area around your nipples and under your arms for lumps or thickenings," he says.

Test your pressure. If you have a history of high blood pressure, it's not a bad idea to have a blood pressure cuff at home, some doctors say. Have your doctor show you how to use and read it right.

See how you see. You can buy an eye chart at most medical supply stores. Hang it on your wall and check your vision from a set distance.

Check your cholesterol. For $15 to $20 you can buy a finger-stick home cholesterol test from most drugstores.

For Mature Adults, Please

At age 50, it's time to add some new tests to your hit parade, Dr. Goldberg says. The main reason is that by this age, women are at increased risk for breast cancer, men for prostate cancer, and both for colon cancer. As you review the following general schedule, keep in mind that factors such as race, your personal health profile and family medical history can change the timing and frequency of your medical tests.

Breast exam: Dr. Aisner recommends annual screening for women over 50. It should include a mammogram and professional breast examination (in addition to monthly self-examinations), he says.

Rectal exam: Nobody wants one. But every 50-plus man needs one every year, says Dr. Goldberg. A digital rectal exam (DRE)—in which your doctor inserts a gloved, lubricated finger into your rectum to feel your prostate—is a man's first line of defense against prostate cancer.

Stool sample: Doctors use a tiny sample of stool to test for any traces of blood—a sign of possible cancer growth or development. This should be done every year, says Dr. Coulehan.

Sigmoidoscopy: Your 50th birthday is a good time to start having this test, and then get it done every five years thereafter, says Dr. Goldberg. A sigmoidoscope is a thin, flexible, lighted instrument that actually lets the doctor look into your rectum and large intestine for polyps, or growths that might signal cancer. The test takes just a few minutes. And don't worry. Doctors insist that the sigmoidoscope is so thin and flexible that although the test is uncomfortable, it's not painful. If you are at higher risk because of family or personal history, your doctor may recommend more inclusive tests such as colonoscopy or a barium enema.

Acing the Test of Life

Doctors have a final piece of advice about medical testing: Don't mistake good grades with good health. "Passing" a battery of tests is not the bottom line. Things like eating less than 30 percent of your calories from fat and staying active are what matter.

"Absolutely nothing is a substitute for good, healthy living," Dr. Coulehan says. "People quibble with me whether their cholesterol levels are 220 or 200 while they're smoking a pack of cigarettes a day."

If you don't take care of yourself, all medical tests do is show you how your unhealthy living is taking its toll, Dr. Coulehan says. "Have a good relationship with your doctor so that you can put your medical tests, your medical history, and your health habits in perspective," he says.

Sleep

Never a Waste of Time

A lot of folks over 50 see sleep as an unproductive waste of time or a sign of sloth. Sleep experts, on the other hand, see it as a restorative daily health tonic, an ally of the alert, the ambitious, and the long-lived.

In fact, researchers suspect and are investigating a direct link between sleep deprivation and disease. There's already at least one study supporting the widespread suspicion among sleep specialists that people who don't sleep very long don't live very long. Several researchers have connected insufficient sleep with less-efficient immune system functioning, possibly via a reduction in the activity of NK cells—the "natural killers" that go after invading viruses.

Disorders and Disdain

A serious sleep disorder such as sleep apnea can quadruple the risk of heart attacks and triple the risk of stroke. But more often the problem with inadequate sleep is a question of basic military strategy. In your war on disease, like any other war, rested troops fight best.

Take stress, for example. While it's still not proved that inadequate sleep causes stress, it certainly sabotages your ability to handle your inevitable daily stress. "If you're poorly rested, you're likely to find stressful situations to be even more so," says sleep researcher Michael Vitiello, Ph.D., professor in the department of psychiatry and behavioral sciences at the University of Washington School of Medicine in Seattle. "And the relationship between stress and health is fairly clear."

Stress isn't the only one of life's little challenges a sleep-swindled brain has a problem with. Your reaction skills also take a hit when you cheat your sleep.

"Relatively small amounts of sleep deprivation will quickly affect your alertness and psychomotor performance," says Michael Bonnet, Ph.D., professor of neurology at Wright State University School of Medicine in Dayton, Ohio, and director of the Sleep Laboratory at the Dayton Veterans Affairs Medical Center. "You become less responsive, especially in a sedentary situation, such as driving."

Small wonder, then, that sleepiness is second only to drunkenness as a cause of fatal single-car accidents. All things considered, getting yourself killed in a car crash is not a recommended strategy for avoiding disease.

So why do so many people shirk their sleep duties? Some suffer from one of the more than 80 disorders dogging our sleep. The most well-known is insomnia—difficulty in getting to sleep or staying there—which haunts women more than men. The most serious, though, is sleep apnea, which can be a killer. It hits most often between 30 and 60, especially those who are overweight. One study found that 24 percent of otherwise healthy middle-aged men had sleep apnea.

With sleep apnea, you literally (and repeatedly) stop breathing when you're asleep. It's actually your body's rescue plan to keep arousing you so that you can breathe again. But the constant waking, even though it's so brief that you won't even remember, deprives you of the sleep you need. Your sleeping hours are virtually worthless; hence, your waking life is virtually nonfunctional. "And that's life-threatening," says Michael Stevenson, Ph.D., a psychologist and sleep specialist at the North Valley Sleep Disorders Center in Mission Hills, California. "It can get bad enough to increase your blood pressure and your risk for stroke and heart attack, not to mention automobile accidents and injuries on the job."

So if you snore (harmless in itself, but also a possible clue to apnea) and you find yourself constantly waking up sleepy and staying that way all day, pay attention. See a sleep specialist, says Dr. Stevenson. Sleep apnea is treatable.

Serious as apnea can be, the most common reason that people of any age don't sleep enough is . . . well, that they just don't sleep enough. We all have friends who insist that they function just fine on limited Zzzs, thank you. But there's a difference between functioning well and just functioning, according to Dr. Vitiello. "I'd never argue with someone who says he can get by on four or five hours sleep," he says. "But his very choice of words condemns him. He's *getting by*."

The A to Z of Zzzs

Sound sleep, then, is an essential element of your overall health strategy. But let's face it, putting long life ahead of live Leno may take some adjusting. As Dr. Stevenson puts it, "You have to work at sleeping well." Here's how.

Get steady. Your "circadian rhythm" is simply the pattern of biological functions (such as the release of certain hormones or changes in body temperature and metabolic rate) that vary with how and when you feel

How Much Is Enough?

How many hours a night should you sleep? Sorry, there's no standard formula. But there are tests you can take to find out. And don't worry: They're strictly pass-fail.

The feelings test: Drowsiness during the day or early evening is a dead giveaway that you need more sleep. "If you fall asleep reading or just sitting quietly before your usual bedtime, you're not getting enough sleep," says Dr. Michael Stevenson of the North Valley Sleep Disorders Center.

The alarm clock test: Did you use your alarm clock this morning? "Anybody who answers yes to that question is at least partially sleep-deprived," says Michael Bonnet, Ph.D., professor of neurology at Wright State University School of Medicine in Dayton, Ohio. If you're allowing yourself the right amount of sleep, you should wake up before the alarm goes off. "Keep going to bed a half-hour earlier each week until you find the point where you don't need an alarm," Dr. Bonnet recommends.

The max-out test: Next vacation, do some sleep research on yourself. A common study technique is to put volunteers in bed for 10 or more hours a night for weeks at a time to see how long they'll sleep when they have more time than they need to do it. Try it. When you wake up, see how long you slept. That's how much sleep you need, says Timothy Roehrs, Ph.D., director of research at the Henry Ford Hospital Sleep Disorders and Research Center in Detroit. If you're like most study subjects, it'll be around 8 hours.

sleepy or alert. The first commandment of circadian rhythm obedience is to keep regular sleeping hours, say sleep researchers. You sleep best when you go to bed at about the same time every night and wake up about the same time every morning.

Haphazard sleeping schedules, on the other hand, can sabotage your circadian rhythm. "Your body temperature does not go up and down as much if you keep a random sleep schedule," Dr. Bonnet says. "So you get into this zombie state where you never feel very alert or very sleepy either."

Stay steady. Why do we sleep late on weekends? Because we can.

Bad idea, Dr. Stevenson says. "The part of your brain that generates sleep doesn't know the difference between Wednesday and Saturday," he points out. "When you sleep in on Saturday and Sunday, you push your sleep cycle forward. It's better to sleep consistently seven days a week."

Catch up on the front end. It'll happen. Overstaying visitors or an evening out will cut into your sleep time. You can make up for some of that lost sleep (but never all of it) the next night. But do it by going to bed earlier, rather than waking up much later than usual, says Dr. Stevenson. Otherwise, you're sleeping right through your circadian rhythm's wake-up call. And then all you're catching up on is lousy, unrestorative sleep. Besides, Dr. Stevenson says, "what matters is how you sleep over the long haul. What you do in a single night is less important."

Ease your way down. You don't bounce a two-year-old on your knee all evening, then throw him straight into the crib and expect him to sleep. He needs to relax first. So do you, if you want healthy sleep. "Give yourself a half-hour or 60 minutes to fade out," Dr. Stevenson says. "You're entering another part of your life, and you can't do it in an instant. You need to withdraw slowly."

You know best what you find relaxing. By definition, it can't be something potentially upsetting. No checkbook-balancing. No doing your income taxes. Television works for some but upsets others. Remember that a lot of tried-and-true sleep-inducers—such as a warm bath or a glass of milk—probably work because you find them relaxing.

Count sheep. We're serious. Dr. Stevenson suggests a sleep-baiting technique you can do once your head hits the pillow. "Keep your eyes open, focus on deep breathing, and try to stay awake rather than try to go to sleep," he says. "Then visualize something you find calming—like fishing on a lake." Or counting sheep? You bet. "That old cliché is actually distracting, relaxing, and kind of hypnotic," Dr. Stevenson says.

Wait until you're sleepy. So you're not sleepy, you say? That's fine, but stay out of the bedroom until you are. That's especially true when you want to sleep but can't. "You start to see your bedroom as this place of torture where you can't sleep," Dr. Stevenson says. "If you're not sleepy, you should get out of there."

In fact, sleep experts urge you to use your bedroom for nothing but sleeping—no television, no writing desk, no rowing machine. Of course, they make an exception for sexual relations.

Keep naps short. There's actually a downward blip in your alertness level around midafternoon, a fine time for a restorative nap. But keep it limited to a half-hour to an hour, says Timothy Roehrs, Ph.D., director of research at the Henry Ford Hospital Sleep Disorders and Research Center in Detroit. Longer naps can actually work against your circadian rhythm.

And any time spent napping is time you won't sleep at night. "A nap is a perfectly good thing if you can deal with that trade-off," Dr. Vitiello says.

Spirituality

Dr. God's Prescription

Want to live forever? Get religion.

The world's major religions may not agree on how we get from here to eternity, but all of them promise eternal life. So it's a nice little cosmic twist that spiritual beliefs may actually delay our journey to the unknown. Numerous studies have suggested that aspects of spirituality contribute to better health, better quality of life, and yes, more years on this mortal coil.

Spirituality is not the same thing as religiosity. True, religious people are spiritual, but spiritual people are not all religious, notes Krista Kurth, Ph.D., a management consultant in Potomac, Maryland, who specializes in spirituality in the workplace. Dr. Kurth's preferred definition of *spirituality* is "the Divine influence working in the human heart."

Note that that's "Divine" with a capital D. For those uncomfortable with the concept of "the Divine," Dr. Kurth offers this definition: "the sense that there is something more than us out there that connects us all." Spirituality, she says, is our link with that something, "our recognition of our connection with the Divine."

Cultivating that sense of connectedness with the Divine has positive health implications for you. Evidence for this doesn't come from clergymen in churches. It comes from scientists in laboratories.

Science Weighs In

Religiously active members of the Church of Jesus Christ of Latter-Day Saints (also known as the Mormons) live longer and have half the death rate from heart disease, cancer, and other debilitating diseases compared to the general population, says James Enstrom, Ph.D., associate research professor in the School of Public Health at the University of California, Los Angeles. Dr. Enstrom knows. He has tracked 10,000 active Mormons for 14 years in order to relate their mortality patterns to their lifestyle. Active Mormons do not smoke, do not drink, and attend church regularly. Sure, abstaining from alcohol and tobacco has a lot to do with their health and longevity. But it's not the whole story.

Church attendance also appears to be a positive health factor. Dr. Enstrom is not sure how church attendance works its magic. But Mormon or not, people who attend church regularly generally are healthier than those who do not attend church, he says. Dr. Enstrom is pretty sure about that because he also followed a large general population sample of nonsmoking people (in an effort to replicate the Mormon lifestyle in a non-Mormon population). What happened? "The nonsmoker who attended church regularly was healthier than the nonsmoker who didn't attend church regularly," he says. Research by other investigators has supported these findings.

But what of the spiritual folks who don't attend church? Do they enjoy better health and a better sense of well-being?

Yes, according to the latest research. For example, the "relaxation response" linked with meditation—a practice with multifarious spiritual origins—provides a plethora of health benefits, says Herbert Benson, M.D., associate professor of medicine at Harvard Medical School and the Beth Israel Deaconess Hospital in Boston and author of *Timeless Healing*. Spirituality also advocates a healthier lifestyle and increases social support, which helps you deal with stress and improves your coping skills.

Positive Energy

Lots of other benefits could come your way if you integrate spirituality into your daily life. People whom Dr. Kurth has studied report:

♦ A sense of deeper meaning, purpose, and direction in life.

♦ A sense of fulfillment. Maintaining a sense of connectedness and direction is hard work but worth it, says Dr. Kurth, because the process of doing it brings this sense of peace and fulfillment.

♦ Renewed energy. "People are so burned out in their work lives and in their lives in general," says Dr. Kurth. "Somehow when one taps into that sense of connecting with the Divine, there is a renewed sense of energy."

◆ An increased feeling of well-being. Psychologists Anne Colby, Ph.D., director of the Henry A. Murray Research Center at Radcliffe College in Cambridge, Massachusetts, and her husband, William Damon, Ph.D., professor of education and director of the Center on Adolescence at Stanford University, conducted a study of people involved in "spiritual work." These were "people who are highly morally committed, people who are devoting their lives to something they really, deeply believe in," explains Dr. Colby. "Helping the poverty-stricken, fighting for civil rights, things like that." Dr. Colby and Dr. Damon found that those who do such work for a long period of time tend to be deeply spiritual and have a very optimistic, resourceful, positive approach to life.

Sometimes you can begin working for others for narrow reasons—perhaps pursuing career or business goals—but eventually adopt another outlook, Dr. Colby and Dr. Damon say. You may start out with selfish motives and end up adopting a broader set of moral goals and a more selfless spiritual perspective simply from the process of doing the work.

Catching the Spirit

Developing your spirituality isn't so much a case of learning as unlearning, Dr. Kurth says. By the time they reach 50, a lot of people have learned to distrust their intuition (that inner voice) and suppress their emotions, for safety's sake.

Men, especially, are often raised that way from birth, but these traits interfere with the spiritual development of both sexes. Here are some "unlearning" tips from Dr. Kurth.

Pause and listen. Don't listen only to your reasoning mind. Listen to your inner urges, nudges, leanings, voices. And give yourself permission to act on them, Dr. Kurth says.

Also, make time to just put the world on "pause," Dr. Kurth says. "We get very caught up with all the events of our lives," she says. "In order to have an intimate connection with some transcendent reality, we have to take time to stop and listen."

Get emotional. "Listen to your emotions and let your emotions and passions inform what you do," Dr. Kurth says. One definition of *enthusiasm* is "being infused with the spirit of God," she says. Often when we are impassioned, we are connecting with our spiritual essence, she says.

Meditate. The simplest, most basic meditation, says Dr. Kurth, is simply to pause for five minutes and focus attention on nothing but your breathing. Breathe comfortably, deeply, naturally. Don't force it. Just relax and follow your breathing for a few moments.

As the body and mind relax in meditation, the brain begins pumping calming chemicals and sending soothing signals that relax your body even more. These signals also stave off or even repair the ravages of stress, a known life-threatener and life-shortener, says Larry J. Feldman, Ph.D., director of the Pain and Stress Rehabilitation Center in New Castle, Delaware. Studies have shown that in the long term, people who regularly practice meditation or some other effective relaxation process develop a much greater tolerance to all sorts of stressors, Dr. Feldman says.

Meet Mother Nature. Take quiet walks in natural settings outdoors, says Dr. Kurth. The beauty, vastness, complexity, and seeming omnipresence of nature can be at once awe-inspiring and relaxing.

Pray tell. Talking over problems in prayer, turning them over to a higher power, is obviously an effort to connect with the Divine. Throughout history many people have found this a helpful spiritual practice, says Dr. Kurth. You might, too.

Make beautiful music. Singing, playing, or listening to inspirational music opens doors to greater spiritual realization, says Dr. Kurth.

Be creative. Working in any of the creative arts can help you discover and develop your spiritual nature. The key here is work that involves inspiration. *Spirit*, says Dr. Kurth, comes from the Latin word meaning "breath," as in "the breath of life." And the word *inspire* comes from the words "in spirit."

Yoga

Stretching and Breathing Away Stress

Yoga claims to be a science, and science itself has shown many of yoga's medical claims to be valid. Surprised? Many in the Western world still are, but the truth is that yoga can help treat a lot of the conditions that can potentially plague 50-plussers.

That includes heart disease, diabetes, back pain, chronic pain, asthma, colitis, arthritis, depressed immune systems, all manner of stress-related illnesses, and more, says Arthur Brownstein, M.D., medical director of the Princeville Medical Clinic and clinical instructor of medicine at the University of Hawaii John A. Burns School of Medicine in Honolulu.

Yoga itself is a complex, several-thousand-year-old, multifaceted system of living drawn and adapted from Hindu teachings. Hatha yoga is the most common style in the West. It consists primarily of focusing attention on the breath and gentle stretches, says Barbara Lang, who teaches yogic breathing at the Duke University Center for Living in Durham, North Carolina.

Saying No to Stress

The greatest and most quickly realized medical benefits seem to derive from the profound calming effect that yoga produces in the mind and body, Dr. Brownstein says. This breaks the debilitating stress cycle in four ways, he says.

◆ Through properly aligning body posture via specific positions (known as poses) and placing mental focus on the efforts

◆ Through slowing, relaxing, and deepening breathing

◆ Through directing attention inward, peacefully, meditatively

◆ Through gently stretching muscles and increasing circulation

A typical hatha yoga class is programmed to take each participant's body through a full range of motion, stretching and strengthening each joint according to its capacity. Regular practice has been shown to ease pain for arthritis sufferers, says Dr. Brownstein. It does this by increasing flexibility, which is a benefit that every yoga practitioner enjoys.

Saying Yes to Yoga

Just as you wouldn't plunge straight into any strenuous exercise without first warming up, you need to prepare for your yoga exercises. Here's how.

See your breath. First, just lie on your back, relax in a comfortable position, and focus on your breathing, says Larry J. Feldman, Ph.D., director of the Pain and Stress Rehabilitation Center in New Castle, Delaware. Experience your breathing getting slower and deeper. Envision it moving in and out. Do this for a few minutes.

This kind of relaxing meditation is perhaps the most important element of yoga for beginners, says Dr. Brownstein. "I tell people, if you do nothing but lie there and breathe and relax during the whole class, you will get something out of it, he says. "It will be a beneficial experience." To add the yoga meditation element to it, simply envision life-sustaining oxygen entering the body and moving into every cell and tissue as you breathe in, Dr. Brownstein says. Feel your muscles relax and tension leave your body as you breathe out. "Let your awareness follow the breath," Dr. Brownstein says.

Bring some towels. To fully concentrate on the exercises, you'll need some small bath towels for your yoga sessions. Roll up one towel and place it beneath your neck as you lie flat on your back—just so it supports the natural curve. Stack folded towels under your head, one at a time, until you find the most comfortable position, the one in which your neck is completely relaxed and not at all strained. You may also wish to place a rolled towel beneath the small of your back for gentle support. Use these in all poses in which lying on your back is necessary, says Dr. Brownstein.

Stop before pain starts. Never go beyond the edge of "comfortable discomfort," Dr. Brownstein says. Never move into pain. Go to the edge of the pain, right to the place where, if you stretch further, it would begin to hurt, he advises. Imagine yourself breathing into that edge, he says.

Be sure to breathe as you stretch. Don't hold your breath as people do when they experience pain. And don't push yourself into the pain. Don't hurt yourself, says Dr. Brownstein. That defeats the whole purpose because you can tear muscle fibers. And if you do feel it's too hard at any time, simply lie on your back and relax and focus on your breathing.

Getting Limber

Loosening and limbering your spine is key to a long life, yogis traditionally claim. Following are two useful yoga techniques that can help you do just that. If you like the gentle stretching and calm inward focus you should experience with these two beginning exercises, consider looking for a class locally. If you have any serious health problems, you will need medical supervision and a yoga instructor who knows how to work with your condition.

Pelvic tilt: Lie on your back, knees bent, feet flat on the floor, arms resting at your sides comfortably. Take a nice, deep breath in, expanding your chest and belly, and exhale. Gently raise your hips off the floor as high as you can without forcing or straining. Your shoulders, upper back, and back of the head should be pressing into the floor. Hold this position for 10 to 20 seconds or as long it's comfortable, allowing the breath to flow in and out of your body on its own. Then, releasing the position as you breathe out slowly, lower your hips back down to the floor and relax. You should work toward repeating this movement up to 10 times.

Spinal twist: Lie on your back. Put your arms out perpendicular to your body, palms up. Bend both knees and bring them toward your chest together. Inhale slowly. As you exhale, lower both knees slowly to the floor on one side of your body. Keep your back flat and arms out. Breathe gently and rest in that position for 30 seconds to a minute. Then inhale, and on the exhalation, slowly bring your knees back to the starting position and repeat the movement on the other side of your body. Do three sets at first. Work up to five.

Vitamins

Just Enough of a Good Thing

Vitamins may be the most convoluted health story of the century. First we discover that without them, we die, slowly and painfully, from deficiency diseases like scurvy and beriberi. Then we figure that, if a little is good, more is even better. Before long we find out that you really can get too much of a good thing, as people succumb to the side effects of vitamin overdose—such as liver damage from too much vitamin D. And now, nearly 100 years after we first heard about vitamins, we're still searching for middle ground.

One thing's for sure: In the proper amounts, vitamins and their sidekick minerals can dramatically improve your health. And one other thing's for sure: Vitamins and minerals alone are not enough for good nutrition. We also need substances known as phytochemicals, such as the flavonoids in red wine that fight heart disease and the carotenoids like lycopene in tomatoes that fight prostate cancer. We need fiber, which keeps us regular, lowers cholesterol, and cuts our risk for colorectal cancer. And we likely need countless other compounds that scientists don't even know about yet. The only way to get all that is from food.

So should you bother with vitamin supplements in your fifties and sixties? Yes, says Katherine Tucker, Ph.D., associate professor of nutrition at Tufts University in Boston. For two reasons: First, we're imperfect. Try as we may, most of us still don't eat well enough to get the Daily Values of all the nutrients we need all of the time, especially as we get older, says Dr. Tucker. Second, there are a few nutrients that can provide us extra protection from conditions like heart disease if we take them in doses higher than what we can get from food. Today, most respected nutritionists recommend loading up on fruits and vegetables and taking a multivitamin/mineral supplement to pick up any slack. Obviously, for the best protection, you should take a multi that has enough of the nutrients you need. Here's what to look for.

E-normous Benefits

If you supplement nothing else, supplement vitamin E, advises Dr. Tucker. You've probably heard by now that vitamin E is an antioxidant. But you might not be aware of just how good this free-radical-fighting nutrient really is. Even researchers have just begun to scratch the surface.

Free radicals are simply oxygen molecules, just like the ones you're breathing in right now, only they've been damaged—meaning that they've lost an electron—via sunlight, pollution, or even your own metabolism. To repair themselves, they steal electrons from your body's healthy molecules, which not only damages your cells but also creates more free radicals. Antioxidants stop this molecular chain of destruction by stepping in and offering their own electrons instead.

Antioxidant action may be most helpful inside your arteries. Scientists have found that free radicals damage your unhealthy low-density lipoprotein cholesterol, making the stuff stick to your artery walls and eventually clogging them up.

Vitamin E is so effective in the fight against this hardening that when British researchers gave more than 2,000 people with partially blocked coronary arteries either 400 or 800 international units (IU) of vitamin E a day for 18 months, these coronary candidates (of either dose) lowered their risk for nonfatal heart attack by 75 percent.

"The benefits of vitamin E against heart disease are pretty well established," says Ichiro Kawachi, M.D., Ph.D., associate professor of health and social behavior at the Harvard School of Public Health. The Daily Value for vitamin E is only 30 IU, a standard that leading health experts consider far below what you need for

Easy-to-Swallow Insurance

The best way to fight cancer, heart disease, and countless other conditions is to eat a diet that's low in meat
and high in fruits and vegetables, says Ichiro Kawachi,
M.D., Ph.D., associate professor of health and social
behavior at the Harvard School of Public Health.

But for those days that a taco shell is the closest you
come to corn, take a multivitamin with 100 percent of
the Daily Value for most nutrients. Better yet, take daily
supplements targeted for the following amounts of
these specific vitamins and minerals, says Dr. Kawachi.

Nutrient	Recommended Amount
Vitamin E	200 to 400 international units
Vitamin C	200 to 500 milligrams
Folic acid	400 micrograms (the Daily Value)
Vitamin B$_6$	2 milligrams (the Daily Value)
Vitamin B$_{12}$	6 micrograms (the Daily Value)
Calcium	200 milligrams (and three to four servings of low-fat dairy foods a day)
Magnesium	100 to 400 milligrams (people with heart and kidney problems should not take supplemental magnesium)
Zinc	15 milligrams (the Daily Value)

disease protection. The problem is that it's practically
impossible to get higher, protective amounts of vitamin E from food alone, since it's mostly found in fatty
oils. You certainly don't want to drink the eight cups

of corn oil that it would take to get 400 IU, so Dr. Kawachi recommends taking a supplement of 200 to 400 IU a day instead.

As a bonus, vitamin E may keep your memory sharp. Though researchers have used only astronomical doses so far (a lot more than anyone should take without a doctor's supervision), vitamin E was able to delay the progression of severe dementia in a group of 341 people with moderately severe Alzheimer's disease, according to a study from Rush Alzheimer's Disease Center in Chicago.

Linus's Legacy

Though the Daily Value for vitamin C is only 60 milligrams, esteemed researcher Linus Pauling took thousands of milligrams of this powerful antioxidant every day, convinced it would fend off everything from the common cold to cancer. Pauling himself lived to be 93, which is pretty impressive, but clinical evidence is still inconclusive about what vitamin C can and can't do.

"We have found that high levels of vitamin C seem to protect against cataracts as well," says epidemiologist Paul F. Jacques, D.Sc., associate professor of nutrition at Tufts University. "But we still need more research to understand what levels are beneficial for most people. So far, it looks like more than two times the Daily Value."

Until we know more, a study at the National Institutes of Health indicates that we need 200 to 500 milligrams of vitamin C a day to keep our systems vitamin C–saturated (we lose vitamin C when we urinate). But since it's easy to get vitamin C from food, experts recommend looking for a supplement with about 200 milligrams.

Folic Acid Frenzy

A once-overlooked B vitamin, folic acid has been shoving its way into the spotlight during the past several years—first as a protective agent against life-threatening birth defects of the brain and spine, then as a potential defender against heart attack and stroke.

The U.S. Public Health Service recommends getting the Daily Value of 400 micrograms of folic acid every day, which can be tough unless you eat a lot of greens, drink fortified orange juice, or eat fortified foods. "Food manufacturers are soon going to be fortifying flour and flour products with folic acid much in the way they add thiamin, niacin, and riboflavin today, which should lead to improvements in heart disease rates," Dr. Tucker says. But until you see folic acid appear on food labels, a multivitamin/mineral supplement containing 400 micrograms of folic acid may help keep your heart healthy.

While you're supplementing folic acid, you may also want to add vitamin B_6 and vitamin B_{12} into the mix, Dr. Tucker says. "There's a concern that by taking a lot of folic acid, you can mask a vitamin B_{12} deficiency, a potentially debilitating condition that becomes more common as we age and our bodies stop absorbing vitamin B_{12} as well as they should," she says. In addition, people who have diets low in folic acid also tend to run low in vitamin B_6, another B vitamin that lowers homocysteine levels. So if you're going to supplement one, you might as well supplement all three. Dr. Tucker recommends looking for a multi with up to 10 milligrams of vitamin B_6 and with 6 to 25 micrograms of vitamin B_{12}.

A Multitude of Minerals

A refined fast-food diet also leaves you lacking in a couple of essential minerals, says Dr. Tucker—magnesium and calcium. Though it doesn't get a whole lot of press, magnesium has been linked to protection from diabetes, arteriosclerosis, hypertension, some headaches, and osteoporosis. Yet Americans routinely consume less than the 400 milligrams (the Daily Value) they should each day. And few get enough calcium without supplementation, Dr. Tucker says. As you know, calcium prevents the bone loss that is so common in women over 50 (and men too). Taking a multivitamin with 100 milligrams of magnesium and 200 milligrams of calcium is smart insurance, she says. However, people with heart or kidney problems should not take supplemental magnesium.

Finally, surveys show that zinc may be the mineral most lacking in diets. That's a serious omission, since zinc helps keep your immune system strong so that you can fight infections and heal wounds. Make sure that you eat enough turkey, oysters, lean beef, or fortified cereals to get what you need each day. Or take a multivitamin/mineral supplement that contains 15 milligrams of zinc. Just don't supplement above that level, according to Dr. Kawachi, or you risk throwing off your body's balance of other important minerals, especially copper, and can lower the body's beneficial high-density lipoprotein cholesterol.

PART 3

A Lifestyle of Longevity

Low-Fat Eating

A Luscious, Rejuvenating Approach to Food

After a two-year, 24,000-mile voyage aboard a 71-foot sailboat, Graham Kerr was stunned by a mutiny in his own kitchen. Kerr, who gained fame as television's "Galloping Gourmet" in the 1960s, his wife, Treena, and their three children had willingly forsaken his delectable but high-fat meals after they discovered that rich foods aggravated seasickness. But the wife and kids revolted against the famed chef's improvised low-fat cuisine as soon as they docked for the final time in 1974.

So while Kerr clung to his newly found low-fat lifestyle, his family eagerly returned to typical high-fat favorites like cheese, eggs, and sausages. The result? Seven years later, Treena suffered a stroke and a heart attack.

Although she fully recovered, Treena was still at high risk for recurrent strokes and heart attacks because she was overweight and her total cholesterol hovered near 350 milligrams per deciliter (mg/dl). So in 1982, she agreed to change her diet. Since then, the couple has stuck to a low-fat lifestyle that consists mainly of fruits, vegetables, and grains. Treena eats no more than 2 ounces of fish, poultry, or red meat daily. Graham's diet allows him to have slightly more, but never more than 6 ounces. By 1995, when she was in her early sixties, Treena had lost 15 pounds; dropped her total cholesterol to 220 mg/dl; raised her high-den-

sity lipoproteins (HDLs), the so-called good cholesterol; and slashed her low-density lipoproteins (LDLs),
the "bad" cholesterol.

"She's done very well," says Kerr, also in his sixties and the author of *Graham Kerr's Best*. "I think
there is no question that you can do wonderful things
if you adopt low-fat eating."

In fact, more and more doctors are convinced

The Skinny on Fat

This table lists the percentage of saturated fat and unsaturated fat in some common cooking oils and fats.
(The percentages do not add up to 100 percent because these fats have small amounts of other fatty
substances.)

Oil/Fat	Saturated (%)	Mono-unsaturated (%)	Poly-unsaturated (%)
11 superb choices . . .			
Canola oil	7	60	30
Safflower oil	9	13	76
Walnut oil	9	23	65
Sunflower oil	11	20	67
Corn oil	13	25	59
Olive oil	14	76	9
Soybean oil	15	24	59
Peanut oil	17	47	32

that eating excessive amounts of fat is second only to smoking as a health threat. A growing arsenal of powerful evidence is proving that cutting way back on dietary fat at any age can prevent or reverse heart disease, short-circuit strokes, and stifle the growth of many cancers, says Michael Klaper, M.D., director of the Institute of Nutrition Education and Research in Manhattan Beach, California.

Oil/Fat	Saturated (%)	Mono-unsaturated (%)	Poly-unsaturated (%)
Rice oil	19	42	38
Wheat-germ oil	19	15	63
Margarine	20	48	32
. . . And 7 ugly ones			
Coconut oil	89	6	2
Butter	64	29	4
Palm oil	50	36	9
Lard	39	45	11
Chicken fat	30	45	20
Cottonseed oil	26	18	53
Vegetable shortening	25	45	20

How Bad Can Fat Be?

Americans love fat. We eat the fat equivalent of six sticks of butter each week. Doing that month after month, year after year, takes its toll by the time you reach 50.

And even more at 60. Of the estimated 13.5 million Americans alive today with a history of heart attack, angina, or both, about 50 percent are age 60 and older. Overall, heart disease and strokes annually kill more than 40 percent of all people who die in the United States. Of the eight controllable risk factors for those two diseases, five—elevated cholesterol and triglycerides, high blood pressure, diabetes, and excessive weight—have been linked to high-fat eating, says Hans Diehl, Dr.H.Sc., M.D., director of the Coronary Health Improvement Project, a lifestyle intervention program based in Loma Linda, California, that has helped more than 15,000 people worldwide reduce their risk of heart disease.

Eighty-three percent of the people who die of heart attack, which can be attributed in part to diet, are age 65 or older.

Heart disease, particularly if it's due to athero-sclerosis (hardening of the arteries caused by fatty buildups in the circulatory system) can at least double your risk of stroke, says Ralph L. Sacco, M.D., director of the North Manhattan Stroke Study at Columbia-Presbyterian Medical Center, an ongoing project examining stroke incidence among 260,000 people living in racially diverse neighborhoods in New York City.

The risk of ischemic stroke, the most common type caused by blood clots that block arteries supplying blood to the brain, may be even higher if you also have heart disease. French researchers who examined 250 men and women in their sixties and seventies found that those who had deposits of fatty plaque narrowing their aortic arches, the main artery leading out of the heart, were up to nine times more likely to have ischemic strokes than those who didn't have such buildups.

"If you have plaque there, more than likely you're going to have it in the arteries leading to or inside the brain, too," Dr. Sacco says.

And Then There's Cancer

Dietary fat also may have a role in up to 40 percent of cancers in men and 60 percent of those that affect women, says Moshe Shike, M.D., director of clinical nutrition at Memorial Sloan-Kettering Cancer Center in New York City and co-author of *Cancer Free*.

Research shows that men in their sixties and seventies who continue to eat lots of red meat are at 2 to 3 times greater risk for colon cancer. They also are more likely to develop rectal cancer and 2.6 times more likely to have prostate cancer than men who limit dietary animal fats. Women older than age 60 who load up on red meat are 2.5 times more likely to develop colon cancer.

Scientists also are learning more about the role of fat in the development of breast cancer. Researchers at the University of Hawaii, for instance, compared the eating habits of 272 postmenopausal women who were being treated for breast cancer with 296 women who lived in the same area but who were cancer-free. They found that overweight women who ate a lot of foods high in saturated fat like sausage, processed cold cuts, beef, lamb, and whole-milk dairy food were at greater risk for breast cancer.

"We know that saturated fats have an impact on

Sorting Out the Lean and the Light

Most folks have mastered the lingo of lipids just enough to know that Minnesota Fats played pool and monounsaturated fats don't. But food labels will include a lot more fatty words and phrases than that. Here are some key ones and what they mean:

Saturated fats are loaded (saturated) with hydrogen atoms. Found primarily in animal foods (meat, poultry, dairy products), these fats tend to raise the level of "bad" low-density lipoprotein (LDL) cholesterol in your blood and increase your risk of heart disease and stroke. Saturated fat has also been linked to several kinds of cancer.

Monounsaturated fats lower the level of LDL cholesterol in your blood and may reduce your risk of heart disease, stroke, and cancer. They are called monounsaturated because they are missing one pair of hydrogen atoms and, therefore, are unsaturated. Olive and canola oils are mostly monounsaturated fat.

Polyunsaturated fats are missing more than one pair of hydrogen atoms. Although they aren't as harmful as saturated fats, they do lower both LDL and "good" high-density lipoprotein (HDL) cholesterol levels and may increase your risk of cardiovascular disease. Polyunsaturated fats also promote cell

hormone levels in the body, and we think that has a role in promoting breast cancer," says Cheryl Ritenbaugh, Ph.D., head of nutrition research at the Arizona Cancer Center in Tucson.

Eating fat also might increase your risk of lung cancer even if you don't smoke, says Michael Alavanja,

division and that can increase your cancer risk. Corn, safflower, and sunflower oils are mostly polyunsaturated fat.

Hydrogenated fats are created when food manufacturers add hydrogen atoms to unsaturated fats so that they solidify and transform into saturated fats. Examples: vegetable shortenings and margarine.

Trans fatty acids are solidified polyunsaturated fats created during hydrogenation. They raise LDL cholesterol levels about as much as saturated fat.

Cholesterol, a fatty chemical compound manufactured by the body, is also found in many foods derived from animals. It helps make important hormones and cell membranes. But excessive amounts of LDL cholesterol narrow your artery walls. HDL cholesterol helps sweep LDL out of the body.

Fat-free. This label indicates less than 0.5 gram of fat.

Low-fat. Has 3 grams or less of fat per serving.

Lean. Less than 10 grams of total fat, 4 grams of saturated fat, and 95 milligrams of cholesterol per serving.

Light. One-third fewer calories or no more than half the fat of the regular product.

Cholesterol-free. Fewer than 2 milligrams of cholesterol and 2 grams or less of saturated fat.

Ph.D., senior scientist at the National Cancer Institute in Rockville, Maryland. In his study of 429 female non-smokers ranging up to age 84, Dr. Alavanja concluded that those who ate the most saturated fat were six times more likely to have lung cancer than those who consumed the least amount of that fat.

"At least seven studies worldwide have shown an effect of saturated fat on lung cancer," Dr. Alavanja says. "It's not conclusive, but the evidence is pointing toward the fact that fat increases the risk of lung cancer among smokers and nonsmokers."

What it comes down to is that you could help prevent and possibly subdue these diseases if you did just one thing: Slash the fat.

"It's very clear that our diet is totally devastating us," Dr. Diehl says. "We know that if we cut the fat content and ate a more plant-food-centered diet, we could drastically cut our risk for most cancers, heart disease, and stroke."

So Why Do We Still Eat Fat?

A surprising number of people—particularly those of us over age 50—haven't gotten the word yet. In fact, one-third of 4,480 people who cook household meals told University of Nebraska researchers that they had never heard that fat was a problem.

"I was very surprised by that finding," says Nancy Betts, R.D., Ph.D., associate professor of nutritional science at the university in Lincoln, who conducted the survey. "The information about fat has been around for a long time. You'd think that by the 1990s everyone would be aware of it, especially the people who are taking care of food preparation for an entire household."

Why are we so perplexed?

Well, you can probably guess that fat exists for a reason. Eating it provides us with essential fatty acids that we need to regulate body temperature, maintain healthy skin and hair, and insulate and protect nerves and vital organs like the heart and kidneys.

The problem is that not all fats are created equal. Monounsaturated fats such as olive and canola oils, and polyunsaturated fats such as corn and safflower oils, are considered healthier than saturated fats, which are found mainly in meats, eggs, and dairy products. Trans fatty acids, another type of harmful fat, are unsaturated fats that have been artificially solidified by food manufacturers to make products like margarines and vegetable shortenings.

Unfortunately, many foods aren't purely unsaturated or saturated. So when you eat a typical American meal, you're likely consuming a mixture of good and bad fats. Therefore, it's possible to unwittingly load up on bad fats even if you chop the obvious ones (such as butter) out of your life.

Why Cut Back Now?

The average American eats about 34 percent of calories from fat. That's down from 43 percent just a few years ago, but a lot of older people continue to consume 40 to 50 percent of their calories from fat, says Cheryl Pingleton, R.D., a dietitian at the Grand Court Lifestyles, a retirement community in Phoenix.

"Many of the people I see are eating a lot of fried foods, creamy salad dressings, and rich desserts," Pingleton says. "They feel as if they've worked their whole lives and now literally want to enjoy the fat of the land."

Enjoying fat too much can lead to serious health problems. If, however, you switch to a low-fat lifestyle, you may quickly feel rejuvenated, particularly if you have a chronic ailment.

"You can lose weight, feel more energetic, have fewer digestive problems, and just feel better about yourself," Pingleton says. "No matter what your age or

Fat-Busting Starts Here

How many grams of fat should you eat each day? First, you need to roughly calculate how many calories you should eat daily based on your age, says Moshe Shike, M.D., director of clinical nutrition at Memorial Sloan-Kettering Cancer Center in New York City and co-author of *Cancer Free*.

To do that, multiply your body weight by 13. (The average person needs to eat 13 calories per pound to do normal daily activities.) Next, subtract 2 percent of that total for each decade starting with your thirties.

So if you are 61 years old and weigh 160 pounds, for example, multiply 160 by 13. That's 2,080 calories. Now deduct 8 percent for being in your sixties. That leaves you with 1,914 calories, your basic caloric need. Now you can use the following chart to figure out the maximum number of fat grams you want to eat per day, depending on whether you're aiming for 30, 25, 20, 15, or 10 percent of calories from fat. Tal-

medical condition—diabetes, gout, high cholesterol, heart disease—low-fat eating is the way to go."

The American Heart Association (AHA) and the National Cancer Institute recommend that no more than 30 percent of total calories come from fat. The AHA says that less than 10 percent of calories should come from saturated fat. Many researchers believe that fat should have an even smaller role on our plates—down to 20 percent or possibly as low as 10 percent of total calories.

"Cutting back on fat will help, and the more dras-

lying your fat grams each day will help you make better decisions when you're reading food labels and preparing meals.

If You Eat (in Calories)	Calories from Fat				
	30%	25%	20%	15%	10%
1,200	40 g	33 g	27 g	20 g	13 g
1,400	47 g	39 g	31 g	23 g	16 g
1,600	53 g	44 g	36 g	27 g	18 g
1,800	60 g	50 g	40 g	30 g	20 g
2,000	67 g	56 g	44 g	33 g	22 g
2,200	73 g	61 g	49 g	37 g	24 g
2,400	80 g	67 g	53 g	40 g	27 g
2,600	87 g	72 g	58 g	43 g	29 g
2,800	93 g	78 g	62 g	47 g	31 g

tically you can cut back, the better off you'll be, with the lower limit being around 7 percent of calories from fat for nutritional adequacy," says Lee Lipsenthal, M.D., medical director of the Preventive Medicine Research Institute in Sausalito, California, where Dean Ornish, M.D., president and director of the institute and author of *Dr. Dean Ornish's Program for Reversing Heart Disease*, is conducting his pioneering research on reversing heart disease. "If you have angina, you'll certainly have less angina. You'll also have less risk of stroke, heart attack, and cancer. And every study that I've ever looked at says it's never too late to make these important changes in your diet."

In fact, according to Dr. Diehl, switching to a low-fat lifestyle even in your later years can help quash the big three killers—heart disease, stroke, and cancer. Here's a look at how dietary fat does its harm and how you can stop or even reverse some of this damage.

The Heart of the Matter

Within five hours of eating a fatty meal like a slice of pepperoni pizza or a bologna sandwich (which are loaded with saturated fat), radical and dangerous changes occur in your body's chemistry, Dr. Klaper says.

First, a tide of fat oozes into the bloodstream and coats red blood cells with a sticky film. "Under normal conditions, blood serum is clear," Dr. Klaper says. "But after you eat a fatty meal, it is thick, white, and greasy. It looks like household glue."

Because they're more sticky, these cells begin to clump together. It's this clumping that eventually forms the blood clots in the arteries, which lead to stroke or heart attack. At the same time, saturated fat raises the harmful LDL cholesterol levels in the blood by suppressing the production of enzymes in the liver that would normally help destroy these compounds.

Adding to your woes, as the body processes the fat, it produces free radicals, the same oxidizing molecules that cause metal to rust and food to spoil. Inside your body, these free radicals cause cholesterol to cling to artery walls and clog them up. Years of eating like that virtually guarantees that by age 60 you'll have at least some atherosclerosis, the underlying condition that can lead to stroke and heart attack.

Arterial rust also makes it more difficult to deliver oxygenated blood, says Dr. Diehl. This starves the tissues and leads to degenerative changes that can cause impotence, hearing loss, degenerative disk disease, memory loss, and vision problems, Dr. Diehl says.

But remember, it doesn't have to happen.

"Atherosclerosis is totally unnecessary," Dr. Diehl says. "But it is reversible, even after age 60. All you have to do is take better care of yourself, particularly how you eat. The simpler your diet, the better your chances of reversing these narrowed arteries and increasing blood flow to more adequate levels once again.

That reversal can happen fast. "In as little as three weeks, most people can eat themselves out of angina symptoms just by switching to a simpler diet that includes very low fat foods," Dr. Diehl says.

Going into Reverse

Several exciting studies have shown that eating a very low fat and low cholesterol diet in conjunction with other lifestyle changes like exercise, smoking cessation, and stress reduction can, as Dr. Diehl says, actually reverse heart disease.

"Our experience has shown that within days of starting a low-fat diet, patients with angina can show an immediate and dramatic decrease in their symptoms," says Monroe Rosenthal, M.D., medical director of the Pritikin Longevity Center in Santa Monica, California. In addition, studies have shown that coronary artery blockages can actually be reversed over a one- to two-year period, he says.

Pritikin researchers, for example, studied a group of 4,587 men and women that included people in their eighties and nineties. After three weeks, those who ate

(continued on page 102)

Minor Metamorphosis Makes a Menu Magnificent

Small changes can make big differences. The daily menus given below (prepared by Nelda Mercer, R.D., of the University of Michigan Medical Center and co-author of *The M-Fit Grocery Shopping Guide: Your Guide to Healthier Choices*) show how. On the left is the typical American diet—2,400 calories, 34 percent of calories from total fat, and 12 percent of calories from saturated fat. The healthier menu on the right provides 2,300 calories, but only 26 percent of calories from total fat and 7 percent of calories from saturated fat. The subtle changes don't sacrifice taste, but make a huge dent in your percentage of fat.

Typical American Diet	The Healthy Alternative
Breakfast	
8 oz orange juice	8 oz orange juice
12 oz coffee	12 oz coffee
1 Tbsp half-and-half creamer	1 Tbsp half-and-half creamer
1 cup puffed rice cereal	1¼ cups ready-to-eat oat cereal
¾ cup 2% milk	1 cup skim milk
	¾ cup strawberries

Typical American Diet	The Healthy Alternative
Midmorning Snack	
12 oz coffee	12 oz coffee
1 tsp nondairy powdered creamer	1 tsp fat-free creamer
1 plain doughnut	1 blueberry muffin
Lunch	
12 oz cola	12 oz instant tea (unsweetened)
1 cup carrot sticks	1 cup carrot sticks
1 oz potato chips	—
Ham-and-cheese sandwich made with:	Grilled chicken sandwich made with:
1 oz regular ham	4 oz grilled chicken breast
1 oz Cheddar cheese	1 oz Swiss cheese
1 Tbsp mayonnaise	2 leaves lettuce
2 slices white bread	1 slice tomato
	1 Tbsp mayonnaise
	1 wheat bun
Afternoon Snack	
1 chocolate bar	1 oz pretzels
	1 medium apple
	12 oz can of diet cola

(continued)

Minor Metamorphosis Makes a Menu Magnificent—Continued

Typical American Diet	The Healthy Alternative
Dinner	
5 oz chicken breast (fried)	1½ cups cooked spaghetti
¾ cup mashed potatoes	¾ cup tomato and mushroom sauce
¾ cup canned peas and carrots	1 oz meatballs
Salad made with:	Salad made with:
1 cup iceberg lettuce, tomatoes, and carrots	1 cup romaine lettuce, tomatoes, and carrots
2 Tbsp ranch salad dressing	2 Tbsp light ranch dressing
1 brown-and-serve roll	1 whole-wheat roll
1 tsp corn oil margarine	1 tsp corn oil margarine
Evening Snack	
1 cup vanilla ice cream	1 cup low-fat vanilla ice cream

a diet that was less than 10 percent of calories from fat and consisted mostly of fruits, vegetables, and whole grains lowered their total cholesterol levels by 23 percent. This reduction sliced their heart attack risk in half.

"There was little difference in drop in cholesterol levels between the young people and the older people," says R. James Barnard, Ph.D., author of the study and professor of physiology in the Department of Physiological Science at the University of California, Los Angeles. "This is clear proof that it's never too late to change your lifestyle and improve your health."

The Ornish Way Works

Even more dramatic results come from Dr. Ornish's landmark work. Dr. Ornish divided 43 men and 5 women with atherosclerosis—many in their fifties, sixties, and seventies—into two groups. The "treatment" group was instructed to go on a strict vegetarian diet deriving fewer than 10 percent of calories from fat. No meat, poultry, fish, or cheese. No nuts or seeds. No chocolate, no coffee, no cooking oils. In addition, they walked for at least 1 hour, three times a week; practiced meditation and yoga daily; and if they smoked, they quit.

Meanwhile, the other group was advised to follow the standard American Heart Association lifestyle program. That is, reduce their fat intake to less than 30 percent of calories, stop smoking, and exercise moderately.

After one year, 82 percent of those in the treatment group had shown reversal of coronary blockage. The average amount of reduction was about 5 percent. But even that modest regression can mean a 100 percent improvement in blood flow, says Dr. Lipsenthal. Those on the AHA diet did not experience these striking results. At best, their disease appeared to progress at a slower rate.

"It's a world of difference. I'm doing things that I never imagined I could do again," says Victor Karpenko, in his seventies and a retired nuclear engineer in Danville, California. When he began the Ornish program in 1987, Karpenko had one artery almost completely blocked, had suffered from persistent angina, and could walk less than a block.

Since then, his total cholesterol has dropped from 290 to 150 milligrams per deciliter, he has lost 30 pounds, his angina is gone, and he regularly hikes in the hills surrounding his home. He also climbs the equivalent of 130 floors on his stairclimber in a half-hour, and he has backpacked in the High Sierras at 8,000 feet with 40 pounds on his back.

"The diet is really the foundation of the whole program," Karpenko says. "I feel so much better now physically and mentally because of it. And it's a diet that really isn't hard to stick to when you consider the benefits."

Little Trims Add Up, Too

But even if you can't see yourself curbing your fat consumption as much as Dr. Ornish suggests, just shaving a modest amount of fat from the obvious sources might have some positive effects.

In the St. Thomas' Atherosclerosis Regression Study in London, for instance, 26 men up to age 66 were put on a diet that limited fat intake to 27 percent of calories and lowered saturated fat to 8 percent of calories. In a similar group, 24 men were allowed to eat their usual English diets, which typically consist of about 40 percent of calories from fat. Three years later, researchers found that 10 men in the dietary group (compared to 1 man in the usual-care group) had small regressions of artery blockages. As a result, the dietary group reported better control of angina and had three times fewer deaths and coronary surgeries and two times fewer heart attacks.

"Anything that you can do to lower your fat is better than doing nothing at all," Dr. Barnard says. "It's like a game of Russian roulette. It just depends on how many bullets you want to stick in that revolver. If it holds six bullets and you eat the typical American diet, then you have five bullets in it. If you want to eat 20 percent, you're down to four. If you go to 15 percent, you're down to three. And if you can manage to get down to less than 10 percent, you may only have one bullet in that pistol, and your risk of these diseases is dramatically reduced."

The Cancer Link: Another Reason to Lower Fat Now

Fat doesn't directly cause cancer. But it promotes it—much like ice on a porch step increases the chances that you'll slip and fall, Dr. Klaper says. Although researchers aren't certain how this happens, they do have plenty of theories. Some suspect that free radicals, produced as the body metabolizes fat, damage a cell's genetic codes and spark cancers. Others believe that fat may interfere with the body's ability to shut down cell growth or that it disrupts the immune system, which may have a protective role against cancer.

High-fat meals also may stimulate production of sexual hormones like estrogen and testosterone that can promote cancer, particularly in the breast and prostate, Dr. Klaper says.

But whatever the reason, it is becoming increasingly clear that the longer you stick to a high-fat lifestyle, the less likely it is that you will remain cancer-free in what should be the best years of your life.

"Eating high-fat foods is like throwing gasoline on

(continued on page 108)

Slash Nearly 100 Grams of Fat Painlessly

Cutting fat out of your foods can be fun and tasty. Here are some simple ways to cut nearly 100 grams of fat from your meals and snacks, according to Cheryl Pingleton, R.D., a dietitian at the Grand Court Lifestyles, a retirement community in Phoenix.

If You Eat:	Switch To:	Fat Savings
Blueberry muffin 6 g fat	A toasted (unbuttered) English muffin with jam 1 g fat	5 g
1 oz bag of potato chips 10 g fat	1 oz bag of pretzels 1 g fat	9 g
3½ oz fried chicken with skin 17 g fat	3½ oz roasted light meat chicken without skin 12 g fat	5 g
2 Tbsp regular French dressing 13 g fat	2 Tbsp reduced-calorie French dressing 2 g fat	11 g
3 chocolate chip cookies 7 g fat	3 fig bars 3 g fat	4 g

If You Eat:	Switch To:	Fat Savings
½ cup rich chocolate ice cream 15 g fat	½ cup peach frozen yogurt 4 g fat	11 g
3 oz corned beef 16 g fat	3 oz lean roast beef (eye of round) 4 g fat	12 g
1 cup cream of mushroom soup 19 g fat	1 cup minestrone soup 3 g fat	16 g
3-in.-square fudge brownie 6 g fat	2-in.-square angel food cake with fresh strawberries 0 g fat	6 g
1 Tbsp margarine 11 g fat	1 Tbsp whipped margarine 7 g fat	4 g
1 Tbsp half-and-half in 2 cups of coffee = 2 Tbsp daily 4 g fat	2 Tbsp evaporated skim milk in 2 cups of coffee = 4 Tbsp daily 0 g fat	4 g
2 oz whole-milk American cheese 18 g fat	2 oz light cheese 8 g fat	10 g
TOTAL: 142 g fat	45 g fat	97 g

a fire," Dr. Klaper says. "You're just fanning the flames of the cancer and helping it spread."

But as with heart disease and stroke, this doesn't have to be your future. In fact, slashing dietary fat might help many of us in our fifties, sixties, seventies, and beyond halt the progression of certain tumors before they become cancerous and prevent recurrences, Dr. Ritenbaugh says.

Derailing Tumors

Cutting back to 20 percent of calories from fat, for example, may reduce your risk of precancerous skin growths and prevent skin cancer in your sixties and beyond, according to researchers at Baylor College of Medicine in Houston. In their study, researchers found that people who continued eating the typical American diet developed three times more precancerous skin lesions, called actinic keratosis, than those who ate a low-fat diet.

Men over the age of 60 who have been cancer-free all of their lives run a 21 percent risk of being diagnosed with prostate cancer, the second leading lethal cancer among American men. But switching to low-fat eating may help stop the growth of microscopic prostate cancers before they have a chance to cause major problems, says William R. Fair, M.D., chief of urologic surgery and chairman of urologic oncology at Memorial Sloan-Kettering Cancer Center in New York City. In his animal studies, Dr. Fair is finding that dipping fat consumption below 20 percent of calories can halt the progression of these tiny tumors.

"I really don't think a low-fat diet could cure a sizable tumor, but if it can halt the progression of a microscopic tumor, then that would be tantamount to a cure," Dr. Fair says.

Cutting back on fat may also stave off colon cancer, according to Harvard University researchers who followed nearly 52,000 male health professionals for two years. Those who ate the least amount of animal fat—about 24 percent of calories—were half as likely to develop precancerous colon polyps as the men who consumed more fat.

"These studies suggest that eating a healthy diet that includes lower amounts of animal fat and higher amounts of fruits and vegetables that have lots of fiber and micronutrients is an important part of what we can do to prevent colon cancer," says Eric Rimm, Sc.D., assistant professor of epidemiology and nutrition at the Harvard School of Public Health.

Women can dramatically reduce their risk of other common types of cancer—particularly breast cancer—if they significantly ease up on fat, Dr. Klaper says.

Researchers put 13 postmenopausal women at the Pritikin Longevity Center in Santa Monica, California, on an eating plan that included less than 10 percent of calories from fat. In three weeks, their blood levels of estradiol, a form of the hormone estrogen linked to breast cancer, fell nearly 50 percent. As a result, the women were far less likely to develop breast cancer at the end of the study, Dr. Barnard estimates.

Even if a woman age 50 or older does get breast cancer, reducing fats may be a good move. Women who have breast cancer might substantially improve their chances of surviving if they are on low-fat diets, according to researchers at the University of Minnesota in Minneapolis who polled 42,000 women between the ages of 55 and 69 on their eating habits. Of the 698 women who developed breast cancer in the next five years, those who reported eating 56 grams of fat a day (almost 2 ounces)

Eat like a Peasant, Live like a King

It's cheap, it's easy, and it's quick. A hamburger and fries at a drive-through? Hardly. It's the traditional Mediterranean diet. From Spain to Sicily, Corsica to Crete, Athens to the Alps, this diet has been a staple of peasant life for centuries. Ranging up to 40 percent of calories from fat, it would seem to be a sure killer. Yet people in this vast region live longer than Americans do, and heart disease and cancer are far less common.

"It's one of the healthiest diets that human beings have developed in the past 2,000 years," says R. Curtis Ellison, M.D., chief of preventive medicine and epidemiology at Boston University School of Medicine.

What's going on? Truth is, researchers aren't absolutely certain why Mediterranean eating habits seem to work. But the success of this lifestyle may have a lot to do with the type of fat that Mediterraneans eat. Of course, most of their foods are low-fat—fresh fruits, vegetables, and grains. These include many of the foods we associate with the sunny Mediterranean: oranges, apples, tomatoes, eggplant, spinach, onions, peppers, and lots of bread. But when it comes to fat, nearly 75 percent of what they con-

had twice the risk of death as women who ate less fat, says Aaron Folsom, M.D., professor of epidemiology at the university and co-author of the study.

"I'm not surprised that lower-fat diets are effective in the prevention of breast cancer as well as its treatment," Dr. Klaper says. "High-fat diets raise the levels of sex hormones like estrogen in the bloodstream, and many breast cancers depend on estrogen to grow."

sume is from heart-healthy olive oil, which is loaded with monounsaturates.

What are the implications of this for 50-plussers? Well, French researchers have shown that people in their sixties who begin living this lifestyle can have a 70 percent drop in heart attack risk. Preliminary evidence also suggests that monounsaturated fats (as in olive oil) may reduce your risk of breast, endometrial, and perhaps lung cancer, says Dimitrios Trichopoulos, M.D., director of the Harvard Center for Cancer Prevention at the Harvard School of Public Health.

Red meat, a prime source of worrisome saturated fat, isn't daily fare in the traditional Mediterranean diet. In fact, it's usually only eaten once or twice a month. Poultry and fish are also eaten less often than in the United States.

But is a Mediterranean diet better than a low-fat diet? "I think both are excellent alternatives to the traditional American fare of meat and potatoes," Dr. Ellison says. "But low-fat is a huge change that is less acceptable to many Americans. Mediterranean eating is a less-radical change, and more Americans are trying it and liking it."

Cutting down on fat also may help women slash their risk of ovarian cancer, a disease that becomes more common as women reach their early sixties, says Harvey A. Risch, M.D., Ph.D., associate professor of epidemiology and public health at Yale University School of Medicine.

Dr. Risch and his colleagues evaluated the eating habits of 450 women up to age 79 with ovarian cancer and 564 without the disease. They concluded that cutting 10 grams of saturated fat a day (about the same amount as in one cheeseburger with all the fixings) could trim the risk of ovarian cancer by 20 percent. And adding 10 grams of vegetable fiber a day—what you would get in about 1 cup of cooked lentils—may take the risk down by another 37 percent.

"It appears possible to cut your risk of ovarian cancer in half by assertive modification of the diet," Dr. Risch says.

How to Start Now

Really cutting back on total fat and sorting out the best low-fat foods from the worst high-fat offenders takes some adjustments, but these changes don't have to be time-consuming or costly or sap flavor from your favorite meals.

Sure changing a lifetime of eating habits can be challenging, especially for people age 50-plus. "But I don't think it's as hard to do as many people perceive," says Sheah Rarback, R.D., an American Dietetic Association spokesperson in Miami. "It doesn't have to be all or nothing. Over time, even small changes in your eating habits can improve your health,"

Here are some basics to get you started.

Keep score. For the next couple of days, jot down on a piece of paper or handy 3-by-5-inch cards all the foods and beverages that you eat and drink. Note the amount and type of fat listed on the nutrition labels. If you're eating in a restaurant, estimate your intake of food, Dr. Shike suggests. This will give you an idea about how much fat you're eating now and how much you'll need to cut back. Every three months or so, do this all over again so that you can see your progress.

Set a goal. Give yourself something to strive for, but make it practical, Pingleton says. Making over a lifetime of eating habits in a week probably isn't realistic. But getting your total fat intake under 25 percent of calories in the next six months is a reasonable goal.

Be bold. Most doctors and dietitians recommend that no more than 30 percent of your calories come from fat. But it seems that the more you slash the fat you eat, the more dramatic the impact on your health. So be adventurous, Dr. Klaper suggests. Experiment with lower levels of fat in your meals. To begin, pick a day of the week and on that day, make a bean dish, pasta, or salad the centerpiece of your meals. If you dine out, try low-fat ethnic foods or vegetarian dishes. Then gradually, over a month or two, increase the number of days of the week you eat like that. All of this will help your taste buds adapt to eating less fat and help you become comfortable with a new lower-fat lifestyle.

Count the grams. Figuring the percentage of fat in a meal can be tricky. An easier way to control fat consumption is to count grams, because that's how fats are measured on nutrition labels, says William Castelli, M.D., epidemiologist, medical director of the Framingham Cardiovascular Institute and former director of the Framingham Heart Study in Massachusetts.

So if you eat 2,000 calories a day and want to keep your fat intake below 20 percent, multiply 2,000 by 20 percent. That's 400 calories. Now divide 400 by 9—which is the number of fat calories in 1 gram. You get 45, the number of grams of fat you're allowing from all the foods that you eat in one day. How much is that? A beef bologna sandwich made with two pieces of meat and a 1-ounce slice of regular Cheddar cheese has about

Frying Isn't the Only Way to Cook

Gerry Bates has an easy time recalling her late husband's favorite dishes: fried chicken, fried catfish, fried eggs . . .

"My husband didn't think something was cooked unless it was fried," says Bates, a registered dietitian, who is the nutritional program manager for the Florida Department of Elder Affairs in Tallahassee. His eating habits contributed to his 1985 death of heart disease at age 59, she says.

But times are changing. A growing number of people in their fifties and sixties are adopting low-fat cooking methods in hopes of avoiding a similar fate or simply to add variety to their meals, Bates says.

"It is surprising to a lot of them that they get away from the frying pan and cook something in a different way and still have it taste good," Bates says.

Here's a glimpse at some of the lean ways Bates says that you can create delicious meals without added grease, butter, or oil.

Steaming and microwaving quickly cook rice, vegetables, and other foods without adding fat. These methods also help retain the nutrients, flavor, and moisture in the food. To steam vegetables, for instance, bring about 1 inch of water to a boil in a large saucepan. Place the vegetables in a steamer basket

36 grams of fat—nearly an entire day's fat allowance in one meal. So use those fat grams thoughtfully, Dr. Castelli says.

Take 20. Try to keep your consumption of saturated fat—the really bad fat—under 20 grams a day (10

and set the basket in the saucepan so that it sits above the water. Cover the saucepan with a tight-fitting lid and cook until the vegetables are crisp-tender. When microwaving vegetables, you need to add only a small amount of water before cooking.

Poaching means cooking food in a simmering liquid, often stock, broth, or water. This healthful alternative to frying works well with boned poultry and firm-fleshed fish like salmon.

Baking and roasting are excellent ways to cook meats, poultry, fish, squash, potatoes, and many other foods. To keep foods moist, be sure to cover them for at least part of the cooking time. Bake meats by using a roasting rack or meat-loaf pan to keep them from sitting in fat drippings.

Braising, also known as stewing, means slowly cooking food in a small amount of boiling water or other liquid. The longer you braise the meat, the more fat leaches into the cooking liquid. When the meat is done, strain the broth into a container and refrigerate it overnight. The next day, skim off and dispose of the fat that has congealed on top and reserve the remaining broth for soup stock. This works well for any combination meat dishes such as chicken and rice, chicken and dumplings, meat stews, or soups made with meat.

grams if you have suffered a heart attack), Dr. Castelli says. Again, read the food labels carefully.

What can you eat and stay under 20 grams? "You could have rolled oats, fruit, and low-fat yogurt for breakfast; a chicken, tuna, or turkey sandwich for lunch; and shrimp cocktail, a 3-ounce filet mignon, vegetables, salad, and fat-free dressing for dinner—and you'd still be under 20 grams of saturated fat for the day," Dr. Castelli says. "Now does that sound like such a miserable experience?"

Make the switch gradually. Cravings for fat won't disappear immediately, but you can retrain your taste buds, says John Foreyt, Ph.D., director of the Nutrition Research Clinic at Baylor College of Medicine in Houston. "You can retrain yourself at any age by making shifts gradually away from high-fat foods."

Make one gradual change a week. If you use whole milk in your coffee or on cereal, for example, try a 50/50 mixture of whole milk and 2 percent milk for a week. Then switch to 2 percent for seven days. Then use a mixture that is half 2 percent and half 1 percent, and so on until you are using skim milk. If skim milk alone doesn't satisfy your taste buds, you can stir in some nonfat powdered milk to improve its texture and flavor, Dr. Foreyt says. You can use the same strategy to wean yourself off cheeses, shortenings and oils, ice cream, and other high-fat traditions.

Reinvent your favorites. The worst thing that you can do is give up your favorite dishes, because you'll feel deprived and may develop cravings that make it harder to stick to a low-fat lifestyle, Dr. Foreyt says. Instead, experiment with low-fat ingredients. "Take your 10 favorite recipes and go into the supermarket and buy all the low-fat substitutes for the ingredients that you would normally use," says Dr. Castelli.

If you prefer not to modify your recipes, then serve the original versions less often—on holidays and special occasions, for instance—and take only half of the portion that you would normally eat, Dr. Foreyt suggests.

Eat with friends. Make your transition to low-fat living a social celebration, Rarback says. Ask a few friends to join a lunch or dinner club. On a rotating basis, one of you makes a low-fat main entrée while the others bring the bread, salad, fruit, or dessert. "It will help all of you experiment with new low-fat recipes, and it is fun to eat together," she says.

Splurge now and then . . . Make high-fat foods like country fried steak a once-a-month treat rather than daily fare, says Michele Tuttle, R.D., director of consumer affairs for the Food Marketing Institute in Washington, D.C. Nobody's perfect, and trying to eat perfectly is frustrating, Tuttle says. "In fact, that's probably the best recipe for failure because the thought that you can never have double chocolate fudge cake again in your life will drive you crazy," she says. "So go ahead and have a little bit with some friends. One dessert split four ways is not a big deal."

. . . But make up for it later. Any one food or any one meal can have some extra fat as long as you compensate for it, Dr. Foreyt says. "Over a week you want your fat consumption to be certainly less than 30 percent of calories and closer to 20 percent of calories if you can get there," Dr. Foreyt says. "So if you eat a hamburger or cheesecake on a Monday, that's fine. But you should adjust your eating plans so that you eat less fat during the rest of the week."

With these essentials in mind, here are some ideas for stocking your pantry, shopping for groceries, eating at home, and dining out that will help you become a savvy low-fat role model for your grandchildren.

The Pantry: Low-Fat Living Starts Here

Filling your pantry with high-fat foods is like asking a compulsive gambler to live next door to a casino. It's too much of a temptation.

"If you don't have the right things in your pantry, you're going to prepare the foods you do have in the same old way, or you're going to be tempted to say 'the heck with it' and go out to eat at a high-fat restaurant," Tuttle says. "So it only makes sense to stock your pantry well."

For low-fat living, here's how to have the right things readily at hand in the kitchen.

Remember the 75/25 rule. "Whenever you open the refrigerator, a kitchen cabinet, or the bread box, 75 percent of what you see should be plant-derived foods, such as pastas, breads, beans, cereals, grains, and fresh, frozen, or canned fruits and vegetables, says Elizabeth Somer, R.D., author of *Nutrition for Women*. "Then the remaining 25 percent can be made up of small amounts of lean meats and low-fat dairy products like milk and cheese. If the bulk of your pantry is like that, then your plate will probably look that way, too."

Consider the pastabilities. Pastas like spaghetti, linguine, and fettucine have earned a bizarre reputation for being fattening. But in reality, these grain foods are almost devoid of fat and are a great source of complex carbohydrates—your body's best fuel.

"If you fill up on pasta, you'll be more inclined to eat less meat, and that will mean that you're eating even less fat," Rarback says. So keep several boxes of your favorite pastas within reach.

But watch your pasta sauce. What fattens up most pastas is what we put on it, says Rarback. A typical white sauce, for instance, is 71 percent calories from fat. And most bottled spaghetti sauces have up to 9 grams of fat in a ½-cup serving.

Instead of those, always keep in your refrigerator a jar of spaghetti sauce that has 5 grams of fat or less to pour over pasta, spread on pizza crust or even on baked potatoes, says Elaine Moquette-Magee, R.D., author of the book series *Fight Fat and Win: How to Eat a Low-Fat Diet without Changing Your Life*.

Count on beans and rice. Dried beans like pinto, navy, lima, and black beans, and grains like brown rice are virtually fat-free and are terrific sources of protein that can reduce or eliminate the need for fat-laden meats in stews, chili, salads, and other traditional dishes, Rarback says. Instead of using 10 ounces of beef in a stew, for example, use 5 ounces and round out the dish with lentils.

Get cracking. Unlike packaged bread crumbs, which have some fat, cracker meal is fat-free, Moquette-Magee says. Cracker meal can be used for coating oven-roasted chicken or fish, as a topping for low-fat fruit crisps and casseroles, or as a filler for meat loaf.

Stock up on low-fat cream soups. Be sure to have in your pantry plenty of low-fat condensed cream soups, like 99 percent fat-free cream of broccoli or cream of chicken, says Evelyn Tribole, R.D., author of *Healthy Homestyle Cooking*. They're great in casseroles and as sauces on meats, poultry, and fish.

Stay away from solids. If you use cooking oils, stock up on liquid olive or canola oils that are loaded with monounsaturated fat. These oils are better for you than solid oils and fats like shortenings that contain lots of saturated fat, says Edith Howard Hogan, R.D., a spokesperson for the American Dietetic Association in Washington, D.C. Better yet, coat your cookware with a vegetable oil cooking spray.

Brown it in broth. Keep defatted chicken broth in your cupboard instead of vegetable oil, Moquette-Magee says. "I use chicken broth all the time to sauté vegetables, pan-simmer meats, or boil and flavor rice," she says. "All it does is keep the food moist and transfer heat. Those are the same things the oil would be doing, except the broth doesn't have all that fat."

Slash fat with a splash from the vine. Alcohol is another good fat substitute to have on hand, Moquette-Magee says. You can use beer and wine to stir-fry meats and simmer mushrooms, green peppers, onions, and other vegetables.

Juice up your meals. White grape, apple, orange, and pineapple juices are all light-flavored alternatives to oil in homemade salad dressings or marinades, Tribole says.

Bring on the prunes. Puréed prunes are one of the best fat substitutes in baked chocolate favorites like brownies and cakes, Tribole says. They're chewy and contribute a naturally sweet flavor to the dessert. A ½-cup can save you more than 800 calories and almost 100 grams of fat compared to a ½-cup of butter. For convenience, Tribole suggests buying jars of baby-food prunes that have already been puréed.

Peel away calories with applesauce. "Applesauce is another great substitute," Tribole says. "You can use it in place of cooking oils or butter in brownies, muffins, and cakes. For every ½ cup of applesauce you use, you'll save about 109 grams of fat and 900 calories."

Go for cocoa. If you bake, keep your pantry well-stocked with unsweetened cocoa powder. It provides rich chocolate taste without the fat of unsweetened baking chocolate, Tribole says. For each ounce of unsweetened chocolate called for in a recipe, substitute 3 tablespoons of unsweetened cocoa powder, she advises.

Keep the cow in the cupboard. Cartons of skim milk that can be stored without refrigeration until opened have no fat and are convenient and cost-effective because they reduce spoilage, Hogan says. The milk contains no preservatives, but is safe because it is pasteurized at a higher temperature than other milk products. You can store it for up to five months in your pantry, she says. These products are available on most grocery shelves. Look for "UHT" (ultra-high temperature) on the label.

Make that fat evaporate. Evaporated skim milk is terrific for sauces and soups because it has the texture and flavor of cream but without the fat, Tribole says. Each cup contains 80 grams less fat and 600 fewer calories than heavy cream.

Use your yogurt. Plain nonfat or low-fat yogurt is a versatile addition to any refrigerator, Moquette-Magee says. It can be used to replace sour cream and make salad dressings, and it is a good, quick add-on to breakfast cereals and desserts.

Pinch-hit for butter. Butter-flavored sprinkles like Molly McButter or Butter Buds add taste to foods without the fat or calories, Rarback says.

Teach old spices new tricks. Low-fat foods may seem less flavorful when you first try them. There are a couple of reasons for that. First, fat adds flavor to some foods, and it's a taste that you're used to. Second, as we age, our taste buds become less acute. So keep plenty of herbs and spices like basil, garlic, ginger, onion powder, tarragon, and oregano in your pantry to add zip to low-fat meals, Rarback says.

"By using some different spices and herbs in

your food, you're going to bring back flavor and zest to the meal and make it more enjoyable while still eliminating fat," she says. Tinker with low-fat foods and spices until you find combinations that you like.

Invigorate with vinegar. "Using a flavorful vinegar like raspberry, tarragon, or rice wine vinegar will allow you to decrease the amount of oil in home-made salad dressings," Rarback says. "So I'd encourage you to have them in your kitchen and experiment with them."

Do a mayo makeover. Regular mayonnaise is 98 percent fat. "It's just egg yolks and oil," Moquette-Magee says. "I can't think of anything worse for you." Try instead one of the light, low-fat or fat-free varieties. If you don't like how they taste on sandwiches, opt for mustard, cranberry sauce, barbecue sauce, or plain yogurt, says Moquette-Magee.

You also might want to try creating your own mayo. Either mix ½ cup of light or low-fat mayonnaise with ½ cup of plain yogurt, or whip ½ cup of low-fat cottage cheese in a food processor or blender.

Have a "biteables" box. Put a variety of low-fat snacks like grapes, dates, celery, rice cakes, and other crunchy, chewy things into a container in your kitchen so that you can quickly satisfy yourself without being tempted to dash out for higher fat goodies between meals, Graham Kerr suggests.

Shopping: Surviving the High-Fat Maze

"If you're the cook in the family, your first line of defense against high-fat living is at the grocery store," Pingleton says.

But while most supermarkets have a tremendous

variety of nonfat and low-fat options, they are also filled with prominently displayed, high-fat enticements.

Here are some ways to get through the grocery store without loading up on fat.

Make a list. This may seem like obvious advice, but some people still don't do it, Somer says. A list will not only save time but also reduce the risk that you'll impulsively throw a high-fat food into your cart, Somer says. So before you go to the store, sit down and plan out what you would like to eat that week.

Don't shop on an empty stomach. "You want your mind working, not your stomach, as you stroll the grocery store aisles," Somer says. "If you're hungry, you're going to be reaching for all the high-fat stuff that you shouldn't be eating." Go grocery shopping after a meal or a snack like low-fat cheese and crackers, she says.

Shop outside in. Generally, the fresher, lower-fat foods like fruits and vegetables are on the perimeter of the store. So shop on the outside aisles first. That way, you'll load your cart with healthier foods and be less tempted to fill it with the more processed, higher-fat products on the inner aisles, says Jayne Newmark, R.D., a nutrition consultant in Phoenix.

Read those labels. Nutrition Facts labels can be your best weapon in your war against high-fat eating. Among other things, each label is now required by law to list the amount of total calories, total fat, saturated fat, and sodium per listed serving size.

When reading the Nutrition Facts label, says Kathy Pompliano, R.D., manager of the M-Fit Supermarket Program at the University of Michigan in Ann Arbor, remember the following rules of thumb: If an item contains 5 percent or less of the Daily Value for a particular nutrient, it is considered "low." On the other hand, if an item contains 20 percent or more of the Daily Value for a particular nutrient, it is considered "high." Look for foods that are low in total fat, saturated fat, and sodium and foods that are high in fiber, vitamin A, vitamin C, and calcium.

Read the ingredients list, too, she suggests. Compare products and choose the one with fewer fat sources listed. Common fat sources include vegetable oil, meat fat, whole milk, butter, cream, and eggs. Check breads and cereals for fiber-rich whole grains, such as whole or rolled oats, or whole, cracked, or stone-ground wheat.

Take a few at a time. Of course, reading every label on every food every time you shop would be tedious and time-consuming. Instead, each time you shop pick out a couple of foods and read those labels very carefully, recommends Mona Sutnick, R.D., Ed.D., a nutrition consultant in Philadelphia and a spokesperson for the American Dietetic Association.

"Today, for example, you could read salad dressing labels and pick one that has little or no fat," she says. "If you like it, you don't have to read salad dressing labels anymore, because you've found one that suits you. That approach will work for virtually every food in the store."

Give hydrogenated foods the heave-ho. Avoid foods like baked goods or margarines that list hydrogenated or partially hydrogenated oils as ingredients. This means hydrogen has been added to unsaturated liquid oils to make them solidify. But adding hydrogen does two things. First, it transforms unsaturated fat into saturated fat, says George Seperich, Ph.D., a food scientist and associate professor of agribusiness at Arizona State University in Tempe. Second, it creates trans fatty acids, molecules that raise LDL cholesterol as much as saturated fat does.

"When I'm shopping and I see the word 'hydro-genated' on the label, that food goes right back on the shelf because I know it is loaded with things that I don't want in my body," Dr. Klaper says.

Water it down. Pick a margarine that lists water as its first ingredient. It will almost certainly be low-fat, Dr. Castelli says.

Whip it up. Whipped margarines also are a good choice because they have more air, and that reduces the fat content, says Gerry Bates, R.D., nutritional program manager for the Florida Department of Elder Affairs in Tallahassee.

Keep vegetables on ice. "For many people in this age group who live alone, buying fresh fruits and vegetables is often a problem because they rot before they're eaten," Rarback says. "Frozen vegetables packed without sauces are a very good alternative. Then a person living alone or a couple doesn't have to worry about spoilage, and they have a fresh-tasting vegetable readily available that they can take out of the freezer and microwave quickly, or use as a base in soups or stews."

Become a cereal-eater. "There didn't used to be a lot of low-fat, low-sodium breakfast cereals, but now there is a multitude of very good ones," says Jeanne Jones, cookbook author and "Cook It Light" syndicated columnist in La Jolla, California. In particular, look for shredded wheat, oatmeal, and puffed rice, corn, or wheat.

Smile when you say low-fat cheese. Most regular cheeses have about 9 grams of fat per ounce. Instead look for low-fat cheeses that have about 6 grams of fat or less per ounce, or part-skim varieties of ricotta and mozzarella that have about 5 grams or less, Moquette-Magee says.

Remember, though, that while nonfat cheeses

taste fine alone or in sandwiches, they don't cook well, according to Kerr.

Reach for nonfat cream cheese. Regular varieties of cream cheese are very high in fat and saturated fat. Look for the nonfat or low-fat varieties to accompany a breakfast bagel, says Pompliano.

Pass on the processing. Make foods that are naturally low-fat your first choice, says Dr. Seperich. That's because many nonfat products—particularly nonfat sweets like cakes and cookies—are highly processed, Dr. Klaper says. Instead of fat, they're packed with gums and sugars that cause the formation of free radicals and drive up triglycerides, a type of fat that increases your risk of heart disease.

People also tend to eat larger amounts of nonfat foods because they don't give the feeling of fullness that fat does. Dutch researchers also have found that fat substitutes can reduce your body's ability to absorb vitamin E and health-promoting antioxidants like carotenoids.

Some nonfat products such as fat-free sour cream, cream cheese, yogurt, and mayonnaise are fine if they are used sparingly on sandwiches or to make other foods like vegetable dips and salad dressings, Dr. Seperich says.

Find a fresh path. Instead of heading straight to the meat department, purchase a new fruit, vegetable, grain, bean, or pasta that you've never tried before, like kiwifruit, bok choy, couscous, Anasazi beans, or ziti, Pingleton says. It will awaken your taste buds and give you another way to experiment with low-fat living.

Gobble up ground turkey breast. Ground turkey or chicken breast are among the leanest meats you can buy, Pingleton says. Be wary, though, if the label doesn't indicate that it is 100 percent breast meat, because the package may include skin and other poultry fat.

If ground turkey or chicken breast isn't available, consider ground beef that's 15 percent fat or less. It's leaner than plain ground turkey, Pingleton says.

Select the "select" meats. The more marbling a meat has, the more tender and tasty it will be. But that marbling is pure fat. Look for the U.S. Department of Agriculture grade on the package. Choose "select" grade meats, which have the least amount of marbling and may be cheaper than other meats, Tuttle says. If that isn't available, get "choice," the next highest grade. "Prime" grades have the most marbling, so save these for special occasions.

Look for loin. Leaner cuts of beef contain the words "round" or "loin," as in "top round" or "sirloin." Lean cuts of pork usually are loins or legs. For ham, choose lower-fat varieties or Canadian bacon, Pingleton says.

As always, go fish. Researchers are backing away from claims that eating five or six servings of fish a week—fish like salmon and tuna, which are rich in a polyunsaturated fat called omega-3 fatty acids—is any more beneficial to your heart than eating one or two servings a week. But those one or two servings will clearly protect your heart better than none at all.

"Fish isn't a magic bullet, but it is a fine choice in the grocery store," says Walter Willett, M.D., Dr.P.H., professor of epidemiology and nutrition and chairman of the Department of Nutrition at the Harvard School of Public Health and author of several classic fish-consumption studies. "It's a healthy food, and from all we know, it is better for you than red meat."

Try eating fish like salmon, trout, or tuna once or twice a week in place of red meats like beef, Dr. Willett suggests.

Be a deli detective. While it's true that many deli

meats and salads are loaded with fat and sodium, there are healthier varieties at supermarkets today, says Pompliano. Look for chicken breast, turkey breast, or other lean and extra-lean meats for a low-fat and low-saturated protein source. To reduce the amount of sodium on these meats, rinse the meat gently under cool water and pat dry before making a sandwich, suggests Pompliano.

If traditional deli items are too hard to resist, ask the deli clerk about lower-fat options. Some delis have fat-free or low-fat macaroni salads and potato salads, says Pompliano.

To really slash the fat that you carry away from the deli, ask the clerk to slice the meat as thin as possible, and instead of ordering it by the quarter- to half-pound, ask for only the number of slices that you think you'll eat that week, Tuttle says. That may prevent overindulging, not to mention wasting food.

Send the oil packing. Tuna and other seafoods packed in oil just add unwanted fat to your meal. Pick water-packed tuna or seafood such as clams canned in their own juices, Jones says.

Dump doughnuts, muzzle the muffins. Because half of the calories in a doughnut comes from fat and a third of the calories in a muffin comes from fat, a bagel is your best choice—it's nearly fat-free."A bagel is a great breakfast food. It is fast, convenient and readily available in most areas," Pompliano says.

Eat a few, but don't go nuts. Eating nuts, which are good sources of monounsaturated and polyunsaturated fats, may protect you from heart disease, according to researchers at Loma Linda University in California. These researchers, who studied the eating habits of 31,000 Seventh-Day Adventists in their fifties, sixties, and seventies, found that those who ate nuts four or more times a week had half the risk of fatal heart attacks than people who munched on them less than once a week.

But keep in mind that the fats in nuts still count toward your daily fat total, and most nuts are chock-full of calories. A cup of peanuts, for example, has about 800 calories. "For the average person nuts can be dangerous because they're like potato chips. It's hard to just have one," Newmark says. If you're going to eat them, avoid doing it by the handful. Instead just use five or six nuts to add flavor or texture to foods like salads or frozen desserts, she says.

Eating at Home: The Personal Low-Fat Touch

By age 70, the average person who cooks for a family has made about 49,000 meals. Unfortunately, most household cooks also have a limited repertoire of about 14 entrée dishes, so they're feeding their families the same high-fat meals day after day, says Kerr. For a low-fat entrée to replace one of those 14—particularly after decades of cooking the same way—you need to personalize the effort.

"Go to some degree of trouble to find out what works well for you," Kerr says. "If you readdress how you prepare food and spice it the way you like it, then it is possible to make the change to low-fat living."

Stick with no-stick. No-stick cookware is worth the modest investment because it has a special coating that allows you to cook or bake without greasing it with fat, Rarback says.

"I know a woman in her sixties who has been using the same cooking pots and pans since her wedding years ago, and there have been a few innovations since then," Rarback says.

Don't drown the pans. If you normally use oil or butter to grease your pans, try dabbing a small spot—about the size of a quarter—onto a paper towel and swabbing it into the pan, Hogan says. That should cut back on the amount you use during cooking. Better yet, use fruit juice or defatted chicken broth instead.

Throw out the frying pan . . . Bake, roast, grill, microwave, or sauté foods that you would normally fry, Dr. Foreyt says. These cooking methods allow fats to run off the meats and be discarded.

. . . But not the chicken. Instead of frying chicken, remove the skin, coat it with a dusting of flour and egg white, dip it in bread or cornflake crumbs, and bake it. "It comes out remarkably well," Tribole says. "That keeps it moist and reduces the amount of fat you're eating significantly."

Be a poacher. Poaching fish in white wine, rather than frying it, trims fat and helps keep the fish flavorful and moist, Rarback says.

Bake those fries. If you crave french-fried potatoes, try this simple low-fat alternative: Cut four medium potatoes into strips, coat them with 1 tablespoon of oil by stirring in a bowl, and bake on a baking sheet in a 450°F oven for 30 to 40 minutes, turning frequently. Sprinkle with paprika or lightly with salt or salt substitute, Dr. Foreyt says.

Shrink the meat. People now in their fifties, sixties, and seventies belong to a generation where it was considered normal (for men, at least) to eat 16-ounce steaks. "But the real serving size that they should be eating is about 3 ounces, which is about the size of a man's palm," Somer says. "So if you eat a 16-ounce steak, you're eating more than three days' worth of meat in one serving."

Use a small amount of meat—2 to 3 ounces after cooking—to complement low-fat meals instead of letting it crowd fruits and vegetables off the plate, Pingleton says. For every bite of meat, take four bites of fruits, vegetables, beans, and grains, Somer says. In any case, try to limit your meat consumption to no more than 6 ounces a day, Tuttle says.

Freeze out TV dinners. Many frozen meals are loaded with fat and sodium, and in some cases take just as much time to prepare as fresh foods, Jones says. In the same 10 minutes that it takes to make fat-laden boil-in-the-bag Swedish meatballs, for instance, you could brown ground turkey breast in a skillet, add some low-fat spaghetti sauce, and pour it over pasta.

Do a macaroni makeover. To lower the fat content of packaged macaroni and cheese, add vegetables like broccoli, carrots, or cauliflower, and use low-fat or skim milk and half as much butter or margarine, Moquette-Magee says.

"Try using 1½ tablespoons of margarine or butter and 2 tablespoons of light sour cream instead of the 4 tablespoons of butter called for," she says. "It's wonderful and you won't notice the difference."

Lighten up puddings. Evaporated skim milk adds body and richness to puddings, but unlike whole milk, it doesn't have any fat, Tribole says.

Ditch the yolks. If your recipe calls for whole eggs, use fat-free egg substitute instead (¼ cup substitute equals 1 whole egg). Since fat content of the substitutes varies, check the label before buying. For baking, however, using two egg whites in place of each whole egg is a better choice, because it reduces the fat yet maintains the flavor and texture of the original recipe, Rarback says.

Soak it in yogurt. Instead of oil-based marinades, try pleasant-tasting plain nonfat yogurt, Rarback says. Allow meat or skinless poultry to soak for several hours or overnight. Marinate fish for only an hour or so because of its delicate texture.

Lose 100,000 fat calories in 25 seconds. "Butter has gone the way of all flesh in our household," Kerr says. "In its place, I've been making fresh cheese from nonfat yogurt. That has actually saved me 100,000 calories a year in fat."

It takes about 25 seconds to prepare, Kerr says. Put a cheesecloth into a hand sieve and scoop in a tub of plain nonfat yogurt. Put a plate on top of the sieve and set it over a bowl in the refrigerator so that the whey can drip out. After 12 hours it should look like thick, creamy, loosely packed cream cheese. If it tastes too sour, add a few drops of maple syrup to sweeten it, Kerr says.

Shred that cheese. Instead of putting a full slice of cheese on a sandwich, grate it or shred it. You'll use less cheese, yet get the same flavor and cut the fat in half, Rarback says.

Cook now, eat later. Once or twice a month make large quantities of low-fat soups, stews, waffles, and other favorites. Then divide them into one- or two-serving packets and store them in the freezer, Pingleton says. Then when you don't feel like cooking, you'll have a ready-made low-fat meal that you can reheat in minutes.

Kick the grease bucket. "A lot of people in this age group like to save the grease from bacon and other fatty foods in a bucket for use in cooking later. Get rid of it," Pingleton urges. That fat is mainly saturated, which causes the most havoc in your body. If you insist on using it, discard the oils that harden on top and use the liquid oil underneath, because it is less saturated, Pingleton says.

Squeeze out the gravy fat. No gravy-lover over 50 is likely to give up gravies. But you can lower its fat. "Put the drippings in the freezer and let the saturated fat harden on top, then discard it," Pingleton says. "Use the broth underneath. It has very little fat and delivers all of the flavor you want in a gravy. Be sure to use skim or low-fat milk, too."

For quick low-fat gravy or sauce, take a can of condensed low-fat cream soup such as cream of chicken or mushroom out of your pantry and mix it with a half-can of water. Then pour the mixture over cooked meat, fish, or poultry and let it simmer for 5 to 10 minutes, Pingleton says.

Flop your vinaigrette. Traditional vinaigrette is made with two parts oil to one part vinegar. Turn that around: Double the vinegar and halve the oil, and you've created an exciting lower-fat salad dressing and marinade, Kerr says. Try this formula with a balsamic or Japanese rice wine vinegar and a tasty olive oil. Throw in a crushed garlic clove and dash of dry mustard and brown sugar for flavor. Whip in a blender and keep it in your refrigerator.

Back away from butter. Most of us over 50 were raised eating lots of butter, Pingleton notes. Here are her suggestions for cutting back on butter: Don't use it in cooking, but add a small amount—about the size of a postage stamp—after the dish is done for flavoring only. On bread or toast, spread it thinly, so that you can still see the bread fiber. If you're making a sandwich, only butter one slice of bread. Better yet, use an all-fruit spread, low-fat mayonnaise, or margarine instead.

"A lot of foods will surprise you by how good

they taste without butter," Tribole says. "You really won't miss it in most cases."

Dining Out: Dodging the High-Fat Temptations

"The same rules you use for eating at home apply when you eat out." Somer says. "You still want to minimize the amount of meat that you eat and focus on fruits, vegetables, and grains."

But restaurant dining requires one key adjustment. "You have to be more vigilant, and you can't assume anything," Somer says.

Call first. Most high-quality restaurants will accommodate you if you give them sufficient notice, Dr. Lipsenthal says. Call a day or so beforehand, explain that you're eating low-fat foods, and ask if they can fulfill some specific requests.

Take a menu with you. If you eat at a restaurant frequently, ask for a copy of the menu to take home with you, Dr. Shike suggests. That way you can study your food choices without feeling pressured to order.

At fast-food restaurants—where many foods are 40 to 55 percent fat—try salads, plain hamburgers, or grilled chicken or ask for a copy of their nutritional information so that you can make wise selections, Dr. Shike says.

Ask for it any way but fried. If a fried entrée is offered on the menu, ask if the chef can bake it, broil it, grill it, or steam it to cut down on the fat, Dr. Shike says.

Ease back on the appetizers. Many appetizers, like buffalo wings, fried zucchini, and creamed soups, are high in fat. If you want something to munch on while you wait for your entrée, ask for bread sticks, grain breads, crackers, pretzels, or fresh vegetables like carrots and celery with honey-mustard dressing (not ranch), and salads with dressings on the side, Pingleton says.

Create a take-home portion. Ask your server to bring a doggie bag when your meal is served. That way you can cut the meal in half and put it in the bag for take-home before you take your first bite, Somer says. You'll not only have a meal for the next day, you'll slash the amount of fat and calories in each serving.

"Don't start eating until you do that, because once you start eating you'll be likely to finish it," Somer says.

Carry a restaurant survival kit. In a small sandwich bag, carry packets of low-fat dressings, herbal teas, spices, hot-pepper sauce, and other essentials that may not be readily available at the restaurant, Newmark says.

Split a meal with a friend. Order soup or salad à la carte with one entrée. It will save you money and reduce the fat in each meal, Somer says.

Get dressings on the side. Many restaurants put more than 3 tablespoons of dressing on their salads, which can add more than 16 grams of fat, Somer says. So always order salad dressings on the side so that you can control the portion. Try to stick with oil and vinegar dressing. It spreads more evenly than cream dressings, so you'll use less of it, she says.

Let go of the extras. Cheese, bacon, olives, eggs, and croutons add unnecessary fat to a salad. Ask your server not to add them, Bates says.

Cut back on the rich sauces. The sauce for fettuccine Alfredo is often referred to as "heart attack on a plate," Dr. Foreyt says. Avoid rich sauces on pasta, meats, or fish or ask for the sauce on the side.

Satisfy the kid within. If you want dessert, ask if you can get a child's portion, Somer says. That will cut some of the fat and still satisfy your sweet tooth.

Topple meat toppings. Choose a pizza parlor that has a salad bar so that you can fill up on fresh fruits and vegetables while you're waiting for your pizza to cook, Somer says. Steer clear of pies that have lots of fatty meats like sausage or pepperoni. Try a vegetarian pizza—ask for extra vegetables and skimp on the cheese—and limit yourself to two to three pieces.

Hold the mayo. Many delis use regular mayonnaise on their sandwiches. Ask if they have a low-fat substitute. If not, ask them to leave it off. If mayo is a must, ask the clerk to just wet the bread with it rather than slathering it on, Moquette-Magee suggests.

Sail clear of tartar sauce. Tartar sauce, which is served with many fish entrées, gets 96 percent of its calories from fat, Moquette-Magee says. So use it sparingly, if at all. "If you order a fish fillet sandwich at a fast-food restaurant and scrape the tartar sauce off the bun, or ask that it not be put on in the first place, you're cutting the fat in that sandwich by 50 percent," she says.

Take a no-thank-you portion. "Years ago, if a child told his mother that he didn't want a particular food, she'd put a little on his plate anyway," Hogan says. "It was called a no-thank-you helping. You can do the same thing now. If you are tempted by a high-fat food, ask for a no-thank-you helping—a tablespoon of it—so that you still get a taste and don't feel deprived."

Wash that sauce away. In restaurants, ask for your vegetables steamed without added oils, butter, margarine, or creamed sauces. If the waiter tells you that the vegetables are already prepared with one of those ingredients, ask if your portion can be put in a colander and rinsed with boiling water to wash away the unwanted add-ons, says Francine Grabowski, R.D., at Cooper Hospital in Camden, New Jersey, and co-author of *Low-Fat Living for Real People*.

Make bacon a special treat. Bacon's another one of those foods that you've probably loved for five decades or more. But just one slice of cooked bacon has approximately 3 to 5 grams of fat, with 80 percent of its calories from fat. Pingleton recommends moving your bacon bites out of the house.

"I tell people not to even buy it or keep it at home," she says. "If you must have it, get it at a restaurant where you're only going to be served 1 to 2 slices instead of the 10 that you would be tempted to eat at home."

Fiber

Roughage—The Smooth Disease Fighter

If your body had a yard sale, fiber would be the junk in the bin marked "free—take it away." It's the last vestige of the food you eat, the waste that remains after your body has wrung out all the goodness it can.

But fiber is far from being an expendable part of your diet. As it passes through your system, this throwaway stuff is actually an important force against cancer, heart disease, and stroke. What's more, it prevents a number of unpleasant side effects of aging:

♦ Fiber stops constipation.

♦ It alleviates diverticulosis, the formation of little pockets in the colon that can trap bacteria, bleed, and become inflamed. This malady affects more than half of all people over age 70.

♦ Fiber reduces hemorrhoid flare-ups.

♦ And a balanced diet including fiber can make your hair and fingernails look better than they have in years.

But those benefits are, well, small potatoes compared to the big-time disease prevention that you get from fiber. Researchers note that people who do nothing more than increase fiber and cut fat see cholesterol levels plummet from over 300 milligrams per deciliter (mg/dl) to under 200. That 33 percent drop in cholesterol translates into a whopping 60 percent lower risk of heart disease and stroke.

High-fiber diets also slash your risk of some forms of cancer. On its way through your body, fiber keeps cancer-causing substances from combining forces to make trouble. And it sends them toward the exit a lot faster.

Fiber doesn't travel alone. A lot of good stuff goes along for the ride. Perillyl alcohol, for instance, is concentrated in fiber. One of a group of compounds called isoprenoids, it is now being tested as an experimental treatment for people with advanced cancer.

Tocotrienols are another kind of cancer-fighting isoprenoids that bind to fiber. Structurally very close to vitamin E, these compounds come in cereal products like oats, rice, and barley, as well as palm and olive oil.

"Isoprenoids actually slow down the growth of tumors or stop their growth entirely," says Charles Elson, Ph.D., a researcher at the University of Wisconsin at Madison. Tumors are always trying to get started in the body, and researchers suspect that isoprenoids routinely prevent a lot of them from forming. And no one ever says thanks.

Dr. Elson notes that plants produce some of these substances when a fungus or an insect attacks. In the laboratory, combinations of isoprenoids offer more protection against disease than individual isoprenoids. "This suggests that you're better off eating a variety of the foods rich in isoprenoids, especially tocotrienols," Dr. Elson says.

Most foods contain a combination of the two types of fiber—insoluble and soluble. Each type fights disease differently, so you get two forms of protection when you take in a mouthful of some fiber-rich foods. Wheat products and vegetables boast lots of insoluble fiber but tend to be stingy with soluble fiber. Heart-protecting soluble fiber shows up mostly in fruits, barley, oats, and beans, and these foods generally contain even more of the cancer-fighting insoluble fiber.

Problem is, if you're like most older Americans, you probably get no more than 14.8 grams of fiber a day. You need 25 to 35 grams for disease protection. Luckily, you can make up the difference easily.

Keep Cancer at Bay with Insoluble Fiber

At first glance, insoluble fiber doesn't seem much like a cancer fighter. It's much more like lawn mulch than food. But studies show that insoluble fiber protects you from colon cancer, and researchers believe it wards off breast, prostate, and pancreatic cancer as well.

Lots of insoluble fiber comes from the substances that form in the cell walls of plants. It's called insoluble because your body can't easily break down this type of fiber during the digestive process.

Insoluble fiber gives your stool its bulk, which helps it move more quickly through your system. That is why foods that are high in insoluble fiber—bran, for instance—are known as nature's own laxatives. In fact, one nursing home found that people who added bran cereal to their breakfasts no longer needed laxatives.

In Finland, diets rich in cereals go along with low rates of breast and colon cancer. In some parts of Africa, where people eat lots of high-fiber foods, there is virtually no intestinal disease—and that includes colon cancer. In laboratory studies, one component of insoluble fiber, phytic acid, actually prevents the beginning of colon cancer.

Here's how insoluble fiber works to protect you.

It dilutes the risk. Lucky you—the same stuff in insoluble fiber that keeps you from getting constipated protects you from cancer, too. Insoluble fiber soaks up water like a sponge. This makes stools bulkier. The extra bulk means that cancer-causing agents get spread out over a larger area. They can't join forces to do as much damage.

It gives a high-speed boost. On the interstate large loads move slowly. But in the intestinal highway, bulk translates into speed. Insoluble fiber gets things moving fast, so there is less time for interaction between the cells that line the colon and cancerous agents.

It creates a cancer-unfriendly environment. Fiber tinkers with the acid levels in your intestines. This changes the way bacteria do their jobs. The end result: more fermentation. While that may give you gas

Get Rid of the Gas

Along with all the benefits, fiber has two side effects that you'd rather do without—gas, and that bloated feeling. Here's how to get fiber without the unpleasantness.

Up your intake gradually. Each week, increase your daily fiber intake by no more than 5 grams. That's the amount of fiber in 2 cups of sliced, unpeeled apples, says Belinda Smith, R.D., research dietitian at the Veterans Affairs Medical Center in Lexington, Kentucky. If you experience discomfort anyway, keep your fiber intake constant for a few days until symptoms clear up. If they still persist, cut back a few grams and wait a few days before making another addition.

Drink up. Fiber draws water to the bowel, says Alan Adelman, M.D., associate professor in the Department of Family and Community Medicine at the Milton S. Hershey Medical Center of Pennsylvania State University in Hershey. So you need to drink 8 to 12 (8-ounce) glasses of water or juice per day. This will also help reduce the buildup of gas.

Soak the beans. "Before you cook them, soak dried beans," Dr. Adelman says. Replace the soaking water when it's time to cook. This helps get rid of the sugars that cause gas.

Add a gas preventer. Try an over-the-counter product containing enzymes such as alpha-galactosidase (Beano), suggests Dr. Adelman.

(okay, nothing is perfect—not even fiber), it also makes it harder for carcinogens to get into your system. Fiber also helps control levels of the intestinal bile acids that play a part in the start-up of colon cancer.

It ties up carcinogens. Substances that lead to cancer of the breast, prostate, and pancreas tend to latch onto fiber. This means that when the body says good-bye to fiber, it also waves *adiós* to any carcinogens that have joined up.

It keeps breast cancer at bay. Insoluble fiber may reduce levels of the harmful estrogen that contributes to the beginnings of breast cancer.

In an Australian study, women who ate 28 grams of fiber a day had half the breast cancer risk of women who ate less than 14 grams a day. In addition, when you eat a lot of fiber, you generally eat less fat. Researchers believe that dietary fat is a big player in postmenopausal breast cancer.

Laboratory experiments also suggest that doubling fiber intake and lowering the amount of fat you eat can drop the tumor rate by 50 percent.

Insoluble Fiber: How to Bulk Up

Insoluble is easy. If you're eating fiber-rich foods, chances are that you're getting an ample amount of the insoluble type. That's because virtually all fiber-rich foods contain more insoluble than soluble fiber. Here is how to make sure that you're getting enough.

Can it. Hey, who needs more work? You get as much fiber benefit from canned beans as dried beans that you soak and cook yourself. Add a can of beans to vegetable and other soups, suggests Belinda Smith, R.D., research dietitian at the Veterans Affairs Medical Center in Lexington, Kentucky.

Maximize your bean benefit. If you prefer dried beans, store them in airtight containers at room tempurature, says James W. Anderson, M.D., a world-renowned professor of medicine and clinical nutrition at the Veterans Affairs Medical Center in Lexington, Kentucky. They'll keep for a year that way. Use glass containers and put them where you can see them, because beans are attractive and you'll be more likely to use them if you see them every time you're in the kitchen. Also, Dr. Anderson recommends soaking beans overnight to prepare them for cooking. but before you do, poke through them to get rid of pebbles or other debris that may have been in the package with them.

Sneak it in. Add fiber to the foods that you normally prepare. For instance, use oat bran instead of white bread as a filler in meat loaf. Add canned kidney beans to lasagna. Introduce beans into casseroles and salads, Smith suggests.

Try instant brown rice instead of instant white rice, says Alan Adelman, M.D., associate professor in the Department of Family and Community Medicine at the Milton S. Hershey Medical Center of Pennsylvania State University in Hershey.

Go whole grain. If you want refinement, take an art appreciation course. Refinement in food is another thing entirely. Refined bread, for instance, loses fiber in the milling process. So choose whole-grain bread products, which can provide 3 grams of fiber or more per slice—meaning you can get 6 grams from one sandwich.

"Refined, processed foods not only lose the fiber, but refining takes out a lot of the trace minerals and possibly the beneficial phytochemicals," notes Rosemary Newman, R.D., Ph.D., professor of food and nutrition at Montana State University in Bozeman.

(continued on page 146)

High Fiber, Low Kitchen Time

If you're used to buying low-fiber, highly processed, off-the-shelf prepared products, switching to high-fiber eating may seem like work. But, says Belinda Smith, R.D., a research dietitian at the Veterans Affairs Medical Center in Lexington, Kentucky, it really can be easy. She recommends the following two-in-one recipe for high-fiber chili and low-fat spaghetti sauce developed by Constance Pittman Lindner for the *Tufts University Diet and Nutrition Letter*.

Start by making the basic meat mixture, then divide it and turn one portion into chili and the rest into spaghetti sauce. The whole process takes well under an hour and leaves you with lots of good eating. Store individual servings in the freezer for a home-cooked meal whenever the mood strikes.

Basic meat mixture: You need: 2 tablespoons olive oil; 2 onions, chopped; 2 cloves garlic, minced; 1 pound ground turkey or chicken; 2 cans (28 ounces each) chopped tomatoes or tomato puree; 1 can (12 ounces) tomato paste; 1½ cups water.

In a large saucepan, heat the oil and add the onions and garlic. Sauté over medium heat for 5 minutes, or until the onions are tender. Crumble the turkey or chicken into the pan. Break up the meat with a wooden spoon and cook for 5 minutes, or until it is browned. Drain off any fat that accumulates in the pan.

Add the tomatoes or tomato puree, tomato paste, and water to the meat mixture. Simmer for 20 minutes. Divide the meat mixture into two portions: Using a slotted spoon, remove two-thirds of the meat and one-third of the sauce for chili and put into another large saucepan. One-third of the meat and two-thirds of the sauce will remain in the original pan for spaghetti sauce.

Chili: You need: 2 cans (16 ounces each) kidney beans, rinsed, drained; ½ green pepper, seeded, chopped; 1½ to 2 teaspoons chili powder; 1½ teaspoons ground cumin; 1 cup shredded low-fat sharp Cheddar cheese.

Add the beans, green peppers, chili powder, and cumin to the chili meat and sauce mixture. Simmer for 5 minutes. Serve sprinkled with the Cheddar. Makes 8 (1 cup) servings. Per serving: 276 calories, 7.1 g fat (23% of calories), 7 g dietary fiber, 38 mg cholesterol, 911 mg sodium.

Spaghetti sauce: You need: 2 tablespoons honey; 1 teaspoon dried basil; 1 teaspoon dried oregano; ½ teaspoon ground black pepper.

To the meat and sauce mixture remaining in the first saucepan, add the honey, basil, oregano, and pepper. Simmer for 5 minutes. Makes 5 (1 cup) servings. Per serving: 325 calories, 8.4 g fat (23% of calories), 6.6 g dietary fiber, 53 mg cholesterol, 1,110 mg sodium.

Phyto-whats? She's talking about protective plant chemicals. In living plants these chemicals guard the plants from harsh weather and insects. In your body, phytochemicals guard against a wide number of diseases, including heart disease, cancer, and stroke.

Read the fine print. Nutrition labels tell you the amount of fiber per serving in a food. But also look at the ingredients list. "In a bread, for instance, the first listed ingredient should be a whole grain," Dr. Newman says. "Better yet, the first three or four listed should be whole grains. That means there are more grains than anything else in the product."

If you get tired of picking up and checking every loaf, concentrate on those with labels that make high-fiber claims, such as "good source of fiber."

Weigh the benefits. Not all high-fiber products are created equal. Say that you want to snack on a high-fiber granola bar. Even if the bar of your dreams has 1 or more grams of fiber, it's a good fiber deal only if the fat and calorie content are low.

"A snack bar with something like 100 calories, 2 grams of fat, and a gram of fiber is fine," Dr. Newman says. "But some have around 300 calories and a lot more fat. That's too much."

Set goals. Don't try to become a fiber-gobbling machine overnight. If you think that you'll have trouble staying the course of a high-fiber diet, set small, realistic goals that you can meet, suggests Smith. Once you have reached those goals, set new ones. To keep yourself on track, keep a diary of what you eat.

Single out singles. Keep your fiber consumption high by lining your kitchen cabinets with easy-to-prepare, fiber-rich staples in packages that are small enough for one or two people. Even if you're an avid cook, says Smith, there will be days when you don't feel like going into the kitchen. Stock up on items such as baking potatoes, canned soups, canned beans, and cereals.

Eat with a friend. Get on the phone and flesh out your social calendar. When there are friends and family to share with, fixing a high-fiber meal seems like no effort at all, Smith notes. Other avenues for social eating: Join community groups or start your own luncheon club.

Soluble Fiber Protects the Heart

Study after study shows that soluble fiber lowers cholesterol, cutting your risk of heart disease and stroke. It may also help clear out your arteries, dropping your risk of high blood pressure.

You get soluble fiber in the outer part of some grains, the white rind in citrus fruits, and the membranes that contain each little section of grapefruit pulp. But in some plants, such as beans or barley, you find soluble fiber throughout.

One-fourth of the fiber that you take in should be soluble, says Dr. Newman. The problem is that most people don't get that much of the soluble type. A lot of foods are gold mines of insoluble fiber but contain almost no soluble materials. For example, you'll get 3 grams of fiber from 3 cups of popcorn. But a mere 0.1 gram will be soluble fiber.

In your body, soluble fiber combines with water, swelling up to create a gelatinous goo that does wonders to protect you from heart attacks and strokes. Here's how it works.

It cuts cholesterol. The higher your cholesterol levels, the greater your risk of heart disease and stroke. The soluble goo gets your cholesterol levels down. Re-

(continued on page 150)

Play the Numbers for Protection

You don't have to play a food lottery, guessing which foods give you the most heart-protecting soluble fiber. Here's a list of the top foods for soluble fiber and the number of grams they contain.

Food	Portion	Soluble Fiber (g)
Vegetables		
Artichoke, cooked	1 medium	2.2
Celery root, fresh, chopped	½ cup	1.9
Sweet potato, cooked	½ cup	1.8
Parsnip, cooked	½ cup	1.8
Turnip, cooked	½ cup	1.7
Acorn squash, baked	½ cup	1.6
Potato with skin, baked	1 medium	1.6
Brussels sprouts, cooked	½ cup	1.4
Cabbage, fresh	1 cup	1.3
Green peas, cooked	½ cup	1.3
Broccoli, cooked, chopped	½ cup	1.2
Carrots, cooked, chopped	½ cup	1.1
Carrot, raw	7½" long	1.1
Cabbage, cooked	½ cup	1.1

Food	Portion	Soluble Fiber (g)
Fruits		
Mango, sliced	1 cup	2.9
Strawberries, whole, capped	1 cup	2.0
Figs	2	1.7
Kiwifruit	2	1.4
Orange	1	1.4
Plums	2	1.4
Pear	1 small	1.1
Grapefruit	½ medium	1.1
Blackberries	¾ cup	1.1
Apricot halves, dried	7	1.1
Apple with skin	1 small	1.0
Cereals		
Quaker Oat Bran	1 cup cooked (½ cup dry)	3.0
Quaker Oat Bran Cereal, ready-to-eat	1¼ cups	3.0
SmartBeat High Fiber Oatmeal,	1 packet, instant	3.0
H-O Super Bran High Fiber Cereal	¾ cup	3.0

(continued)

Play the Numbers for Protection—Continued

Food	Portion	Soluble Fiber (g)
Kellogg's Bran Buds	⅓ cup	3.0
Quaker Oatmeal, cooked	1 cup	2.0
Health Valley Healthy Crunch	½ cup	1.4
Raisin bran	1 cup	1.2
Quaker Instant Oatmeal	1 packet	1.0
Nabisco 100% Bran	⅓ cup	1.0
Kellogg's All-Bran	½ cup	1.0
Post Oat Flakes	⅔ cup	1.0
Kellogg's Common Sense Oat Bran	¾ cup	1.0
Cheerios	1¼ cups	1.0
Grains		
Pearl barley	¾ cup cooked	1.8

searchers believe that once the soluble fiber reaches the small intestine, it interferes with absorption of fat. "The total amount of fat in the diet is probably the major factor in cholesterol control," Dr. Newman says. "In addition, soluble fiber may trap bile, which must

Food	Portion	Soluble Fiber (g)
Oat flour	¼ cup	1.6
Rye flour	¼ cup	1.3
Wheat germ	4½ tablespoons	1.0
Legumes		
Large lima beans, canned	½ cup	5.7
Kidney beans, cooked	½ cup	2.8
Cranberry beans, cooked	½ cup	2.7
Butter beans, cooked	½ cup	2.7
Baked beans, canned, cooked	½ cup	2.6
Black beans, cooked	½ cup	2.4
Navy beans, cooked	½ cup	2.2
Lentils, cooked	½ cup	2.0
Pinto beans, cooked	½ cup	1.9

be replaced. The replacement material is cholesterol, which is drawn out of the blood and tissues." That cholesterol-laden bile heads on down the intestinal highway and out of the body.

But the cholesterol-lowering benefits don't stop

there. Elsewhere on the digestive route, bacteria break down soluble fiber to create short-chain fatty acids. When these are absorbed back into the body, they restrict the body's ability to synthesize cholesterol, reducing your blood's cholesterol levels still more.

Researchers note that some people can lower cholesterol much more cheaply and just as effectively with fiber than with cholesterol-lowering medication. At the University of Minnesota, researchers looked at 10 studies of oat bran and found that eating just 3 grams of soluble fiber a day (what you would get in 1 cup of ready-to-eat oat bran cereal) can drop cholesterol levels by 2 to 3 percent. In people whose levels were over 230 mg/dl, cholesterol declined more steeply, an average of 6 to 7 percent. And it seems that the more oat bran people eat, the more cholesterol goes down. In one study, 6 to 9 grams of soluble fiber brought cholesterol levels of over 260 down by 23 percent.

Dr. Anderson recalls that he began eating oat bran in 1977. A pioneer in oat bran research, he couldn't even get the stuff from food suppliers. Oat bran's main use in those years? Face powder.

But he found that just a bowl of cereal and three to four oat bran muffins a day lowered his cholesterol from 285 to 175 in five weeks. He also lost 8 pounds in that same time. He has been researching (and eating) oat bran ever since.

It cleans out your arteries. Researchers theorize that soluble fiber may also be an arterial housecleaner, helping to reduce the risk of the plaque buildup in your arteries that can lead to heart attacks and strokes. Soluble fiber helps lower the level of cholesterol that circulates in your body—and that automatically drops your risk of an artery-clogging buildup.

It controls blood sugar. Soluble fiber improves the body's ability to maintain normal blood sugar, by slowing absorption of starchy foods. This helps forestall plaque buildup in the arteries, which can lead to a heart attack or stroke.

It fights high blood pressure. Researchers studied 850 Yi people, members of an ethnic minority in southwest China. They found that the Yi diet, high in oats and buckwheat, resulted in lower blood pressures and lower levels of the harmful low-density lipoprotein cholesterol.

It slashes cancer risk. In one laboratory study, researchers used a modified form of pectin, a soluble fiber. They found that this special kind of pectin helped prevent cancer from spreading. It kept cancer cells from sticking to the walls of the lungs, keeping lung tumors from getting a start.

In Search of the Soluble

Most foods contain much more insoluble fiber than soluble. But you can increase your intake of soluble fiber by making small changes in how you approach foods that you're probably already eating.

Leave the liquid. The liquid that comes with canned beans contains a lot of dissolved soluble fiber (the reason why it is soupy instead of watery). Unless you have salt-sensitive high blood pressure or congestive heart failure, the salt in the liquid should not bother you. Save the liquid and combine it with soups. Or, for a low-salt or no-salt substitute, cook

Prescription for Prevention

Eating more fiber can substantially lower your cholesterol levels, greatly reducing your risk of heart disease and stroke. High-fiber diets also slash your risk of some forms of cancer, including breast, colon, pancreatic, and prostate cancer.

Do:

■ Eat wheat products and vegetables for insoluble fiber.

■ Get soluble fiber from fruits, oats, and beans.

■ Increase your fiber intake by adding beans to soups, lasagna, casseroles, and salads.

■ Eat brown rice instead of white rice and replace refined flour with whole-wheat flour.

■ Choose whole-grain bread products.

■ Drink 8 to 12 (8-ounce) glasses of water or juice each day. Fiber draws liquids out of your system.

Don't:

■ Add a high-fiber psyllium supplement if you're on other medications without first checking with your doctor.

your own beans and save the leftover liquid, says Dr. Anderson.

Put away the peeler. The peels of many fruits and vegetables are rich in soluble fiber. Don't peel apples, pears, peaches, or potatoes. Eat the white inner rind of oranges, which is high in pectin. For grapefruit sections, spoon out the membrane with the pulp for extra soluble fiber, Dr. Anderson says.

Eat it whole. While you get concentrated nutrients from fruit juice, you lose out in the fiber department. An 8-ounce glass of extracted carrot juice contains just 2 grams of fiber, compared with the 14 grams you would get from the six carrots (1 pound) that went into the juicer, says Dr. Adelman.

Get supplemental protection. "A lot of people find that it's easier to take a soluble fiber supplement than to adjust their diets," says Dr. Adelman. The main ingredient in fiber supplements like Metamucil is psyllium, which comes from the ground-up seed husks of a plant grown in India. It has been used as a laxative for more than 60 years. You get the most benefit if you take psyllium with a meal.

While taking a supplement is the easy way out, it may not be the best way to reward your taste buds. "My patients who use a supplement tell me that it tastes like powder mixed with water," Dr. Adelman says. "They make it palatable by mixing it with orange juice or apple juice."

Psyllium is also available in cereals. In one study people with mildly high cholesterol levels ate Bran Buds, a cereal high in psyllium, for two weeks. Their cholesterol levels dropped by 8 percent.

Don't supplement without your doctor's okay, since psyllium can interfere with other medicines that you may be taking.

Make substitutions. Look for products containing substances such as TrimChoice, formerly known as Oatrim, a fat substitute that is made from oat flour, which is rich in soluble fiber. Produced by Mountain Lake Manufacturing, it appears as hydrolyzed oat flour in cheese, baked goods, confections, and meat, as well as a variety of other low-fat products.

While it is touted for its low-fat benefits, Oatrim also cuts cholesterol. In a U.S. Department of Agriculture study, 24 people with high levels of cholesterol who ate products containing Oatrim experienced a 16 percent drop in total cholesterol in five weeks. Their levels of protective high-density lipoprotein cholesterol were unchanged. To add to the benefits, blood pressures went down and their blood sugar levels became more stable.

Take it in stages. To maximize soluble fiber's cholesterol-busting power, work your way up through three levels of consumption, Dr. Anderson suggests. Stay at each level for four to six weeks.

At Level I, adjust your diet so that you take in 10 grams of soluble fiber a day. You will probably get a 5 to 10 percent drop in cholesterol levels. Then move to Level II, consuming 15 grams of soluble fiber per day for a 10 to 15 percent cholesterol reduction. Finally, at Level III, combine 15 grams of soluble fiber with a psyllium supplement (under your doctor's supervision). This will give you a 15 to 20 percent cholesterol reduction.

The Power of Plants

Scientists Cheer for Fruits, Vegetables, and Grains

Imagine an array of well-armed forces battling heart disease, cancer, and stroke, catching cancerous invaders and throwing them out of your system before they destroy healthy cells. Shrinking any tumors that get started. Sending blood pressure tumbling down. Cleaning out the fat in your arteries. Keeping your arteries clear of the blood clots that lead to strokes. Protecting cells against DNA damage. Even slowing down the aging process.

Sounds like the antics of superheroes in your grandchildren's video games? Actually, it's what goes on in your body when you eat fruits, vegetables, and grains. Scientists have discovered that when you eat food made from plants, you get the benefits of all those powerful defenses. They come from *phytochemicals*, a term that simply means chemicals in plants. Scientists once thought that these largely nonnutritional, noncaloric substances were useless, just along for the ride.

But the picture is changing. Experts, sifting

through the thousands of phytochemicals in plants, are learning that those you consume can help ward off cancer, heart disease, and stroke. In fact, more than 200 studies have shown that diets high in fruits and vegetables cut cancer risk. That becomes even more important as you get older and your risk of heart disease, cancer, and stroke increases.

Think of phytochemicals as a smoothly functioning bureaucracy. Most phytochemicals work in groups, but no one knows exactly what each one does. Most have unpronounceable names and produce a cascade of chemical reactions that resemble a Rube Goldberg drawing.

Sometimes protective phytochemicals make their presence known: You can see their calling cards in the bright orange color of carrots or sweet potatoes. Or you get a whiff of phytochemicals in action when you come nose-to-clove with garlic. You taste them in the sharp bite of freshly cut watercress. But many are undetectable.

Researchers theorize that some antioxidant phytochemicals evolved to protect plants from oxygen (since plants feed on carbon dioxide, with oxygen as waste), as well as wind, weather, and insects. "These substances keep plants from oxidizing under the hot sun's ultraviolet radiation," says Suzanne Paxton Pierson, a pharmacy doctor and president of Preventive Nutrition Consults in Woodinville, Washington. And, she says, they protect bulb plants that grow underground from an onslaught of microbial and insect hazards.

"These chemicals are there to protect the plants, not you," says James A. Duke, Ph.D., herbalist and ethnobotanist in Fulton, Maryland, and author of *The Green Pharmacy*. But, notes Dr. Duke, "you can borrow the protective benefits."

Slash Your Cancer Risk

Up to 33 percent of potential cancers might be prevented just by eating a diet rich in fruits and vegetables, according to scientists at the National Cancer Institute.

"We can save more than 150,000 lives a year, right now, with no treatments, no medical costs, no long-term recovery—if people just eat the foods that protect them," says Edward Miller, Ph.D., professor of biomedical sciences in the Department of Biomedical Sciences at Baylor College of Dentistry in Houston, who researches oral cancer.

"Studies worldwide show that phytochemicals protect against cancer," says Paul Lachance, Ph.D., chairman of the food science department at Rutgers University in New Brunswick, New Jersey, and an internationally known researcher in the field. But, he cautions, "there is no panacea phytochemical, no one thing you can take or eat for protection."

If you eat lots of plant foods (and thus plenty of phytochemicals), you have a lower risk for cancers that attack the lungs, bladder, cervix, mouth, larynx, throat, esophagus, stomach, pancreas, colon, and rectum. Scientists also believe plant foods may help protect you from breast and prostate cancer.

In the laboratory, phytochemicals keep cancer-forming substances and defective cells—which are turning into cancers—from getting a foothold or spreading. Some phytochemicals contain hormones that disrupt the growth of breast cancer and prostate cancer cells.

How I Did It: She Knows Beans

Diagnosed with breast cancer at age 49, Grace Maloney recalls, "I knew I would beat it. I just put one foot in front of the other mentally. But, back then, I didn't really make any big changes in my life, with one exception—I stopped smoking."

But when the Jackson Heights, New York, resident reached menopause, she did change her diet. "With menopause, I noticed that I put on another 10 pounds," says Maloney, now in her sixties. "That wasn't healthy, so I knew that I had to change."

Her downfall wasn't a sweet tooth. It was cheese and other high-fat foods. "It was a real sacrifice to give up those foods," she sighs, recalling a special treat—cheese and pâté.

Switching to more fruits and vegetables made her life a lot easier. "I've always hated cooked vegetables," she says. "In fact, I cook them for my husband, but I can't stand to eat them. So I tried them raw. I discovered that I liked raw carrots and fresh string beans."

She added tomatoes to her assortment and stocked up on fruit. "I've always loved fruit, and it was wonderful to have an excuse to buy more," Maloney says. She started buying watermelons, cutting them up and storing them in the refrigerator, along with

Cure Cardiovascular Problems

Phytochemicals also go right to the heart of a key health issue for those over 50. "The 60-to-80 age group has a much greater risk of heart disease than younger people do," notes Dexter Morris, M.D., vice chairman

her vegetable assortment. "I'd just nosh on that when I wanted a snack," she says. "Pretty soon, eating fruits and vegetables got to be a routine."

But she hasn't given everything up. "I have my wine with dinner every night," she says. "My husband, Robert, and I eat out twice a week. We try to order sensibly, but I figure that because I eat carefully almost all the time, I'm entitled to an occasional treat. The other day at a French restaurant, I even had pâté."

Maloney made even more lifestyle changes to keep her heart healthy. "I'm doing a lot of bicycle riding, just for flexibility," she says. "Although I ignore it, I have arthritis of the spine. I've found that movement helps my arthritis. Plus, I do weight-bearing exercises. And I started playing tennis an hour a day on the handball wall. The wall never yells at me, and I never have to wait for it to show up."

The effort has paid off. Now when she travels, she has more stamina. "I didn't behave myself when I was young, and it's nice not to have to pay too much for your past sins when you get older," Maloney says. "It has been a sacrifice, but I'm glad for the result. I don't think that I look my age, and I feel great. It keeps me going."

of the Department of Emergency Medicine and a heart researcher at the University of North Carolina at Chapel Hill School of Medicine. "If your diet is rich in fruits and vegetables, you can reduce risk."

Some plant chemicals help your cardiovascular

system by neutralizing harmful low-density lipoprotein (LDL) cholesterol that, if left unchecked, can lead to hardening of the arteries. Others act on the walls of your blood vessels to lower your blood pressure. Or they make blood platelets less sticky and less likely to clot so that you're not as vulnerable to strokes.

In a study begun in 1973, researchers kept track of 1,883 men ages 35 to 59 who had high cholesterol levels. Over the next 20 years, the men who had the highest levels of carotenoids (a phytochemical) in their blood had 60 percent fewer heart attacks and deaths.

Fight Free Radicals

Many phytochemicals also do double-duty as antioxidants, neutralizing free radicals, which are unstable molecules that damage or destroy the body's healthy cells.

Free radicals have been linked to more than 60 diseases and medical problems. Beyond heart disease, cancer, and stroke, these include premature aging, stiff joints, wrinkled skin, arthritis, diabetes, and liver cirrhosis. Not only does your body churn out these harmful free radicals routinely, they also come in from the outside, from such things as cigarette smoke, pollutants, medications, pesticides, and household cleaners.

So the free-radical-fighting antioxidant properties of many phytochemcials are clearly welcome. And antioxidants are particularly important as you climb out of your fifties because they reduce the effects of aging, says Joanne Slavin, Ph.D., professor in the Department of Food Science and Nutrition at the University of Minnesota in St. Paul.

Phytochemical research is a relatively new field, so there's much to be studied and discovered. Here's a breakdown of the major phytochemical groups that seem to provide the most protection and how scientists think they work.

Organosulfur Compounds: Scents That Protect

The aromatic clout and pungent flavor of plants in the allium family—garlic, onions, leeks, chives, and shallots—are actually signs that protective phytochemicals are at work. These organosulfur compounds, which you also get in cruciferous vegetables such as broccoli and cauliflower, help protect you against cancer and heart disease.

Cancer. Foods rich in organosulfur compounds could be called dietary anticarcinogens, according to John Potter, M.D., Ph.D., head of the Cancer Prevention Research Program at the Fred Hutchinson Cancer Research Center in Seattle. Studies have shown that some of the powerful organosulfur compounds in these plants, such as diallyl disulfide, block or suppress carcinogens. Plus, they help the body intercept and eject cancer-causing agents before they can do any damage.

Another important organosulfur compound, alliin, works as a powerful antioxidant, disposing of the free radicals that damage healthy cells and play a part in both cancer and atherosclerosis. In animals, alliin interferes with tumor growth and prevents the molecular changes that lead to cancer.

Some of these chemicals also help the immune system stay strong, increasing the number of your body's infection-fighting T cells. Researchers at the

Fight Disease While You Eat

Ever think that you could protect yourself from disease every time you put food to your lips? You can, if you eat foods rich in phytochemicals. Here's how to get more of the foods that protect you from cancer, heart disease, and stroke.

Keep it varied. No one knows why, but vegetables grown in different plots of ground can have very different concentrations of beneficial chemicals. How do you compensate for those differences? "Vary what you eat," says Leon Bradlow, Ph.D., director of the Murray Rayburn Laboratory of Biochemical Endocrinology at Strang Cancer Research Laboratory in New York City. By choosing lots of different fruits and vegetables, you ensure yourself maximum phytochemical coverage.

Minimize meats. If a slice of meat usually occupies half your dinner plate, slowly cut back until your meat serving is the size of a deck of cards or smaller, and the rest of the space is filled with vegetables, pasta, or rice, says John Potter, M.D., Ph.D., head of the Cancer Prevention Research Program at the Fred Hutchinson Cancer Research Center in Seattle. If you make your changes gradually, the shift will be easier to tolerate.

Count on mistakes. Tell your family and friends

University of Minnesota School of Public Health looked at the eating habits of more than 41,830 Iowa women ages 55 to 69. Those who ate garlic, a particularly rich source of organosulfur compounds, had a one-third reduction in risk of colon cancer.

that you're trying new foods for health and enlist their psychological support. "Learning new styles of cooking takes time, and you will screw up," says Dr. Potter. "It's easier if your friends and family are tolerant of your failures."

Make it a party. Get together with friends for "moving dinners," perhaps held once a week at a different person's home. That way, you can all learn together, Dr. Potter says.

Crack open a cookbook. Get ideas for new foods by checking out cookbooks from the library or buying a few. Look for books that promote fruits and vegetables and other plant foods, suggests Dr. Potter.

Eat what you like. "If you don't like something, you probably won't eat it," says Dexter Morris, M.D., vice chairman of the Department of Emergency Medicine and a heart researcher at the University of North Carolina at Chapel Hill School of Medicine. If you only like tomatoes and hate other vegetables, just eat more tomatoes. "There are probably enough different kinds of phytochemicals in every vegetable to do you some good," he says. "It's not like there is only one kind in a tomato and another kind in a carrot. There are mixtures in all. It's more important to eat vegetables than to worry about which ones."

In other studies researchers note that the bacteria-fighting organosulfur compounds may also fight off cancer by disarming *Helicobacter pylori*, a bacteria found in the stomach that can lead to stomach cancer.

As a bonus, Danish scientists have discovered that chemicals in garlic not only block the growth of cancer cells but also delay the normal aging process of healthy cells.

Heart disease and stroke. Organosulfur compounds found in onions, garlic, and other members of the allium family defend your heart. "When you eat a hearty meal, you get an influx of fats into the bloodstream that make your blood more likely to clot," says Isabella Lipinska, Ph.D., a nutritional counselor for the Cardiac Rehabilitation Program at St. Elizabeth's Medical Center in Boston. "The alliums, particularly onions, will help your body manufacture substances to get rid of the fat quickly." By doing that, they lessen your risk for heart disease and stroke.

Organosulfur compounds contribute to lower blood pressure without the common side effects, such as headaches and impotence, that some people get from prescription medication. Experts theorize that these compounds dilate the muscle cells in the arteries, opening up blood vessels and lowering blood pressure. They may also help the blood circulate to the smaller vessels more efficiently, lowering blood pressure even more.

These phytochemicals also decrease levels of harmful LDL cholesterol that can narrow artery walls. And they increase levels of the beneficial high-density lipoprotein (HDL) cholesterol that keeps your arteries free of plaque and protects against heart disease and stroke.

Scientists in Australia examined the results of eight trials with a total of 415 people. Those who consumed a commercial dried garlic powder for one to three months lowered their blood pressure. Project researchers speculate that if long-term studies of garlic eaters sustain this same rate of lowered blood pressure, the results might be 30 to 40 percent fewer strokes and 20 to 25 percent less coronary heart disease.

Another study measured cholesterol levels, revealing an 11 percent drop in harmful LDL cholesterol and a 6 percent drop in total cholesterol in people who took 900 milligrams a day of garlic powder tablets (the equivalent of about three cloves) over a 12-week period. That's important because researchers estimate that every 1 percent drop in total cholesterol could translate into a decrease in heart attack risk of 2 percent.

You get protection against stroke from these phytochemicals, too. At Brown University, men ages 30 to 70 who had cholesterol levels of 230 to 290 consumed 700 milligrams of garlic a day. Total cholesterol and LDL cholesterol levels declined by 8 percent. The levels of beneficial HDL cholesterol did not change.

Here are some ways to get the most benefit from organosulfur compounds. You should check with your doctor before you increase intake if you are on anticlotting medicines or aspirin, according to Dr. Lachance.

Get souped up. As you get older, your body doesn't absorb food as easily, a problem compounded if you have dentures and don't chew your food properly. Dr. Lipinska advises using a blender to liquefy vegetables, then making cream of vegetable soups, complete with onion and garlic.

Put away two to three a day. "For health benefits, based on retrospective epidemiologic studies, eat two to three cloves of garlic a day," advises Dr. Paxton Pierson.

Yu-Yan Yeh, Ph.D., professor of nutrition science at Pennsylvania State University in University Park, conducted a study of men ages 35 to 55 with high LDL ("bad" cholesterol) levels. They received supplements equal to two to three cloves, and their LDL cholesterol levels dropped. Still, Dr. Yeh says, "it's better to incorporate fresh garlic into daily cooking and to eat healthy foods instead of taking a supplement. You get extra benefits from vegetables you eat with garlic."

Pass up the riches. Adding garlic or other foods rich in phytochemicals may tempt you toward the wrong kinds of food. A garlicky sauce, for instance, is hardly a wise choice if it's also rich in butter or other animal fats, notes Dr. Yeh. "The benefits won't offset the health hazards of rich food," he says.

Sauté for health. "You'll get the most benefit out of alliums (garlic and its relatives) by chopping them up and then sautéing them in a little oil," says Dr. Yeh. The chopping activates some phytochemicals while heat gets others going. "Use olive oil or canola oil, because they're high in monounsaturated fat and don't seem to contribute to higher LDL cholesterol levels the way other oils do," he says.

Say good-bye to heartburn. Garlic and other alliums don't agree with everyone's digestive tract. If you get heartburn, try deodorized garlic such as aged garlic extract, says Dr. Yeh. People who participated in one study consumed the deodorized supplemental equivalent of three cloves a day. They got the benefits, and no one felt the burn.

Keep it cooked. Avoid raw garlic because, like other bulb vegetables, it grows underground in close contact with bacteria that may be harmful to you. (So don't mix raw garlic in oil, for instance, and store it in the refrigerator.) Raw garlic also gives some people intestinal irritation, Dr. Yeh says.

Use condiments for flavor only. Condiments such as onion or garlic powder may add flavor to your food, but processing techniques have probably cost them just about all of their protective benefits. So just be aware that the payoff doesn't go any farther than your taste buds.

Use it or lose it. The enzymes that activate protective phytochemicals get busy when you chop or press the garlic, but they dissipate within 12 to 24 hours. So you'll get the most benefit when it's freshly chopped, according to Dr. Lachance. If you cut up a garlic clove and save it for another day, all you'll get is the taste.

Isothiocyanates: Leaves That Stem Cancer

You get plant chemicals called isothiocyanates in leafy green vegetables such as watercress, arugula, cabbage, Chinese cabbage, and brussels sprouts, as well as broccoli and cauliflower.

These compounds help the body get rid of cancer-causing substances. "They take the trash out, to put it in the simplest terms," says Stephen Hecht, Ph.D., professor of cancer prevention at the University of Minnesota Cancer Center in Minneapolis. "Fewer carcinogens reach their cellular targets." These chemicals also make it difficult for cancer-causing substances to zero in on the DNA (genetic material) of healthy cells. In the laboratory, they have kept tumors from forming and have detoxified carcinogens.

In a laboratory experiment, watercress-eating rats that ate a diet containing an isothiocyanate from watercress and a carcinogen from tobacco were 50 percent less likely to develop lung tumors than those exposed only to the carcinogen.

Here's how to get the most benefit from the iso-thiocyanates in your food.

Eat it raw. "Isothiocyanates are released when you chew the raw vegetable or chop it up," says Dr. Hecht. "You know it's happening because of the sharp taste. Cooking reduces some of the compounds, but the vegetables still contain a lot of beneficial chemicals."

Keep it fresh. While the phytochemicals in these vegetables are fairly stable, you'll get more if you eat fresh vegetables, Dr. Hecht says. If, for example, you chop up watercress or broccoli and use it the next day, the taste will be subdued—and the benefits will be slightly less, according to Dr. Duke.

Put it high on the list. "The National Cancer Institute recommends at least five helpings a day of fruits and vegetables," Dr. Potter says. "While you won't be immune to cancer if you eat a lot of cruciferous vegetables, they do contain a large number of compounds that we strongly suspect to be anticarcinogens."

Eat the leaves. "Phytochemicals are most concentrated in the broad leaves of many vegetables in order to protect the plant, although we also see some concentration in seeds," says Dr. Duke.

Indoles: Part of the One-Two Punch

Like Laurel and Hardy, indoles and isothiocyanates go together. Eat the leafy greens of cruciferous vegetables like broccoli, cauliflower, and cabbage, and you get the benefits of both, says Dr. Duke.

To get the most overall benefits from indoles, eat the equivalent of a quarter head of cabbage a day or an equal amount of broccoli (about half a bunch), brussels sprouts, or cauliflower. "We have found the highest levels of indoles in savoy cabbage, the crinkly looking type, and in purple broccoli," says Leon Bradlow, Ph.D., director of the Murray Rayburn Laboratory of Biochemical Endocrinology at Strang Cancer Research Laboratory in New York City.

Cancer. Indoles protect against breast cancer because they alter the body's estrogen metabolism. But it's not for women only—it has the potential for use as a treatment for prostate cancer.

"In humans, they stop the growth of small virus-caused tumors. In animals, these vegetables prevent breast cancer," Dr. Bradlow says. "This makes us optimistic that we'll see similar results in humans. We already know that people in China and Korea, who eat cabbage all their lives, have much lower breast cancer rates than people in the West."

You get added benefits from broccoli, a rich source of indoles. It also contains sulforaphane, a phytochemical that prevents mammary tumors in rats.

Heart disease and stroke. Because indoles are phytoestrogens (estrogen-like substances from plants) they may help lower the risk of heart disease and stroke. Estrogen has been linked to lower levels of harmful LDL cholesterol and may even help control high blood pressure and reduce the blood's tendency to clot.

Isoflavones: Tofu to the Rescue

Isoflavones are a group of plant estrogens found in soy products that can bring remarkable health benefits to those in their fifties, sixties and beyond. "In countries where people consume a lot of soy, the rate of breast and prostate cancer is very low," says Clare Hasler, Ph.D., director of the Functional Foods for Health Program at University of Illinois at Urbana-Champaign.

Cancer. The powerhouse isoflavones in soy are genistein, daidzein, and equol. In laboratory tests they keep cancerous cells from growing. Some studies on animals show genistein also keeps tumors from growing and getting the blood supplies they need. And, in fact, when leukemia cells divide, genistein also helps them to return to their original healthy state.

In laboratory studies the phytoestrogens in soy reduce the number of mammary tumors in rats and prevent the growth of human breast cancer cells. Researchers also think that phytochemicals such as isoflavonoids may slow the growth of prostate cancer.

In a Japanese study, the diets of 142,875 women were followed for 17 years. Breast cancer risk was lowest in women whose diets included miso soup, made from soybean paste. Researchers theorize that the isoflavones do the job.

Studies also show that soy consumption is tied to a lower rate of colon and rectal cancers. Soy also is a good source of saponins, another group of phytochemicals that, in the laboratory, fight cervical, pancreatic, gastric, colon, breast, and prostate cancers.

Heart disease and stroke. Studies have shown that soy can bring down your cholesterol levels from the high-risk range to the moderate- or even low-risk range, according to Dr. Hasler. "Soy contains a variety of chemicals that probably interact. Even independently, some of them do lower levels of harmful cholesterol," says Susan Potter, R.D., Ph.D., associate professor of nutrition at the University of Illinois at Urbana-Champaign.

Scientists believe that plant estrogens in the diet lead to the low levels of heart disease in Asian countries. They speculate that phytoestrogens slow down atherosclerosis, protecting the arteries.

Soy may taste bland, but it is unique among plants. The important protectors, genistein and daidzein, are only found to any significant extent in soybeans and the foods that come from them. These two phytochemicals may keep LDL cholesterol from oxidizing so that it can't easily attach to artery walls. Genistein may also keep artery walls from thickening and keep platelets from clumping together, reducing the risk of heart disease and stroke.

University of Kentucky researchers reviewed 38 previous studies and concluded that soy protein lowers LDL cholesterol and triglyceride levels but does not affect levels of the beneficial HDL cholesterol. In some experiments soy-rich diets have reduced total cholesterol by 10 percent and LDLs by 13 percent. Cardiologists estimate that a cholesterol reduction of 10 percent lowers your risk of death by 30 percent.

Dr. Susan Potter conducted a study to examine the blood cholesterol and bone density of women ages 50 to 70. Findings showed that women who consumed 40 grams a day of soy protein isolate, the powerful stuff in soy foods, ended up with a drop in LDL and an increase in HDL cholesterol levels.

"We also found that bone density improved in those women taking a soy protein isolate with slightly higher levels of isoflavones," she says. "Soy consumption may possibly be an alternative to estrogen therapy."

Unfortunately, the typical American diet is virtually soyless. Use these methods to increase your soy consumption.

Go ahead, try tofu. Tofu isn't the most appealing food to look at, but it absorbs the taste of spices and other foods you cook it with. So you can easily transform the bland into the sublime.

Look for Asian main-course and soup recipes. For grilling and sautéing, use extra-firm tofu, which won't crumble. Add small cubes of tofu to salads, says Dr. Hasler. Add a light dressing or a topping of nuts or seeds and you won't even know the tofu's there.

Keep it firm. Fermented soy products such as tempeh are available in dense, firm blocks. Researchers theorize that fermented soy products are easier for your body to use. Tempeh, firmer than tofu, is perfect for grilling or stir-frying.

Stick to low-fat. Look for low-fat (1 percent) tofu, tempeh, and soy milk products. Avoid high-fat varieties, advises Dr. Hasler.

Drink bean milk. "I drink soy milk," says Dr. Hasler. "The beany flavor is great on whole-grain cereals or granola." Soy milk also comes in vanilla and carob flavors. You can find it in some grocery stores. Soy protein can also be found as a supplement in health food stores.

Eat a burger. Some vegetarian hamburger substitutes are made with soy products. Check the label, says Barbara P. Klein, Ph.D., professor of foods and nutrition at the University of Illinois at Urbana-Champaign. Look at the fat content as well; some contain more than their fair share. If you just can't do without your meat, try one of the vegetarian sloppy joe mixes available at grocery stores and use half meat and half soy substitute.

Lay off the sauce. You won't get much help from soy sauce—it contains very little soy, says Dr. Lachance. Most products are also loaded with salt, which can raise your blood pressure. Other condi-

Visit an Exotic Aisle

Adjusting your diet for disease prevention calls for changing your shopping habits as well. And that means being prepared to steer your grocery cart off the beaten path.

Fill 'er up with produce. At the supermarket, head straight for the fruits and vegetables section and fill up your cart there, suggests Isabella Lipinska, Ph.D., a nutritional counselor for the Cardiac Rehabilitation Program at St. Elizabeth's Medical Center in Boston. That way, you'll be less likely to overdo it in the aisles with less nutritional foods.

Find strength in numbers. Lots of cities have co-op food stores, where members buy food in bulk and split up the distribution chores. Usually, you get top-quality fruits and vegetables at a lower price. If you and your friends organize a combined "buying and cooking" club, you'll reap benefits in taste, health, and finances, notes John Potter, M.D., Ph.D., head of the Cancer Prevention Research Program at the Fred Hutchinson Cancer Research Center in Seattle.

Buy it off the truck. Frequent farmers markets, where local produce is often tastier, suggests Dexter Morris, M.D., vice chairman of the Department of Emergency Medicine and a heart researcher at the University of North Carolina at Chapel Hill School of Medicine. With some extra charm in your shopping expedition and a tastier time in the dining room, you'll be more likely to stick to the fruits-and-vegetables habit.

ments, such as Bac-Os, contain soy, but in such small amounts that they won't do you any good.

Make a substitution. When you bake, trade 25 percent of your regular flour for soy flour. You'll get those soy benefits, and most recipes will come out the same, says Mark Messina, Ph.D., a nutritionist and soy expert in Port Townsend, Washington, and author of *The Simple Soybean and Your Health*.

Lignans: A Little Flax'll Do Ya

Lignans are powerful plant estrogens that are most plentiful in flaxseed, something that you probably don't normally include in your diet. You do get small amounts in cereals and vegetables.

"Some baking companies add small amounts of flax, or linseed, to give breads and other baked goods a nutty flavor," notes Dr. Hasler. "You can get products made with flax in health food stores, too."

"This is a new area for research, and we don't know that much about it yet," cautions Dr. Hasler. She suggests that if you want to add flax to your diet, do so very slowly, perhaps sprinkling a little fortified flax (no more than a teaspoon) on your breakfast cereal. It's available at health food stores.

Cancer. Lignans, especially in flaxseed, also seem to prevent breast cancer, at least in the laboratory. In addition to working as phytoestrogens, providing the body with estrogen, lignans are antioxidants, helping to prevent cell damage and stop cancers before they start.

Heart disease and stroke. As antioxidants, lignans may help prevent the dangerous LDL cholesterol damage that can lay the groundwork for heart disease.

In a study at the University of Western Ontario, rats ate flax and flaxseed oil—and their blood pressures held stable, while blood pressures rose in the rats that got no flax in their diets. In another study, people ate three slices of bread containing flaxseed and 15 grams of ground flaxseed a day and saw drops in LDL cholesterol levels and in the clotting action of their blood.

Carotenoids Show Their Colors

You see evidence of carotenoids in the bright red, orange, and yellow pigments of some plants. They're also in leafy green vegetables. You'll find them in carrots, tomatoes, sweet potatoes, cantaloupe, winter squash, parsley, pink grapefruit, Swiss chard, spinach, beet greens, pumpkin, watermelon, broccoli, mangoes, oranges, papaya, and tangerines. They're also in fish liver oil.

Cancer. "Study after study shows that diets rich in carotenoids fight disease," says Dr. Lachance. In one, a high-carotenoid diet reduced the risk of lung cancer in nonsmokers. Researchers studied the diets of 1,197 people in Hawaii. Those who ate a variety of fruits and vegetables and consumed high amounts of three carotenoids had less lung cancer. The European Institute of Oncology in Milan looked at rates of oral cancer in Beijing, China, and found that carotenoid consumption reduced risk.

In a survey of 3,000 northern Italians, people who ate seven or more servings of raw tomatoes a week ended up with a 50 to 60 percent lower risk for cancers of the mouth, esophagus, stomach, colon, and rectum. Researchers also think that carotenoids reduce the risk of cancers of the cervix and pancreas.

A particularly powerful carotenoid, lycopene, comes in tomatoes and everything made from them, including pizza sauce and ketchup. (Watermelon, guava, and pink grapefruit also have lycopene.)

In the laboratory, tomato juice extract has prevented the formation of cancer-causing compounds. An Israeli study showed that lycopene knocks out human endometrial, breast, and lung cancer cells in the laboratory. It also affects the systems that allow the cells to grow into tumors. And researchers at Harvard Medical School found that people who ate tomatoes, tomato sauce, tomato juice, and pizza— all foods rich in lycopene—had lower rates of prostate cancer.

But lycopene isn't the only carotenoid that protects. Beta-carotene is another potent disease preventer. You get it in sweet potatoes, carrots, apricots, spinach, collard greens, cooking pumpkins, and cantaloupe.

Your body converts beta-carotene into some vitamin A and retinoic acid, which thwarts precancerous and cancerous cells while it enhances T cells, a key part of your body's immune system. As antioxidants, beta-carotene and lycopene root out the dangerous free radicals that can turn cells cancerous.

Researchers note that beta-carotene seems to help reduce the risk of cancers of organ linings, including colon cancer. Researchers think that precancerous colon polyp tissue that contains beta-carotene is less likely to turn malignant. In a combined Swiss and Italian study, beta-carotene in the diet protected against endometrial cancer.

The carotenoids work together, too. In a study conducted by the University of Hawaii, diets rich in beta-carotene, alpha-carotene, and lutein resulted in lower risks of lung cancer in a study of more than 1,200 people. You get lutein in broccoli, green peas, celery, spinach, kale, collard greens, Swiss chard, mustard greens, red peppers, okra, and romaine lettuce.

Heart disease and stroke. Researchers agree that the more carotenoids you eat, the lower your risk will be for chronic heart disease. "They work as antioxidants and prevent the formation of LDL cholesterol," says Dr. Morris.

Try these methods to get the biggest boost from carotenoids.

Use a little fat. "Since most of the carotenoids are fat soluble, eat them with other foods that contain a hint of fat," says Dr. Morris.

Go for color. Reds, oranges, and deep greens tell you that carotenoids are present, even in fruits and vegetables where you might not expect them. For instance, red-leaf lettuce has more carotenoids than iceberg lettuce, and you get more carotenoid benefit from pink grapefruit than from white grapefruit. If you're a meat-and-potatoes sort of person, put some yams or sweet potatoes on your plate for an extra carotenoid boost. (Not that there's anything wrong with white potatoes—they are a good source of potassium, an important mineral, says Dr. Lipinska.) If your lunch features a piece of broiled chicken and potatoes, add a slice of red pepper or tomato, she adds.

Snack on vegetables and crackers. Raw vegetables plus a high-fiber, low-fat cracker or two give you the most phytochemical benefit, Dr. Lipinska says. The small amount of fat in the cracker enables your body to take in fat-soluble phytochemicals as well as the water-soluble kind. Make your snack even more beneficial by choosing a bright orange or green vegetable, high in carotenoids.

Concentrate. You'll get more carotenoids from

Prescription for Prevention

When you eat a diet rich in fruits, vegetables, and grains, you stoke up your defenses against heart disease, cancer, and stroke. You may cut your disease risk in half.

Do:

■ Wheat products and vegetables for insoluble fiber.

■ Eat at least five helpings a day of fruits and vegetables.

■ Choose bright orange or dark green vegetables.

■ Add vegetables rich in organosulfur compounds to soups. Choose garlic, onions, leeks, chives, shallots, broccoli, and cauliflower, for example.

■ Enjoy raw vegetables with a cracker to get the benefits of both water-soluble and fat-soluble phytochemicals.

■ Eat the leaves, seeds, and peel, where many phytochemicals are concentrated.

■ Drink milk made from soybeans and try soy-based vegetarian hamburger substitutes.

■ Drink tea, which is rich in phytochemicals, instead of coffee.

Don't:

■ Add more than just a teaspoon of flax to your cereal.

■ Rely on canned fruits, which lose valuable nutrients during storage.

some concentrated products, says Dr. Morris. Tomato paste, ounce for ounce, contains twice as many carotenoids as do fresh tomatoes, for instance. Tomato puree contains 20 percent more.

Keep your own hue. Carotenoids are fat soluble, which means that your body stores them until they are used. If you take in too much, the side effects will be obvious to everyone you see. "You can turn orange." Dr. Morris says. "This doesn't happen if you get carotenoids in food, because you'd have to eat an awful lot. But it's easy to take too many supplements."

Beyond keeping your normal skin tone, Dr. Morris says, you're better off getting your carotenoids from food—not from a bottle—for other reasons: It's hard to know the quality of supplements and how well your body can use the substances they contain. And researchers haven't yet figured out whether the carotenoids themselves help your body or whether other substances linked with them in fruits and vegetables are providing the real benefit.

Flavonoids: Can't-Miss Protection

You're in luck—flavonoids occur in just about every plant, from apples to onions to soy. Even black tea (the kind that you get at the grocery store) and Japanese green tea contain flavonoids.

Cancer. "Flavonoids dissipate the substances that cause cancer," Dr. Lachance says. "They prevent—they don't cure."

Studies at Rutgers University have shown that, at least in laboratory mice, green tea blocks the development of cancer tumors by 90 percent. Black tea, says Dr. Lachance, performs only a little less impressively. Green tea is also one of many flavonoids that double as powerful antioxidants. Researchers have found that the process used to make the green tea leaves activates a key antioxidant, epigallocatechin gallate. In the lab, it prevents tumors of a broad range of cancers.

Research indicates that some flavonoids, such as quercetin in onions and kaempferol in leeks and garlics, fight off the earliest stages of cancer. In a Dutch study involving 58,279 men and 62,573 women ages 55 to 69, scientists found that onion eaters decreased their risk of stomach cancer.

Heart disease and stroke. In a Canadian laboratory study, a flavonoid called purpurogallin protected the heart against the injuries that occur during a heart attack. Another Dutch study followed 805 men ages 65 to 84 over a 25-year period. Those who ate a flavonoid-focused diet (mostly from black tea, but also from onions and apples) had a 58 percent drop in risk of dying of a heart attack. Average daily tea consumption? About 3.4 cups.

That study was part of a larger, seven-country study which revealed that, all in all, a high-flavonoid diet was the reason for a 25 percent variance in coronary heart disease among the countries studied. Researchers in Israel discovered that red wine, which is high in flavonoids, lowers LDL cholesterol levels, which when raised leads to hardening of the arteries. Laboratory research shows that flavonoids can reduce the tendency of blood platelets to stick together and cause clots.

To get the most of flavonoids, try these tips.

Look to the vine. Researchers are actively scrutinizing "the French paradox," the fact that people who drink wine regularly seem to have lower rates of heart disease even when they dine on rich French cuisine. "We think that the chemicals in wine are potent antioxidants, and they may keep blood from clotting," says Andrew Waterhouse, Ph.D., a researcher in the department of viticulture and enology at the University of California, Davis. The people who benefit, studies show, drink just a little wine on a daily basis.

Turn to tea. Dr. Lachance says that tea will give you an effective dose of flavonoids—but you have to drink it regularly. "I drink a cup of coffee in the morning and then drink black tea the rest of the day," he says. "I drink around a half-dozen cups. It's safer than coffee, too, because it's not as stimulating."

Triterpenes, Monoterpenes: Cancer Squeezers

Triterpenes are a group of compounds that include limonoids, found in the seeds, fruit, and juice of citrus plants. Monoterpenes also are found in citrus but in the skin or peel. Monoterpenes are also present in caraway seeds in the form of D-carvone.

Cancer. "We're excited about these substances as possible anti-cancer agents because people consume them at high levels anyway," says Dr. Miller. "We used to think that vitamin C was the protective component in citrus, but studies suggest other agents. For this reason it's better to drink the glass of orange juice than to take a vitamin tablet."

Epidemiological studies show that citrus consumption is linked to protection against a whole slew of cancers—oral, esophageal, and pancreatic, among others.

In laboratory rats, some of the phytochemicals in citrus reduce the number of tumors by up to 60 percent. This is only at very high dosages and with side effects. They also help your body increase the production of enzymes that dispose of cancer-causing substances.

Dr. Miller is studying limonoids, a group of cancer-fighting phytochemicals that fend off oral cancer in animals. Two substances, limonin and limonin 17-beta-D-glucopyranoside, actually block and suppress tumors.

Heart disease and stroke. A University of Wisconsin at Madison study shows that monoterpenes can decrease the harmful LDL cholesterol that contributes to heart disease and stroke.

It's definitely worth making the effort to get monoterpenes into your diet because you get a lot of other good things from citrus, too (such as vitamin C and fiber). Here are two ways to do it.

Make salad surprising. Combine fruits to make a fruit salad (avoid canned fruits—they lose vitamin C during storage). Buy a variety of fruits and, every day, serve them in different combinations—a slice of plum, apricot, peach, and apple, for example.

Use the peel. Use orange or lemon peel as a flavor enhancer in fruit drinks and carbonated beverages. It's rich in protective d-limonene. For limonoids, keep away from the watered-down citrus drinks or the carbonated citrus drinks. Eat the actual fruit or drink the real juice, recommends Dr. Miller. In one study, researchers applied orange-peel oil to skin tumors and found that the tumors grew much more slowly.

Tannins: Stains That Sustain

You might think of tannins as colorful concoctions used in dying, making inks, and even in the tanning process. One tannin, ellagic acid, is in the kinds of foods that stain your clothing—strawberries, raspberries, blackberries, and loganberries. And it may make a lasting impression on your body, too, by protecting you from cancer.

Cancer. Research on tannins (and ellagic acid, in particular) is under way in laboratory studies. Researchers believe ellagic acid may keep cancerous substances from altering the DNA of healthy cells. In the laboratory, it neutralizes cancer-causing substances and helps prevent cancers in tissues of the lung, liver, skin, and esophagus.

Heart disease and stroke. In the laboratory, ellagic acid works as an antioxidant, preventing oxidation of the fats that turn into LDL cholesterol.

Here are some ways Dr. John Potter suggests for getting tannins into your system.

Go straight to the source. Grape juice may be a sweet refreshment, but you're better off eating the grape itself to get the benefit of the phytochemicals clustered in the grape peel.

Get jamming. You're better off eating the whole fruit and nothing but the fruit. But if your tastes run to jellies, take a close look at the contents listed on the label. Pick products listing a higher content of real fruit.

Top it off. Find inventive ways to work berries into your daily eating pattern. Use berries to top off desserts like sherbet, for instance, or sprinkle them over a slice of melon.

The Top Foods
for Your Health

From Almonds to Yogurt, Your Edible Allies

The pharmacy is not where folks over 50 find the best stuff for warding off cancer, heart disease, and stroke. Cheap, good-tasting, disease-preventing substances are right there in the everyday, garden-variety foods available in any grocery store.

The secret lies in eating a wide variety of the right foods that contain an assortment of disease-fighting substances. That way, you create a protective mosaic of vitamins, minerals, enzymes, and other substances that help you stay disease free. So be sure you get the five-plus servings of fruits and vegetables recommended by the National Cancer Institute and leading nutritionists.

The following foods stand out as top-notch disease fighters, easily found in the supermarket.

A note about serving sizes: The standard serving size for cooked vegetables or chopped raw vegetables is ½ cup and, for raw leafy vegetables, the serving size is 1 cup. For fruit a serving is one medium apple, banana, or orange or ½ cup of chopped, cooked, or canned fruit. A serving of cooked cereal, rice, pasta, or cooked dried beans is ½ cup.

A note about the Daily Value: The Daily Value is the amount of a nutrient that scientists figure you need each day if you eat a 2,000-calorie diet. If you eat more or fewer calories, your Daily Value will be higher or lower accordingly.

A note about vitamin A: Actual vitamin A is found in animals, not plants. A source of vitamin A in our bodies, however, is beta-carotene, which is found in plants. Throughout this chapter you will note that certain vegetables or fruits are a good source of vitamin A because, through a simple process, the body converts beta-carotene into a usable form of vitamin A.

Almonds

Not what you would expect to head up a list of healthy foods, almonds weigh in like sumo wrestlers in calories and fat. But fortunately, most of the fat is monounsaturated, the kind that may actually reduce high blood pressure and cholesterol.

Cancer. Almonds deliver copper to power up your immune system, which needs more of a boost as you get older. A serving of almonds (the amount that fits in your hand, about an ounce, or 24 whole kernels) gives you 13.5 percent of the Daily Value for copper. Plus, they provide some fiber (1.9 milligrams) and calcium to help lower your risk of colon cancer.

Heart disease and stroke. In one study, people eating 3½ ounces of almonds a day reduced cholesterol levels by 20 points. Almonds are a good source of riboflavin, which has been associated with lower heart disease rates. In addition, a handful of almonds is high in magnesium—it provides 21 percent

187

of the Daily Value, which may help prevent blood clots and lower blood pressure.

Apples

Whole, sliced, juiced, cooked, or sauced, apples deliver protection from disease.

Cancer. Take a bite and take in some glutathione, which may be a tongue-twister to say, but it's a mouth-saver to eat. The glutathione in apples cuts the risk of oral and throat cancer by up to 50 percent in comparison to the risk in people who don't eat apples. It also makes your immune system work as though it belongs to someone much younger. The problem is that as you approach 60 your blood levels of glutathione may be 17 percent lower than people under 40. This antioxidant is available only from raw vegetables and fruits, so eat your apples raw. (You'll have to think of another excuse to eat apple pie.)

Apples are also a great source of another mouth-saver—vitamin C, which helps guard your mouth against cancer. And they provide you with flavonoids, antioxidants that help stop cancer's start-up process. A medium-size apple, with peel, gives you a little more than 2.5 grams of total fiber, protection against both cancer and heart disease.

Heart disease and stroke. When researchers in the Netherlands studied 805 men ages 65 to 84, they found that the apple eaters had a 32 percent lower risk of dying from heart disease, in part because of flavonoids concentrated in the apple peel.

Researchers think that the vitamin C in apples also performs such feats as lowering your blood pressure, which could help protect your arteries and heart. Vitamin C also helps prevent oxidation of blood cholesterol and, therefore, slows clogging of the arteries. Apples are high in flavonoids, which have antioxidant properties. One small apple with skin gives you 1 gram of soluble fiber, which can aid heart health.

Apricots

The taste is tart, but the benefits are sweet. This little low-fat, low-cal, zero-cholesterol fruit packs a lot of protection in the form of beta-carotene, dietary fiber, and vitamin C. And remember that apricots in the dried form contain even greater concentrations of their beneficial nutrients.

Cancer. A serving of three fresh apricots boosts your body's defenses as a source of more than half of the Daily Value of vitamin A. People who eat a lot of vitamin A/beta-carotene have lower rates of breast, cervical, and uterine cancer. They may also get protection against cancer of the esophagus, stomach, colon, and mouth. Vitamin A also helps keep invaders out by strengthening the mucous membranes that line the digestive, respiratory, reproductive, and urinary tracts.

The vitamin C helps lower your risk of cancer of many vital organs. More than 1 gram of insoluble fiber is in a ½-cup serving of canned apricots, and there are 5 grams of total fiber in ¼ cup of dried apricots, which helps fend off colon and breast cancer.

Heart disease and stroke. Proof that good things come in small packages, seven dried apricot halves give you 1.1 grams of soluble fiber to help bring down high cholesterol and high blood pressure.

189

Apricots provide potassium, which helps lower high blood pressure. One serving of three fresh apricots is the source for more than half the Daily Value of vitamin A, which may protect you from the harmful low-density lipoprotein (LDL) cholesterol buildup that can lead to hardening of the arteries. Stroke victims in Belgium fared better when their diets included lots of sources of vitamin A.

Artichokes

The ancient Romans paid more for artichokes than any other garden vegetable. Perhaps they were thinking about taste rather than disease protection. But you can think of both.

Cancer. A ½-cup serving of artichoke hearts gives you 4.5 grams of total dietary fiber for protection against colon cancer. Plus, you get 10 percent of your Daily Value of copper to boost your immune system. And 14 percent of the Daily Value of vitamin C helps protect you against a variety of cancers.

Heart disease and stroke. One medium cooked artichoke gives you 2.2 grams of soluble fiber for heart health. Its vitamin C also fights the hazardous LDL cholesterol and other fats in the blood by keeping them from latching onto artery walls where they can do their dirty work.

A serving provides almost 11 percent of the Daily Value for folate (the natural form of the supplement folic acid), which helps prevent rises in homocysteine levels. Elevated homocysteine may increase the risk of heart disease. Researchers estimate that if people took in more of the B vitamin folate, between 13,500 and 50,000 deaths from coronary artery disease could be prevented every year. A ½-cup serving of artichoke hearts provides you with more than 12 percent of your Daily Value of magnesium, which may prevent the blood clotting that increases your risk of a heart attack or stroke. It also helps lower blood pressure.

Asparagus

It's a stand-up kind of vegetable. Next time you see a bunch of asparagus upright in a pan of water in the grocery store, think about how these low-cal, cholesterol-free little green spears stand up to disease.

Cancer. According to research, asparagus could actually help block tumor development. Obviously, you wouldn't want to go on an all-asparagus diet, but these laboratory findings make it clear that your body will benefit from a regular helping of these great defenders. In the laboratory, compounds in asparagus keep cells from mutating and keep tumors from forming.

Weighing in with 1.4 grams of insoluble fiber, a single serving of cooked fresh asparagus (about six spears) beefs up your defenses against colon cancer. Asparagus also provides vitamin C to protect you from a variety of cancers and copper to help strengthen your immune system.

Asparagus is a very good source of an antioxidant called glutathione, which has been found in animal studies to inhibit tumor growth. Asparagus gives you almost 33 percent of a day's requirement for folate, which keeps your cells healthy. Studies show that people who eat a diet rich in folate have lower levels of cancer of the cervix, colon, and rectum, and folate may help prevent cancer of the esophagus.

Heart disease and stroke. The ingredient list for asparagus reads like a who's who of heart protection: It's a source for nearly 10 percent of your Daily Value of vitamin A, which helps prevent buildup of the harmful LDL cholesterol in your arteries. At the same time, people with high amounts of beta-carotene have higher levels of the protective high-density lipoprotein (HDL) cholesterol than people with low amounts of beta-carotene.

As you get older, it becomes harder for your body to absorb the B vitamins, so after the age of 50 you have to take in more than you used to. B vitamins are plentiful in asparagus: Folate and vitamin B_6 protect your heart, partly by lowering levels of the harmful amino acid homocysteine. Homocysteine is associated with high risk of heart attack and stroke. Riboflavin boosts the other B vitamins.

The soluble fiber in asparagus lowers the levels of LDL cholesterol and fats in your blood.

Avocados

Avocados contain a lot of protective nutrients, but they're also high in fat. One avocado leaves you with almost 31 grams of fat. And that's a bigger problem now that you're older and trying to slow the buildup of the body fat that leaves you more at risk for heart disease, some cancers, and excessive weight. But there's a silver lining: About two-thirds of the fat is monounsaturated, which may actually lower cholesterol levels. Plus, you can use mashed avocados or guacamole as a healthier mayonnaise substitute.

Cancer. Heading up the protective roster are 5.3 grams of insoluble fiber—a lot of protection from colon cancer. You get as much insoluble fiber from one avocado as you do from 5 tablespoons of toasted wheat germ.

A standard serving, half of an avocado, gives you 14 percent of the Daily Value of vitamin B_6. If you're low on vitamin B$_6$, your immune system gets sluggish—something you can't afford to have happen as you get older. But studies show that increasing your intake of vitamin B$_6$ will reverse that slump. You also get 14 percent of the Daily Value of copper, important to help shift your immune system into high gear. Beta-carotene in avocados helps disable cancer-causing agents before they strike. Avocados also provide vitamin C to guard against a variety of cancers and glutathione to help strengthen your immune system.

A serving of avocado provides more than 15 percent of the Daily Value of folate. Researchers think that this nutrient protects healthy cells from cancerous invasion. High levels of folate are also linked to low rates of cancer of the cervix, colon, rectum, lung, and possibly of the esophagus. In the laboratory, substances in avocados even keep tumors from getting started.

Heart disease and stroke. In one study people who ate ½ to 1½ avocados each day reduced cholesterol levels from an average of 236 milligrams per deciliter (mg/dl) of blood to 217. Even better, the levels of the beneficial HDL cholesterol, which lowers your risk of heart attack, didn't go down.

Researchers note that certain B vitamins can reduce heart disease risks by 10 to 25 percent. And avocados are loaded with B vitamins, including folate and vitamin B$_6$. Studies show that folate and vitamin B$_6$ may help keep the levels of homocysteine low, which means lower risk of heart disease. Homocysteine tends to accumulate in the blood of people who eat meat, and it may harm artery walls. Half an avocado gives you more than 9 percent of the Daily Value for magnesium, which also bolsters heart health.

Go Light on Meat

Unless you count skinless chicken breast and fish, you won't see meat on the list of top 100 foods for health. Meat tends to be high in calories, fat, and iron. But some lean cuts have a place in a healthy diet. Here are the top meat-dish choices for women and men over age 50. All give you over half your Daily Value of protein.

Eye round roast. A lean 3-ounce serving (the size of a deck of cards) has 143 calories, 59 milligrams of cholesterol, and just over 4 grams of fat. Protective nutrients include vitamin B_{12}, zinc, niacin, vitamin B_6, potassium, riboflavin, and magnesium.

Top loin steak. One lean 3-ounce serving with fat trimmed, contains 168 calories, 65 milligrams of cholesterol, and 7 grams of fat. Protective nutrients include vitamin B_{12}, zinc, niacin, vitamin B_6, potassium, riboflavin, and magnesium.

Lamb foreshank. One lean 3-ounce serving gives you 159 calories, 88 milligrams of cholesterol, and 5 grams of fat. Protective nutrients include vitamin B_{12}, zinc, niacin, riboflavin, magnesium, and potassium.

Pork tenderloin. One lean 3-ounce serving gives you 139 calories, 67 milligrams of cholesterol, and 4 grams of fat. Protective nutrients include vitamin B_{12}, riboflavin, vitamin B_6, zinc, and magnesium.

Avocados are rich in soluble fiber, which helps control cholesterol. Plus, avocados contain potassium, which helps to lower blood pressure and reduces your risk of stroke.

Bananas

Voted America's favorite fruit, bananas are almost fat-free.

Cancer. The B vitamins—one banana has 33 percent of the Daily Value of vitamin B_6—help strengthen your immune system to fight off cancer-causing interlopers.

Scientists think that a healthy helping of other substances in bananas—vitamin C and the powerful antioxidant glutathione—can help cut your risk of cancer of the mouth and strengthen your immune system. When glutathione was added to the white blood cells of both older and younger people, it increased their infection-fighting ability. The benefit was especially strong in the white blood cells from the older people. The 1.4 grams of insoluble fiber, found in one banana, helps reduce your risk of colon cancer. In the laboratory, substances in bananas keep tumors from developing.

Heart disease and stroke. In a study of 859 men and women, those who ate just one potassium-rich fruit, such as bananas, per day had a 40 percent lower risk of stroke.

Folate, a B vitamin that protects against cancer, also safeguards your heart by lowering levels of the harmful amino acid homocysteine, a risk factor in heart disease and heart attack. Vitamin C increases beneficial HDL cholesterol while it reduces harmful LDL cholesterol and triglycerides. You get 17 percent of the Daily Value of vitamin C from one banana.

Barley

Barley has been a staple of good health from time immemorial, even getting a thumbs-up in the Bible, which describes the good land as one of "wheat and barley." With that kind of endorsement, what are you waiting for?

Cancer. One serving of barley (½ cup cooked) gives you almost 2 grams of insoluble fiber to fight cancer.

Heart disease and stroke. A ½-cup serving of cooked barley gives you 1.2 grams of soluble fiber, which is great news for your heart.

Beans

The butt of many jokes, beans are superheroes of disease protection. Take your pick: black, garbanzo, cranberry, navy, pink, pinto, kidney, white, or yellow. You can't beat them.

Cancer. Research shows that women who eat a diet rich in beans have lower rates of breast cancer, thanks to substances in beans that block estrogen. Natural chemicals in green and wax beans, and even in the juice from beans, keep cells from mutating. They also destroy enzymes that give cancer its start.

Beans boost your immune system. One-half cup of canned garbanzo beans (chick-peas), for instance, gives you 10 percent of your Daily Value of copper and 8.4 percent of your Daily Value of zinc. You get protection from colon cancer with almost 4 grams of insoluble fiber in ½ cup of cooked beans.

Heart disease and stroke. A high-bean diet cuts the risk of heart disease because it lowers cholesterol levels. Even bean sprouts help your heart. In one study people with very high cholesterol levels ate 1½ cups of cooked beans daily for three weeks and made no other dietary changes. Their cholesterol levels fell by an average of 60 points.

One-half cup of cooked garbanzo beans gives you 1.3 grams of soluble fiber, the heart-protecting stuff. And 35 percent of the Daily Value of folate further cuts your risk of heart disease and stroke. Plus, you get magnesium and potassium. These nutrients help prevent blood clots and reduce high blood pressure.

Beets

On the surface, beets don't look all that remarkable. But research reveals that beets are rich in the protective plant compounds known as phytochemicals.

Cancer. Sure, beets have an impressive lineup of vitamins, minerals, and fiber. Just ½ cup canned beets gives you a very beneficial 1.5 grams of insoluble fiber and 6.4 percent of the Daily Value for folate to protect your cells and DNA coding.

But that isn't what has been impressing lab researchers. What's in the beet? At least 11 (and probably more) phytochemicals that fight cancer, including genistein, a substance that keeps estrogen from linking up with cancer cells to start tumor construction. It also keeps blood vessels from getting supplies to tumors. But beets have even more cancer-fighting properties that researchers have yet to explain.

Heart disease and stroke. One serving (½ cup) gives you more than 0.5 gram of the soluble fiber that helps lower your cholesterol levels and keeps plaque in the arteries from getting out of hand. Plus, you get 6.4 percent of your daily needs for the ever-important folate, lowering your risk of heart disease.

Don't forget the green stalk and leaves that top the beet itself. One-half cup of the cooked greens (especially when they're young) will give you 2.2 milligrams of beta-carotene, 2 grams of dietary fiber, plus some calcium, to lower mild blood pressure and cholesterol, magnesium to ease heart arrhythmia, and vitamin C to lower blood pressure and prevent oxidation of blood cholesterol. What's more, that same serving of beet greens provides 9 percent of the Daily Value of copper—a boon to your immune system.

Blackberries and Blueberries

Black or blue, you can't go wrong. Ever notice that when blueberries are exposed to acid (in lemon juice or yogurt, for example), they turn red? Exposed to baking soda, they turn a little green. But fear not—the change in color won't affect the change in protection.

Cancer. Blackberries pack more fiber than any other summer fruit (3.6 grams in ½ cup). Blueberries and blackberries contain important cancer fighters, including the phytochemicals catechins, flavonoids, and phenolic acids. Blackberries also contain ellagic acid, which neutralizes three different cancer-causing agents. Blackberries are high in vitamin C, which helps reduce your risk of cancers of the breast, cervix, esophagus, lung, mouth, pancreas, rectum, and stomach.

Heart disease and stroke. One-half cup of blackberries gives you more than 25 percent of the Daily Value of vitamin C. (Blueberries contain a little less vitamin C.) The vitamin C in these berries helps keep your HDL cholesterol levels high, which lowers the risk of your arteries becoming plagued by plaque.

Breads and Cereals

The name of the game is whole grain. Get out your reading glasses and check the fine print on packages. Look for the words "whole wheat" as the first ingredient on your bread wrapper—that means the bread contains whole-wheat flour.

Other good ingredients to look for are things like oat bran, soy flour, seeds, nuts, or whole grain. About 22 nutrients are diminished due to processing. And manufacturers only put a few nutrients back in. For example, enriched flour has had niacin, riboflavin, thiamin, and iron added to it.

Cancer. Two studies have found that something in oats keeps cells from mutating, but they haven't yet identified the compounds that provide the protection.

The consumption of breads and cereals made from whole grains may help lower the risk of colon cancer. Insoluble fiber speeds up the time it takes food to travel through the intestinal tract. So potential cancer-causing substances may be moved out of the body more quickly. Or, it could be that insoluble fiber lowers colon cancer risk because the fermentation of the fibers in the colon lowers the pH levels. Lower pH in the colon has been associated with lower colon cancer risk.

Heart disease and stroke. One slice of whole-wheat bread contains about 2 grams of dietary fiber. Fiber lowers cholesterol levels partly because it slows the absorption of cholesterol. Oats, rye, and barley are good sources of soluble fiber.

While there's little calcium in breads, yeast makes it easy for your body to take full advantage of what's there, according to a study at Creighton University in Omaha, Nebraska. Some bread and cereal products are fortified with vitamins and minerals for added protection against disease. Look for cereals fortified with folic acid, the supplemental form of folate, as well.

Broccoli

This is the workhorse of the food world. A serving (½ cup) of chopped raw broccoli contains only 12 calories and just a tiny bit of fat. Cooking destroys a few nutrients, but broccoli is worth its weight in gold in just about any form.

Cancer. One serving (½ cup) of cooked broccoli gives you 97 percent of the Daily Value of vitamin C, an effective fighter against cancer of the breast, cervix, esophagus, lung, mouth, pancreas, rectum, and stomach.

You also get a sizable portion of folate to help keep your cells healthy and able to fight off cancerous agents. Researchers have found that folate plays an important role in cell division. It also helps keep the genetic coding in DNA intact. People whose diets are rich in folate have lower rates of cervical, colon, rectal, lung, and possibly esophageal cancer.

Cancer-fighting substances in broccoli also include such tongue twisters as flavonoids, isothiocyanates, sulphoraphane, indoles, carotenoids, dithiolthiones, glutathione (in uncooked broccoli), monoterpenes, plant sterols, phenolic acids, glucobrassicin. (Whew!) In fact, researchers have cataloged—and they're not done yet—more than 30 substances in broccoli that seem to have cancer-fighting abilities.

Heart disease and stroke. A lot of the cancer-fighting substances also help your heart. Vitamin C can prevent the LDL particles in blood from becoming oxidized, which helps lessen the risks for heart disease. A 13-year study of men with high cholesterol levels revealed that the higher their carotenoid levels were, the lower their risks were for heart disease and strokes. Flavonoids lower your risk of heart disease and heart attack. Carotenoids shoot down harmful LDL cholesterol.

Cooked broccoli gives you 1.2 grams of heart-saving soluble fiber, which lowers LDL cholesterol levels and helps control blood sugar.

Broccoli is a source for a high amount of vitamin A, which may help decrease your risk of heart disease. Unlike some foods, broccoli contributes calcium that your body can use easily, which is important because calcium helps reduce mild high blood pressure and reduce harmful LDL cholesterol. The higher your LDL levels, the bigger your risk of heart disease.

Cabbage

In Lewis Carroll's *Through the Looking Glass*, a talking walrus speculates about cabbages and kings. It might have sounded like nonsense to put the two together, but the walrus had a point. Cabbage is a king of disease protection.

Any way you slice it, coleslaw it, steam it, boil it, or soup it, cabbage is a powerful disease-fighting food. And savoy cabbage, the crinkly stuff, is the leader of the protective pack.

Cancer. Researchers at the Strang-Cornell Cancer Research Lab in New York City found that women

How to Be a Crack Snacker

Remember: The terms *snack* and *junk food* are not at all the same. Here's how to satisfy your munchies and get disease prevention at the same time.

Plant the seeds. Seeds don't seem like healthy foods. They're pretty high in fat. But, in moderation, they offer you a lot of protection from cancer, heart disease, and stroke.

Sunflower seeds. They're a good source of fiber and vitamin E, an important nutrient that in supplement form protects against heart attacks, cancer, and stroke. Although it's hard to get vitamin E in most of the foods you eat, eating foods that contain vitamin E can only help in the fight against heart disease. A ¼-cup serving provides almost 3 grams of fiber. But here's the problem: You also get almost 16 grams of fat from that ¼ cup.

Sesame seeds. There's that trade-off again: High calories, high fat (1 ounce gives you 13 grams). You also get iron that you probably don't need, since your body stores more iron as you get older. On the positive side, in a 1-ounce serving, you get almost 4 percent of the Daily Value of calcium, 20 percent of the Daily Value of copper, almost 5 grams of fiber, almost 25 percent of the magnesium that your heart needs daily, and 115 milligrams of your potassium needs,

who eat lots of cabbage and other cruciferous vegetables have lower levels of a kind of estrogen that stimulates breast cancer. The estrogen declined just five days after the women started eating more cruciferous vegetables. And the levels stayed down for the three

helping to control your blood pressure. Plus you get an assortment of riboflavin, niacin, and folate (the natural form of the supplement folic acid).

Ice the fruit. Make fruit ices. Put a serving of your favorite fruit in a blender and mix it until smooth. Pour it into a bowl or shallow pan and put it in the freezer. Stir every 15 minutes or so to break up ice crystals and keep it from freezing solid too fast. It will take 1 to 1½ hours (and six to eight vigorous stirrings).

Pop the corn. Three cups of air-popped, unbuttered popcorn—enough to get you through even the longest movie—gives you 92 calories, 1 gram of fat, and more than 3 grams of fiber.

Soiree with sorbet. If you're on the prowl for a healthful after-dinner treat, try fruit sorbet with some fresh fruit thrown in. Not only will you stoke up on the goodness of the fruit, you also will take in less fat and cholesterol than you would with ice cream.

Pear it down. Grate a crispy Bosc pear and put it on hot breakfast cereal for a taste treat. Slice the Comice pear and use it in cereals or even for dessert.

Eat potato chips. Do what? Surprise—fat-free potato chips are readily available these days, so you can have the snack that you crave without the high fat, sodium, and calories. Look for brands with zero fat and low sodium and calories.

months of the study. Those who ate the equivalent of one-third of a head of cabbage daily got the most benefit. Researchers attribute the drop to one substance, indole-3-carbinol.

The list of heavy-duty cancer fighters in cabbage

also includes flavonoids, indoles, monoterpenes, phenolic acids, plant sterols, and sulforaphane. This long list of the hard-to-pronounce natural chemicals stops cancer at every stage of its development. Some substances keep cancerous agents from getting the slightest toehold in cells. Others keep healthy cells from mutating, block tumor development, or cut off the blood supply to tumors.

Cruciferous vegetables such as cabbage also contain glutathione, which helps counter cellular destruction by free radicals.

Heart disease and stroke. One cup of shredded raw cabbage gives you 37.6 percent of the vitamin C that you need each day, increasing your protective HDL cholesterol and lowering hazardous LDL cholesterol levels.

That cup of shredded raw cabbage provides some folate, which helps decrease the risk of heart disease.

Cantaloupe

One of the food world's Southern belles, cantaloupe looks sweet but gets tough in your system. You get a mouthful of protection in every bite.

Cancer. You get a healthy 1.5 milligrams of beta-carotene from ½ cup of cubed cantaloupe or about 2.5 milligrams from a quarter of a melon.

Plus, that ½ cup of cubed cantaloupe gives you a little over 50 percent of the Daily Value of two heavy hitters against cancer: vitamin A and vitamin C. And folate weighs in for the fight against cancer. (Folate may help ward off cancer of the cervix, colon, rectum, lung, and possibly the esophagus.) It also helps keep cells healthy and DNA—the substance that makes each person different—from getting damaged and passing on mutations to new cells. Glutathione may cut your risk of oral cancer and helps your immune system work as well as it did when you were a whole lot younger.

Heart disease and stroke. Beta-carotene may help clear your arteries of the harmful LDL cholesterol that can clog up the works and run up your risk of heart disease and stroke. In one major study, people whose diets included high levels of beta-carotene had half the number of fatal heart attacks and strokes as those whose levels were low.

Its potassium helps lower your blood pressure. Cantaloupe provides more than 56 percent of the Daily Value of vitamin C, which increases the good cholesterol, drops the bad, and helps lower your risk of developing arterial plaque.

Carrots

In the 1800s, an art critic predicted a revolution in painting, all because of the way Paul Cézanne painted some simple little carrots. The result? Modern art. Now carrots are at the center of another revolution—the discovery of important disease fighters.

Cancer. The orange color highlights the carrot's protective compounds. Bright oranges, yellows, reds, and greens signal the presence of carotenoids, a powerful class of cancer-fighting substances. A single raw carrot gives you more than 12 milligrams of the carotenoid called beta-carotene, which in turn provides 405 percent of the Daily Value of vitamin A. Scientists note that beta-carotene may actually reverse cancers of the cervix and uterus that have started. And it protects against cancer of the lung, breast, cervix, uterus, esophagus, stomach, colon, and mouth. Vitamin A is an essential component of the mucous membranes that line the digestive, respiratory, urinary, and reproductive tracts, your body's first lines of defense against many invaders.

Researchers at Johns Hopkins University in Baltimore discovered that people who have little beta-carotene in their blood have four times the risk of developing lung cancer. The Harvard Nurses' Study found that women who eat less than one serving a day of foods rich in beta-carotene have a 20 percent higher risk of breast cancer.

Carrots contain other helpful substances, including limonene, to protect against cancer of the mouth. In studies limonene has actually reduced the size of tumors. So far, more than 50 cancer-fighting compounds have been isolated in Bugs Bunny's favorite food.

Heart disease and stroke. Beta-carotene and its chemical cousin vitamin A do wonders for your heart. Studies show that people who get a lot of this nutrient suffer fewer heart attacks. One theory is that the beta-carotene may keep dangerous LDL cholesterol from attaching to artery walls. In the Physicians Health Study, men who took in high levels of beta-carotene had half as many strokes and fatal heart attacks as those who didn't. One-half cup of cooked carrots also gives you 1.1 grams of soluble fiber, which lowers blood cholesterol levels.

Carrots carry vitamin B_6 for possible heart protection and some copper to help maintain heart structure. One raw carrot gives you 11 percent of the Daily Value for vitamin C.

Cauliflower

The plain Jane of the vegetable world, cauliflower looks and tastes, well, pretty colorless. But the lackluster exterior is just a front—the substances in cauliflower go a long way toward protecting you from disease.

Cancer. Researchers have identified a bunch of substances that are powerful cancer fighters (and bestowed upon them names that would bring any Pictionary game to a halt). Some of these substances help the body counteract substances that cause mutations in DNA. Others make it hard for cancer-causing agents to zero in on healthy cells. And they cut off supplies to tumors. Talk about leading the resistance. Cauliflower is a good source of glutathione, an antioxidant, which in the lab has increased the ability of white blood cells to divide.

You also get the usual suspects for cancer prevention: insoluble fiber, folate, and vitamin C. A cup serving of raw cauliflower has 2 grams of insoluble fiber, and ½ cup of cooked cauliflower has almost 1 gram. There's also some vitamin B_6 in a serving of raw cauliflower, which keeps your immune system strong.

Heart disease and stroke. Here's a good lineup for protection: vitamin B_6, which helps lower your risk of heart attack and stroke, plus folate, an important B vitamin that helps reduce your levels of homocysteine, an amino acid linked to plaque buildup in the arteries, heart attack, and stroke.

One-half cup of cooked cauliflower has nearly 0.5 gram of soluble fiber, which lowers LDL cholesterol levels and heart attack risk. It also provides about 40 percent of the Daily Value of vitamin C, which helps increase levels of the good HDL cholesterol while it shoots down the bad LDL stuff.

Celery

A dieter's delight, a serving of celery (three stalks or 1 cup diced) gives you only 19 calories, less than 0.1 gram of fat, and no cholesterol.

Cancer. Studies have shown that compounds in

celery actually neutralize toxic substances and prevent tumors from developing. There's a group of chemicals called the phthalides that may protect you from stomach cancer. When researchers in Minneapolis looked closely at one form of the chemical, 3-n-butyl phthalide, they found that it (along with another substance in celery, sedanolide) interferes with the development of tumors and helps activate an enzyme that detoxifies harmful substances in the body's tissues.

You also get protection from cancer thanks to insoluble fiber, folate, vitamin C, and vitamin B_6.

Heart disease and stroke. Butyl phthalide may also lower blood pressure by helping to relax the muscles that line the blood vessels. In the laboratory the chemical seems to reduce stress hormones that cause blood vessels to constrict and blood pressure to rise. The vitamin C in celery also helps raise your beneficial HDL cholesterol levels, lowering your risk of heart disease and stroke.

Cherries

"Life is just a bowl of cherries," goes the song first belted out by Ethel Merman in 1931. Eat them and you'll sing a song of disease protection.

Cancer. A cup serving of sour cherries gives you almost 1 milligram of protective beta-carotene and is a source of 26 percent of the Daily Value for vitamin A, which may combat cancer-causing substances and disable them before they can invade your body's cells. Scientists discovered that a diet high in beta-carotene-rich foods helps reduce the risk of lung cancer in smokers and nonsmokers.

One-half cup of canned red sour cherries gives you almost 1 gram of protective insoluble fiber. There is some vitamin C in canned sweet cherries. And vitamin C protects you from cancer of the breast, cervix, esophagus, lung, mouth, pancreas, rectum, and stomach. There is also some cancer-fighting beta-carotene. Sour cherries contain more beta-carotene than sweet cherries, and they're lower in calories, too.

Heart disease and stroke. Vitamin C in cherries also helps raise your beneficial HDL cholesterol levels and lower your risk of heart disease and stroke. At the same time, it cuts the amount of the harmful LDL cholesterol and triglycerides that leave you vulnerable to a plaque buildup in your arteries. Its potassium helps keep your blood pressure under control.

Chestnuts

You probably remember a song about chestnuts, open fires, and holidays. Mel Tormé penned the lyrics in 1946. As a disease fighter, chestnuts will help you enjoy many holidays to come.

Cancer. Just eight chestnuts give you 9 grams of dietary fiber for protection against colon cancer and only 1.5 grams of fat. Additionally, chestnuts contain copper to protect your immune system and vitamin C to help lower your risk of cancer of the breast, cervix, esophagus, lung, mouth, pancreas, rectum, and stomach.

Heart disease and stroke. Heart helpers in chestnuts include potassium; magnesium; vitamin C; and the beneficial B vitamins folate, riboflavin, and vitamin B_6. Altogether, you end up with lower blood pressure, less risk of a clot that could lead to a heart attack or stroke, lower levels of the harmful LDL cholesterol, and higher levels of the protective HDL cholesterol.

Chicken Breast

It's a deal you shouldn't pass up: This part of the chicken (without the skin) gives you half the fat that you would get from a trimmed, choice-grade T-bone steak.

Cancer. Your immune system gets a boost, thanks to zinc and vitamin B_6. Chicken breasts are rich in niacin, which some scientists think may help prevent cancer.

Heart disease and stroke. Half a breast gives you a lot of vitamin B_6, which, when combined with folate, can drop your risk of heart disease by 10 to 25 percent, doctors say. You also get smaller amounts of other B vitamins such as riboflavin. Chicken provides potassium, which helps lower high blood pressure; and magnesium, which may also protect your heart by helping lower blood pressure.

Chicory Greens

Time to do a little exploring of the unfamiliar. On your next visit to the vegetable aisle of your supermarket, keep an eye peeled for chicory greens, also known as curly endive or, simply, endive. If your cashier picks it up and asks, "What's that?" you can reply, "It's protection against disease."

Cancer. You get 72 percent of the Daily Value of vitamin C in 1 cup of raw endive, decreasing your risk of a variety of cancers. Almost half of the Daily Value of folate is found in endive, which helps protect you against cancer of the cervix, colon, rectum, lung, and possibly the esophagus. Folate also helps keep cells healthy, making it harder for cancerous invaders to attack. Plus, the calcium in endive seems to give you protection from colon cancer.

Heart disease and stroke. Why leave the tried and true to experiment with this strange food? Because it's a hotbed of heart protection. A rich supply of vitamin C means that your levels of good HDL cholesterol get a boost while you beat down levels of the harmful LDLs and blood fats. Chicory greens also give you 18 percent of the Daily Value of calcium, which may help lower high blood pressure and LDL cholesterol levels, and potassium, which helps lower high blood pressure.

Chinese Cabbage and Bok Choy

They come from different groups within the oriental cabbage family, but both protect you from diseases that kill.

Cancer. Researchers note that people in Asia have lower rates of some forms of cancer. They theorize that compounds such as indole-3-carbinol in cabbages change the body's estrogen metabolism and stop the growth of small virus-caused tumors.

These cabbages give you some fiber. A 1-cup serving of shredded raw bok choy gives you 0.7 gram. And it gives you the important B vitamin folate, which may protect against cancer of the cervix, colorectum, lung, and possibly the esophagus. You also need folate to keep your cells healthy.

One-half cup of boiled bok choy is a source for more than 42 percent of the Daily Value of vitamin A, which strengthens your body's defenses against cancer. Almost 8 percent of the Daily Value of calcium in that ½ cup of bok choy helps lower your risk of colon cancer. Your body absorbs calcium from bok choy slightly more easily than it does calcium from milk.

Heart disease and stroke. You get potassium to help lower your blood pressure. Vitamin A lowers your risk of stroke—one theory is that it keeps LDL cholesterol from getting a grip on artery walls. Plus, with ½ cup of boiled bok choy, you get 37 percent of the Daily Value of vitamin C to further lower LDL and harmful fat levels in the blood and increase the beneficial HDL cholesterol.

Clams

Remember when people used to call money "clams"? Well, for their disease-preventing benefits, clams are worth a lot—especially since, when canned, they're less expensive than a lot of other seafoods. But don't go overboard: One 3-ounce serving of canned clams gives you 23 milligrams of iron or 264 percent of your requirements for iron. Men and postmenopausal women should aim for 9 milligrams or less of iron a day. Your body stores more iron as you age, so you don't want to risk too big a buildup, which potentially can be serious.

Cancer. One serving gives you 29 percent of your Daily Value of copper and almost 16 percent of your Daily Value of zinc to help strengthen your immune system. You'll also get more than 31 percent of your Daily Value of vitamin C, which helps reduce your risk of cancer of the breast, cervix, esophagus, lung, mouth, pancreas, rectum, and stomach. And the calcium in clams helps cut down your risk of colon cancer.

Heart disease. You get big-time heart protection from the B vitamins. One serving of clams gives you more than 1,400 percent of your Daily Value of vitamin B_{12}, plus some folate. Researchers theorize that these B vitamins can lower your risk of heart disease by 10 to

25 percent. They help reduce levels of homocysteine, an amino acid linked to high risk of heart disease.

Researchers say that clams and some other foods from the sea are high in omega-3 fatty acids, which may protect the heart. Omega-3's seem to lower the body's production of triglycerides, fats in the blood that are harmful in excess amounts. Plus, omega-3's help get the triglycerides out of the bloodstream. Scientists have linked low levels of triglycerides to high levels of the HDL cholesterol that may help protect you from heart disease.

Collards

A member of the cabbage family closely related to kale, collards give you disease-fighting benefits along with a mild taste.

Cancer. Indoles, isothiocyanates, sulforaphane, and quercetin—that's not the name of some blue-chip law firm. It's a lineup of cancer-preventing substances that get into your system when you take a bite of collards.

You also build up your body's first line of defense with vitamin A, which helps strengthen the membranes that line your body's vital organs and helps keep cancerous invaders at bay. A serving of collards provides a decent amount of the antioxidant vitamin E, which protects red blood cells and cells of the lungs. A deficiency of vitamin E may cause the initiation of some cancers.

Some studies show that the consumption of high levels of vitamin E decreases the levels of prostaglandin E_2, a substance that limits the efficiency of the immune system. Although these studies used supplements, food sources of vitamin E like collards help.

Heart disease. Collar heart disease with collards. One serving (½ cup, frozen, chopped, and cooked) provides more than 3 grams of beta-carotene, plus it's a source for 101 percent of the Daily Value of vitamin A. These important nutrients may help keep your arteries from getting clogged up with dangerous cholesterol. It also contains more than 37 percent of the Daily Value of vitamin C, which helps increase the protective HDL cholesterol while it lowers the harmful LDLs that can clog your arteries. Collards are also a source of vitamin E. A lack of vitamin E has been associated with the early stages of heart disease.

Corn

In Mitchell, South Dakota, people know how to show some appreciation for corn. Each year, the outside of the Corn Palace in Mitchell is covered in patterns, colors, and designs, all made from ears of corn. It's a big building. More than 3,000 bushels go into the project. And why not? In terms of disease protection, corn deserves a palace.

Cancer. Scientists have identified substances in corn that fight off cell mutations, the first step in cancer production. You get a number of other cancer protectors, too. One ear gives you almost 9 percent of the folate that helps your cells stay healthy. High folate levels are also linked to lower rates of cancer of the cervix, colon, rectum, lung, and possibly the esophagus. Vitamin C cuts your risk of cancer of the breast, cervix, esophagus, lung, mouth, pancreas, rectum, and stomach. Almost 2 grams of insoluble fiber protect against colon cancer.

Heart disease and stroke. Potassium in corn helps lower high blood pressure. You get a helping of the heart-protecting B vitamins and more than 14 percent of the Daily Value of vitamin C to help keep HDL cholesterol levels high and the harmful LDL stuff on the low side, in addition to helping to prevent the buildup of plaque in your arteries.

Cranberries

In pies, sauces, or juices, cranberries do more than give a tang to your taste buds. Most people probably think of cranberries only at Thanksgiving and Christmas, but they provide year-round disease protection.

Cancer. It's time for a reprise on the song of disease prevention called ellagic acid, a polyphenol. In the lab this substance fights cancer of the lung, skin, esophagus, and liver. It decreases the number of tumors and even keeps cancers from forming. Among fruits and nuts tested for ellagic acid content, cranberries have high amounts. Polyphenols also work as antioxidants to fight cancer-causing agents and may even counteract some of the effects of aging.

Cranberries also belt out 1.2 grams of insoluble fiber per ½ cup of chopped raw berries to protect against colon and breast cancer.

Heart disease and stroke. A serving contains more than 0.5 gram of soluble fiber, which helps keep high blood pressure down. Plus, it has 12 percent of your Daily Value of vitamin C, which keeps your arteries clear of the nasty fats and cholesterol that clog things up and lead to heart attacks and strokes. Also, the same polyphenols that protect you from cancer may help stave off heart disease.

Cucumbers

Cool as a cucumber, so the saying goes. But cucumbers are definitely hot stuff when it comes to disease prevention.

Cancer. Chlorogenic acid may be the substance in cucumbers that makes them a powerful weapon against cell mutation. Cucumbers contain other important chemicals that protect you from cancer—coumarins, phenolic acids, monoterpenes, and triterpenes. About a third of a cucumber (an average serving) gives you close to 9 percent of the Daily Value of vitamin C to help protect against cancer of the breast, cervix, esophagus, lung, mouth, pancreas, rectum, and stomach.

Heart disease and stroke. The boost from vitamin C also helps keep your levels of protective HDL cholesterol high.

Figs

The fig leaf provided Adam and Eve with coverage of one kind. And figs still keep you covered against disease. Two fresh medium-size figs contain only 74 calories and less than 0.5 gram of fat.

Cancer. Two fresh medium figs give you almost 1.5 grams of insoluble fiber to protect you from colon and breast cancer. A serving of five dried figs gives you almost 4 grams of insoluble fiber. Those five dried figs supply you with 15 percent of the Daily Value for copper to help your immune system stay strong and fend off invaders. The calcium in figs helps protect against colon cancer.

Heart disease and stroke. You get a lot of cholesterol-lowering soluble fiber from two fresh figs (1.7 grams). Plus, the potassium in figs helps lower your blood pressure.

A serving of five dried figs gives you even more: more than 3.5 grams of soluble fiber, more than 13 percent of the Daily Value for calcium, and 11 percent of the Daily Value of the heart-saving vitamin B_6.

Flounder and Family

From a health standpoint, you just can't go wrong with flounder or its popular relatives sole, turbot, and fluke. Beyond providing nutrients that protect you from disease, they're also low in fat. One average serving of 3 ounces weighs in with 1.3 grams of fat and 100 calories.

Cancer. These flat-bodied bottom-feeding fish are full of disease prevention. One 3-ounce serving (the size of a deck of cards) gives you vitamin B_6 to keep your immune system working effectively.

Heart disease and stroke. Flounder have a good amount of omega-3 fatty acids, which may help lower your risk of heart attack by lowering triglyceride levels. You get the heart-protecting B vitamins, namely vitamin B_6 and B_{12}. These nutrients reduce your risk of heart disease by up to 25 percent. Add to that magnesium to help prevent clots that can cause heart attacks or strokes. Magnesium also helps bring down high blood pressure.

Garlic

In World War II, Russian soldiers used garlic as an antiseptic. Not the sort of information that you'd care to share over dinner, but it should give you an inkling that garlic powers up more than your breath.

Cancer. In lab animals garlic reduces tumor growth by 60 percent. Researchers note that it even keeps cells from mutating. Antioxidants in garlic help keep harmful substances in the body from damaging healthy cells. The anti-tumor-promoting activity in garlic may be due to ajoene, quercetin, or other phytochemicals in the bulb. In the lab, researchers at Penn State University showed that a compound in garlic, DATS, slowed the growth of lung cancer cells. Aged garlic extract inhibited the growth of human breast cancer cells in the test tube.

Heart disease and stroke. Study after study has shown that people who eat one-half to one clove of garlic a day see their cholesterol levels drop by an average of 9 percent.

When scientists studied the results of eight previous garlic powder tests, they found that in half the tests, the people who ate garlic powder had a significant reduction in blood pressure readings.

A study at Tulane University Medical Center in New Orleans found that people who took a special garlic tablet experienced a 6 percent drop in their total cholesterol levels compared to those who did not take the tablet.

Grapefruit

It wasn't given the scientific name *Citrus paradisi* for nothing. Grapefruit is the fruit of paradise in terms of disease protection.

Cancer. Lycopene, carotenoids, limonene, flavonoids, glutathione, terpenes. Sounds like the mutterings of a mad scientist. But these natural chemicals all show cancer-preventing promise, and you get a healthy dose of them in ruby red grapefruit. This is especially good since your lycopene levels decrease as you age.

All grapefruit contain terpenes, substances that encourage enzymes in your system to block carcinogens. Grapefruit of all colors are also rich in vitamin C to protect you from cancer of the breast, cervix, esophagus, lung, mouth, pancreas, rectum, and stomach. Half of a white grapefruit gives you nearly 69 percent of the Daily Value of this important nutrient (you get about 13 percent more from red). You'll get extra fiber if you eat your grapefruit like an orange. Eat the membrane that encases each segment as well as the pulp. You get 1.3 grams of insoluble fiber from half a pink grapefruit with the membrane, to fight off colon and breast cancer. If you spoon the grapefruit out, without eating the membrane, you'll still get 0.5 gram of insoluble fiber.

Heart disease and stroke. The amount of the flavonoid naringin found in half a grapefruit may help prevent excessive clumping of red blood cells in your arteries. That same serving size of any grapefruit equips you with just over a gram of the soluble fiber to help lower your cholesterol. It also contains some potassium, which downs another hazard to your heart by reducing high blood pressure. The vitamin C helps lower the harmful LDL cholesterol levels to keep arteries clear of the plaque that paves the way for heart attacks and strokes. It also helps keep protective HDL cholesterol levels high.

Grapes

Dionysus, the Greek god of wine, supposedly sailed in a ship outfitted with grape vines flowing from the mast. Gods didn't need disease protection, but you do. And the grape provides it.

Cancer. Grapes are a good source of flavonoids, substances that scientists theorize may fight cancer. Plus, there's vitamin C to further cut your risk. Vitamin C seems to lessen the risk of certain cancers, including those of the cervix, breast, lung, mouth, pancreas, rectum, and stomach.

Heart disease and stroke. Flavonoids in grapes protect you from heart disease. In a study of 805 men ages 65 to 84, researchers found that those whose diets were highest in flavonoids had a 32 percent lower risk of dying of heart disease than those who ate the least. Researchers believe that flavonoids keep blood platelets from clumping together and forming a clot.

One-half cup of grapes (that's about 16 grapes) gives you a good amount of vitamin C, which helps raise the good cholesterol, lower the bad, and keep arteries clear. You get more than 0.5 gram of heart-protecting soluble fiber, which helps lower cholesterol.

Green Beans

They're just immature beans, still in the pod (or just out of it). Left in the garden, they would eventually grow up to be Great Northern, kidney, or pinto beans, depending on the variety. But immaturity is a plus (with beans, anyway). They're richer in beta-carotene and vitamin C than dried mature beans.

Cancer. Researchers have found that juice from the beans keeps cells from mutating.

Beta-carotene, which becomes vitamin A in our bodies, works as an antioxidant, fighting cancer-causing substances that your body produces and that come from things like car exhaust and tobacco smoke. In one study of lung cancer in nonsmokers, high intakes of the carotenes in green vegetables and fruits, which include beta-carotene, seemed to help protect against lung cancer. Vitamin A helps disable hazardous substances that can cause cancer—before they go to work in your body. A ½-cup serving of beans also gives you 1 gram of insoluble fiber to help prevent colon cancer.

Heart disease and stroke. Green beans are a source for some vitamin A, which does double duty. Not only does it help protect you against cancer, but it also helps lower your risk of heart attack and stroke. Beta-carotene, which gets converted into vitamin A, works as an antioxidant that may help keep the harmful LDL cholesterol from forming. This is the stuff that forms plaque buildup on artery walls and can pave the way for heart attacks and strokes.

Guavas

These tropical fruits are available in varying quantities, almost all year-round, especially during the late fall and early winter.

Cancer. Guavas look like limes with smooth skin, but they contain six times more vitamin C. In one fruit you get more than 275 percent of the Daily Value of this important nutrient to help sideline your cancer risk.

One guava also gives you more than 4 grams of insoluble fiber to help reduce your risk of colon and breast cancer.

Heart disease and stroke. In one doctor-supervised study, 120 people on medication to lower their blood pressures cut out the medicine and scarfed down several guavas a day. Their blood pressures went down and their levels of cholesterol and triglycerides dropped even further on guavas than on medication.

A guava gives you nearly 1 gram of soluble fiber and is a source of 14 percent of the Daily Value of vitamin A and vitamin B_6 to cut cholesterol, drop blood pressure, and help keep your heart healthy.

Honeydews

Whether at a summer roadside stand or in the grocery store, people looking for honeydew melons do a strange dance as they pick up melon after melon to shake them and poke them. And it's worth going to all the trouble because honeydews protect you.

Cancer. One-half cup of cubed honeydew provides you with 35 percent of the Daily Value of vitamin C, an antioxidant that helps protect your body from various cancers.

Heart disease and stroke. Just a sliver of this melon packs a punch: Its vitamin C helps keep the heart-protecting HDL cholesterol levels high while sending the harmful LDL levels into the cellar. Studies show that high levels of vitamin C keep your arteries from getting clogged and make you less vulnerable to strokes and heart attacks. Honeydew also provides potassium, which helps lower your blood pressure.

Kiwifruit

What taste would you get if you crossed a banana with a strawberry and added a touch of tartness? The kiwifruit—a brown, fuzzy-skinned fruit with emerald green pulp that hails from California and New Zealand.

Cancer. Kiwifruit are packed with vitamin C—in an ounce-for-ounce contest, the kiwi even beats out oranges. One large fruit gives you almost 150 percent of the Daily Value of that cancer-fighting nutrient. You also get a gram of insoluble fiber to guard against colon and breast cancer. Research has found that substances in the kiwifruit also keep cells from mutating. Studies show that high intakes of vitamin C lower the risk of breast cancer.

Heart disease and stroke. Vitamin C may be the food world's workaholic. Not content with protecting against cancer, it also helps your heart by lowering the levels of harmful fats and triglycerides in your blood. This means less buildup of debris to narrow arteries and increase your risk of a heart attack or stroke. Kiwifruit are loaded with vitamin C.

Plus, you get more than 0.5 gram of soluble fiber and some other nutrients that keep your heart healthier: 6.8 percent of the Daily Value of magnesium, plus some potassium to help lower blood pressure.

Kohlrabi

Kol-rah-bee. If you think that pronouncing kohlrabi is a brainteaser, just wait until you get a load of the science-speak that sums up how substances in this wonder food can protect you.

Cancer. On the cancer front, let's sample this strange use of the English language: Antimutagenic, desmutagenic, and inducers of glutathione-S-transferease. Translation: All are methods by which your body fights off tumor initiation.

You also get the usual lineup of protection that comes with any cruciferous vegetable. One-half cup cooked kohlrabi contains 74 percent of the Daily Value of vitamin C to help protect you from cancer of the breast, cervix, esophagus, lung, mouth, pancreas, rectum, and stomach. You also pump up your immune system with copper and vitamin B_6. If you like to nibble your kohlrabi raw, a 1-cup serving provides some folate, which may protect against cancer of the cervix, rectum, colon, lung, and possibly the esophagus.

Heart disease and stroke. Beyond weighing

in with the vitamin C that helps block the formation of the LDL cholesterol that can build up in your arteries, kohlrabi helps lower your blood pressure with potassium.

Lemons

"I would like a medium dry vodka martini—with a lemon peel. Shaken and not stirred, please." Leave it to James Bond, master of high-tech weaponry, to figure out the protective qualities of even the lowly lemon and its peel.

Cancer. That spray from the lemon twist releases limonoids, powerful substances that, in animal studies, prevent oral cancer. But the twist isn't the only way to get protection. You can grate the zest (the colored part of the peel) and use it as a flavor enhancer.

Lemons put the squeeze on cancer: Flavonoids inhibit the hormones that promote cancer. Monoterpenes work as antioxidants to neutralize harmful substances. Phenolic acids keep dangerous nitrosamines from forming. Terpenes help enzymes block carcinogens.

Vitamin C gets into the act, too—eat a wedge, one-quarter of a lemon, and you get close to 13 percent of the Daily Value, lowering your risk of oral cancer. And you pick up just under 0.5 gram of dietary fiber to guard against colon cancer.

Heart disease and stroke. Lemons fight heart disease with a payload of vitamin C, which helps prevent cholesterol from building up to block your arteries.

Lentils

Whether you chose red, brown, or green lentils, this bean is such a star that it deserves to shine on its own, rather than get lumped with the rest of the beans.

Lentils are often sold as "dahl," but this isn't the best buy for protection, since the fiber-rich outer skins have been removed.

Cancer. One-half cup serves up more than 4.6 grams of insoluble fiber to help protect against colon cancer. You also get almost 45 percent of the Daily Value of folate, which may protect you against cancer of the cervix, colon, rectum, lung, and possibly the esophagus. Folate also helps your cells stay healthy, making it harder for cancers to attack, and keeps the important DNA intact. Plus, you get 12.5 percent of the Daily Value of copper and 8.4 percent of the Daily Value of zinc to help strengthen your immune system.

Heart disease and stroke. This little bean is a beacon of heart protection. In one study people with high cholesterol who added 1½ cups of lentils or other legumes to their diets each day for three weeks experienced an average 60-point drop in cholesterol. Add to that some soluble fiber to help lower your LDL cholesterol and 9 percent of the Daily Value of vitamin B_6, which may help keep homocysteine levels low. The magnesium and potassium in lentils work together to lower high blood pressure and keep blood from clotting, which could lead to a heart attack or stroke.

Lettuce

Lettuce is a mixed bag in terms of benefits. You don't get many nutrients from the pale green stuff that most of us put on our sandwiches, although even that contains protective substances. The more exotic lettuces with big, dark leaves give you a lot of protection. Rule of the green thumb: The darker green the leaf, the more protection you'll get from it.

Cancer. Scientists have found that even the juice of lettuces contain substances that fight cell mutation and interfere with the development of tumors.

Romaine lettuce, with broad, dark leaves, is a noble cancer fighter. One-half cup, shredded, gives you more than 9 percent of the Daily Value of folate. This valuable B vitamin may protect you against cancer of the cervix, colon, rectum, lung, and possibly the esophagus. It also helps cells stay healthy and able to fight off cancerous agents.

Romaine also gives you 11 percent of the Daily Value of vitamin C, reducing your risk of cancer of the breast, cervix, esophagus, lung, mouth, pancreas, rectum, and stomach. More good news: Endive does just as well.

Heart disease and stroke. One-half cup of romaine packs 81 milligrams of potassium. Arugula is a heavyweight in beta-carotene, a substance that may block harmful LDL cholesterol and that reduces your risk of stroke, with 2 milligrams in a 1-cup serving.

Lobster

Who says that healthy eating can't be fun? Steamed or boiled, lobster contains 0.5 gram of fat and just 83 calories per serving.

Cancer. Eat lobster and you do a favor for your immune system as well as your taste buds. Three ounces of lobster (about the size of a deck of playing cards) gives you 83 percent of your Daily Value for copper and more than 16 percent of your Daily Value for zinc, both of which keep your immune system at its best. Calcium in lobster helps in the fight against colon cancer.

Heart disease and stroke. Lobster's the catch

of the day in terms of heart protection. A rich helping of omega-3 fatty acids may help lower your risk of heart attack by lowering triglyceride levels. Plus, you get a lot of nutrients that may help lower high blood pressure: 5 percent of the Daily Value of calcium, more than 7 percent of the Daily Value of magnesium, and some potassium.

High levels of homocysteine in the blood are linked to high risk of heart attack. Some B vitamins such as B_{12}, plentiful in lobsters, counteract them. You get 44 percent of the Daily Value of vitamin B_{12} in a serving.

Mangoes

A taste sensation, mangoes remind some people of a fruit assortment of apricots and melons. Others characterize it as a cross between peaches and pineapple. But however you describe it, you get the taste of a fruit cocktail in just one fruit.

Cancer. Vitamins A and E turn out to be heavyweights in cancer protection, protecting your body from cancer-causing substances such as nitrosamines. Vitamin E lodges in cell membranes, where it fights off cancerous agents. And just half a mango is an excellent source of vitamin A, providing you with almost 78 percent of its Daily Value and almost 6 percent of the Daily Value for vitamin E.

A serving of half a mango gives you more than 2.3 milligrams of beta-carotene. Researchers have also discovered that a diet high in beta-carotene-rich foods protects both smokers and nonsmokers from lung cancer. You'll find about 5 percent of the Daily Value for copper in half a mango, boosting your immune system.

Heart disease and stroke. Half a mango gives you 1.5 grams of the soluble fiber that keeps high blood pressure down. The same nutrients that lower your cancer risk also help your heart: Vitamin E helps disarm fats before they can latch onto artery walls and clog up the works. Vitamin A and beta-carotene also work to protect your arteries from the plaque buildup that leaves you at risk for heart attacks and strokes. In addition, you get 46 percent of the Daily Value for vitamin C, which helps decrease the risk of stroke among elderly people.

Milk

It has a well-deserved rep for building bone, but that's not all it does. Skim milk deserves a place high on your list of protectors against cancer, heart disease, and stroke.

Okay—you've tried it, and it tastes watery and looks worse. You can fix that. Try decaf café latte. It's pretty much hot milk with a little espresso mixed in. Less than 80 calories and 0.5 gram of fat are in it, plus you bone up and protect your heart with 264 milligrams of calcium.

Or give the milk a richer taste and creamier look by stirring 2 to 4 tablespoons of instant nonfat milk powder into each cup of skim. You also get extra calcium that way.

Cancer. The skim in skim milk isn't something to take lightly. One study links high rates of breast cancer in mice to a high-fat and low-calcium diet.

Beyond cutting out the fat for cancer protection, skim milk provides calcium, which may reduce your risk of colon cancer; and zinc, which helps your immune system stay strong. Skim milk is a source of vitamin A and beta-carotene, which may help disarm the cancerous agents that invade your cells. One study suggests that beta-carotene, derived from foods, reduces the risk of lung cancer in nonsmokers.

Heart disease and stroke. One cup of skim milk fortified with vitamin A gives you almost 10 percent of the Daily Value for vitamin A and a little beta-carotene, which may help keep cholesterol from attaching to your artery walls and increasing your risk. (Buy milk in cardboard cartons that block the light—fluorescent lights in supermarket display cases can cost you up to 90 percent of vitamin A after 24 hours.)

Skim milk makes a three-pronged attack on high blood pressure: You get more than 30 percent of the Daily Value of calcium (which many researchers believe to be a countermeasure to mild high blood pressure), close to 7 percent of the Daily Value of magnesium, and more than 405 milligrams of potassium. Calcium may also help lower levels of the harmful LDL cholesterol.

You also get a sampling of the B vitamins riboflavin, B_{12}, and B_6, which are important for reducing your risk of heart disease, heart attack, and stroke.

Mushrooms

The mushroom may be a lowly fungus, but it has been a favorite of royalty since ancient Egypt. And it defends your body nobly with antibacterial and medicinal substances.

Cancer. Mushrooms contain antibacterial substances that help keep tumors from growing.

Shiitakes are also rich in other nutrients. Four cooked mushrooms (72 grams) give you almost 33 percent of the Daily Value of copper to make your immune system's defenses, well, mushroom. You also get almost 2 grams of dietary fiber to help protect you from colon cancer and heart disease, and you receive more than 6 percent of the Daily Value of zinc to help protect your immune system.

Button mushrooms also give you immunity-building protection: ½ cup gives you 8.5 percent of the Daily Value of copper.

Heart disease and stroke. Just four cooked shiitake mushrooms equip your system with more than 84 milligrams of potassium, lowering your blood pressure. Its vitamin C does double duty against both cancer and heart disease as it raises your blood levels of beneficial HDL cholesterol and drops the levels of the harmful LDL cholesterol and triglycerides, or fats, in the blood. You end up with a lower risk of the plaque buildup in the arteries that can lead to a heart attack or stroke. You also get small amounts of the heart-helping folate and vitamin B_6, which have been shown to lower the production of homocysteine—a substance that activates a clotting system, making blood more prone to adhere to arterial walls. Regular mushrooms, served raw, aren't nearly as powerful as cooked shiitakes, but with a quarter cup of them you still end up with a very respectable 42 milligrams of potassium to fight heart disease.

Mussels

Mussels muscle up your body's protective systems.

Cancer. One serving of 3½ ounces of cooked mussels provides vitamin A, which may help strengthen your body's defenses and protect against lung cancer. Its vitamin C helps ward off cancer of the breast, cervix, esophagus, lung, mouth, pancreas, rectum, and stomach. Almost 18 percent of the Daily Value of zinc and a helping of copper assist your immune system.

You get almost 19 percent of your Daily Value of folate, which may lower your risk of cancer of the cervix, colon, rectum, lung, and possibly the esophagus.

Heart disease and stroke. Mussels are rich in the omega-3 fatty acids, which may help keep your cholesterol levels low and fight heart disease. Some studies have found that vitamin A and beta-carotene block the harmful LDL cholesterol and lower your risk of stroke. Vitamin C keeps the beneficial HDL cholesterol levels high and also helps knock down the nasty LDLs and triglycerides, fats in the blood. Potassium weighs in with almost 266 milligrams, keeping your blood pressure low.

The innards of these deep blue shells are rich in the B vitamins. High levels of B_{12}, B_6, and folate in the blood have been shown to lower the production of homocysteine—a substance that activates a clotting system, making blood more prone to adhere to arterial walls. So getting the proper daily dose of these vitamins helps lower your heart disease risk. Mussels contain almost 19 percent of the Daily Value of folate, 397 percent of the Daily Value of the important vitamin B_{12}, and 5 percent of vitamin B_6. These tasty mollusks also contain more than 24 percent of the Daily Value of riboflavin, which has been shown to control cholesterol levels.

Nectarines

The name probably comes from the Greek word for "drink of the gods." The nectarine should be celebrated for its disease-fighting capabilities as well as its taste.

Cancer. Researchers working with the National Cancer Institute found substances in nectarines that help prevent cancers from getting started and growing.

Your immune system will like the taste of nectarines—one fruit is a source of copper, vitamin B_6, and vitamin A to help keep cancerous agents away. More than 12 percent of the Daily Value of vitamin C is in a nectarine, which helps protect you against cancer of the breast, cervix, esophagus, lung, mouth, pancreas, rectum, and stomach. And it has close to 2 grams of insoluble fiber to help you cut your risk of colon and breast cancer.

Heart disease and stroke. Eat a nectarine and give high blood pressure a downward thrust, thanks to more than 288 milligrams of potassium. Nearly a gram of soluble fiber helps you send your cholesterol down, too. Vitamin C helps lower the levels of LDL cholesterol that tend to build up plaque in your arteries.

Olive Oil and Canola Oil

Wait a minute—how can oils be on a healthy foods list? Easy.

Cancer. Next time you measure out a tablespoon of olive oil, look at it this way: You're getting almost 8.5 percent of the Daily Value of vitamin E, which helps your infection-fighting T cells do their job. You're also keeping the rest of your immune system up to par. Plus, vitamin E seems to reduce the risk of oral cancer.

Heart disease and stroke. When researchers at the University of Milan examined the relationship between the Mediterranean diet and low rates of heart disease, they decided to investigate oleuropein, a component of olive oil. They found that it blocks the start-up of chronic heart disease.

Canola oil is rich in omega-3 fatty acids (the same stuff that makes fish the dish of protective choice) that may combat cholesterol and protect you from heart disease.

Both olive and canola oil are good sources of vitamin E. Several large studies have shown that vitamin E reduces the risk of heart disease by preventing the oxidation of cholesterol and the formation of blood clots. Although these studies used vitamin E supplements, foods that contain vitamin E can always help.

Not surprisingly, both of these oils are high in monounsaturated fat, the kind that doesn't clog up your arteries. In fact, it's been linked to lower levels of both cholesterol and blood pressure.

Onions

Shakespeare had nothing nice to say about onions. In "A Midsummer Night's Dream," a character advises, "Eat no onions nor garlic, for we are to utter sweet breath." Maybe that's good advice for a romantic evening, but not for a disease-free life.

Cancer. Onions come in all shapes, sizes, and colors. You'll get more cancer protection from red onions because they contain the most flavonoids, substances that studies show help fight cancer.

But any onion contains a wealth of cancer protection. Compounds in onions block or suppress carcinogens, help keep cells from mutating, and interfere with tumor growth. They have even been reported to protect against radiation damage.

Heart disease and stroke. The flavonoids in onions may lower blood pressure. They also help neutralize the LDL cholesterol that leads to clogged arteries (and increases your risk of a heart attack or stroke).

Oranges

Christopher Columbus carried orange seedlings with him across the Atlantic. What would Florida and California look like if he had forgotten that part of his cargo?

Cancer. Orange juice is loaded with limonoid glucosides, natural chemicals that reduce the growth of cancer in animals. You also get glutathione, which may lower your risk of oral and throat cancer and help your immune system work more efficiently. Eat an orange

A Dash of Protection

Spices that wake up those bland foods also protect you from cancer, heart disease, and stroke. Try these.

Chilies. Hot peppers, the source of dried chilies and cayenne, contain capsaicin, a chemical that fights bacteria and mutes your system's pain receptors. Chilies are rich in vitamin C. One-half ounce of the red variety gives you more than 57 percent of the Daily Value.

Curry. Turmeric, the characteristic flavor in Indian curry dishes, contains curcumin, which in the lab prevents cancerous lesions of the skin, breast, and colon. It also helps keep blood platelets from sticking together and causing clots, and helps stop fats from oxidizing into harmful cholesterol.

Horseradish. A cousin to broccoli and cauliflower, fresh horseradish contains beta-carotene and vitamin C, along with the phytochemical isothiocyanate that gets the body's protective enzymes working to root out cancerous agents. Fresh is best. Prepared horseradish is not very nutritious.

Parsley. Two sprigs offer more than 4 percent of the Daily Value of vitamin C, 2 percent of the Daily Value of vitamin A, and a little fiber. They're also a good source of the protective flavonoids and beta-carotene. You benefit most from dried parsley, with its concentrated nutrients like copper and magnesium.

and get almost 2 grams of insoluble fiber to help prevent colon and breast cancer. You take in more than 116 percent of the Daily Value of vitamin C to protect against cancer of the breast, cervix, esophagus, lung, mouth, pancreas, rectum, and stomach. Look for calcium-fortified orange juice, which may combat colon cancer.

Heart disease and stroke. One cup of calcium-fortified orange juice gives you about 33 percent of the Daily Value of calcium. In some studies, calcium has been shown to also help lower your blood pressure. Plus, that healthy dose of vitamin C lowers the bad LDL cholesterol levels and raises the good HDL levels. And just a ¾-cup serving gives you almost 0.5 gram of the soluble fiber that protects your heart.

Oranges give you 237 milligrams of potassium to help keep your blood pressure in check. Eat the white part just under the outer peel and the center core of the orange for an extra dose of heart-protecting flavonoids, a group of phytochemicals.

Oysters

"Why, then the world's mine oyster, Which I with sword will open," wrote Shakespeare. Crack open that stubborn little shell, and you will discover an abundance of disease protection, too.

Cancer. Oysters help make your immune system a hard shell for cancer to crack. Six medium steamed oysters provide you with 159 percent of the Daily Value of copper and 509 percent of the Daily Value of zinc. Talk about defenses. Plus there's vitamin C to contribute to the cause of protection. They are also a source of vitamin A, which may cut your risk of cancer.

Heart disease and stroke. Oysters defend

your heart, too. Just six oysters give you a lot of the important B vitamins that reduce risk of heart disease: 245 percent of the Daily Value of vitamin B_{12}, plus some riboflavin. Vitamin B_{12} is harder for your body to absorb as you age, making it especially important that your diet gives you enough.

Magnesium in oysters helps prevent the blood clots that can lead to a stroke. Oysters also provide potassium, which can help lower high blood pressure.

Papayas

Sweet and refreshing, these large fruits contain little black, peppery-tasting seeds (and, yes, they're fine to eat—some people actually use them as a substitute for capers).

Cancer. One serving, about 1 cup of cubed papaya, gives you 144 percent of your Daily Value of vitamin C, important to help cut your risk of cancer of the breast, cervix, esophagus, lung, mouth, pancreas, rectum, and stomach. It's also a source of beta-carotene and vitamin A, which may help strengthen your body's defenses. You get more than 13 percent of the Daily Value of folate to help ward off cancer of the cervix, colon, rectum, lung, and possibly the esophagus. Folate helps keep cells healthy so that they're less easily invaded by carcinogens.

Heart disease and stroke. Vitamin C raises the levels of HDL cholesterol, protecting you from heart disease and heart attacks. It also lowers the harmful blood fats that attach to artery walls and increase your risk of a heart attack or stroke.

Vitamin A gets into the act and has been found in some studies to block LDL cholesterol before it can become a permanent (and unwelcome) fixture in your arteries. Vitamin B_6 helps lower levels of the harmful LDL cholesterol, decreasing your risk of heart problems.

You also get a little magnesium to reduce the blood's tendency to clot where it shouldn't. Calcium in papayas may help lower mild high blood pressure and LDL cholesterol levels. And a serving of papaya gives you 359 milligrams of potassium, which helps keep high blood pressure down, too.

Peaches

When settlers from Spain came to the New World, they brought peaches with them. "Just peachy," you might say, especially when you consider what peaches do to protect you.

Cancer. In the lab, substances in peaches make it hard for cancerous tumors to get started. Peaches contain glutathione, which may reduce the risk of oral and throat cancer.

One fruit gives you nearly a gram of insoluble fiber, lowering your risk of colon and breast cancer. Its vitamin C protects important organs from cancer. Vitamin A in peaches may help keep cancerous agents from getting into your system.

Heart disease and stroke. One peach gives your heart all-purpose protection. It's a source of more than 9 percent of your Daily Value of vitamin A, which may help keep the harmful LDL cholesterol from getting a lock on artery walls.

Peaches provide you with more than just one LDL-fighting weapon—think of it as gang warfare on your behalf. Along with vitamin A, vitamin C clobbers the LDL cholesterol that leads to clots. It also increases the levels of the HDL cholesterol that keeps the bad stuff from getting a grip. Potassium in peaches protects against high blood pressure.

Pears

If you're shaped like a pear, you're in luck: Your risk for disease is lower than your apple-shaped friends. For those of you who don't sport the pear shape, and for those "pears" who want to remain healthy, eating pears (the fruit) has some considerable disease-fighting effects.

Cancer. In the laboratory, substances in pears prevent cell mutations and may trip up cancer's first steps in your body. In one medium pear, you get more than 3 grams of insoluble fiber to protect against colon cancer and a helping of copper to help keep your immune system up to par.

Heart disease and stroke. A pear gives you almost 2 grams of soluble fiber to protect your heart. Add to that more than 350 milligrams of potassium to help drop your blood pressure.

And about 11 percent of the Daily Value of vitamin C is found in a pear, which cuts harmful LDL cholesterol and raises the beneficial HDL cholesterol levels. (You'll get less benefit from canned pears because they have been peeled. The canning process also saps away some of the vitamin C.)

Peas

Remember the story that you read to your children about the princess and the pea? If her highness had been thinking about disease prevention, she would have banished the servant who put the pea under the mattress instead of on the dinner table.

Cancer. While the princess of the story did discover the pea, today's researchers remain puzzled.

Peas do seem to prevent cells from mutating, although no one yet has a clue why that happens.

But we do know that peas are a good source of vitamins A and C. One-half cup of snow peas gives you about 64 percent of the Daily Value of vitamin C, protecting you from cancer of the breast, cervix, esophagus, lung, mouth, pancreas, rectum, and stomach.

Heart disease and stroke. Peas give you princely protection—one serving, about ½ cup of green peas, provides almost 17 percent of the Daily Value of vitamin C to help slash the LDL cholesterol that leads to clots. This nutrient also helps raise levels of the HDL cholesterol that keeps the LDLs from getting a grip. They are also a good source of vitamin A, which may help keep LDL cholesterol from attaching to arterial walls. There's some vitamin B_6 and folate, which help lower the blood levels of homocysteine, a substance that activates the blood's clotting system. The magnesium in peas helps lower mild high blood pressure, and the soluble fiber keeps cholesterol down.

Pecans

Yes, they're really high in calories. Of the nuts that you are likely to see in the grocery store, only macadamia nuts pack in more. They're high in fat, too, although 55 percent is monounsaturated, the kind of fat that doesn't contribute to clogs in the arteries. But pecans also wield some mighty weapons against cancer, heart disease, and stroke.

Cancer. Pecans' ellagic acid, in a study using laboratory mice, has been shown to be a powerful adversary that fights cancer of the lung, skin, esophagus, and liver. It detoxifies carcinogens and scavenges substances that carcinogens need to do their nasty work.

It might even keep cancerous substances from damaging DNA.

One ounce of pecans—that's about a handful—also gives you almost 18 percent of the Daily Value of copper, an essential nutrient for your immune system. It provides almost 11 percent of the Daily Value for zinc, another key mineral for immunity.

Heart disease and stroke. That single ounce of pecans does a lot for your heart. You get 105 milligrams of potassium and more than 9 percent of the Daily Value of magnesium to lower high blood pressure. Magnesium also helps keep your blood from clotting. The monounsaturated fat in pecans helps lower cholesterol and high blood pressure.

Peppers

You know John Wayne didn't talk much in films—just mowed down villains and saved the town (or country). Bell peppers are a lot like that. They don't get the attention, but boy do they come to the rescue.

Cancer. Red peppers are really just green ones that got to spend more time on the vine—and in the process stocked up on extra nutrients that protect you.

You get more vitamin C in one red pepper than you do in two oranges. Low vitamin C levels have been linked to a higher risk of developing breast, cervical, esophageal, lung, oral, pancreatic, rectal, and stomach cancer. Plus, you get 2.5 milligrams of beta-carotene (more than in a cup of apricots and nine times more than in a green bell pepper). Researchers have found that beta-carotene may help cut your risk of oral cancer. You also get carotenoids and flavonoids for added anti-cancer protection.

Heart disease and stroke. The flavonoids that protect against cancer also help you steer clear of heart disease and stroke. In a five-year Dutch study, older men with diets high in flavonoids had a lower risk of heart attack and stroke.

Peppers are loaded with other nutrients for your heart: ½ cup sweet green peppers gives you 74 per-

Prescription for Prevention

When you get right down to it, your best recipe for prevention of heart disease, cancer, and stroke—next to quitting smoking, of course—is right in your own kitchen: in foods you can buy cheaply and prepare easily.

Do:

■ Eat foods from plants. Fruits, vegetables, grains, nuts, and seeds are low in cholesterol and high in natural substances that fight disease.

■ Eat a variety of healthy foods. You'll get a wide assortment of protective substances from a diversified diet.

■ Emphasize fresh, not processed foods. You'll get more nutrients that way.

Don't:

■ Overcook your vegetables. While some protective compounds are impervious to heat, others aren't.

■ Overindulge in nuts and other foods that are high in protective substances but also high in calories.

cent of your Daily Value of vitamin C to help keep your arteries clear of debris.

Eating peppers gives you some vitamin B$_6$ and folate, which a study involving older adults found may reduce the risk of heart disease.

Persimmons

Persimmons are the Jekyll and Hyde of the food world: Bite into an unripe persimmon, and you'll get a taste more bitter than three-day-old coffee. When ripe, persimmons turn sweet and spicy.

Cancer. One medium-size Japanese persimmon weighs in with a lot of disease protection. You get more than 2 milligrams of beta-carotene, and they are a source of almost 73 percent of the Daily Value of vitamin A. Several studies have shown that these nutrients may protect against cancer. You get 9.5 percent of the Daily Value of copper to help your immune system, and more than 6 grams of dietary fiber to lower your colon cancer risk.

Heart disease and stroke. The vitamin C in persimmons helps keep the levels of the HDL cholesterol high while it decommissions the harmful LDL cholesterol. Your arteries get the benefit: There is less plaque buildup, which can lead to a stroke or heart attack. Persimmons also have some potassium, helping to lower high blood pressure.

Pineapple

Pop quiz: Where do pineapples come from, really? South America. By the time Columbus arrived, they had spread to the Caribbean. Other explorers soon carried them to China and the Philippines. Finally, they landed happily in Hawaii.

Cancer. This globe-trotting fruit packs a lot of

disease-preventing power. Researchers working with the National Cancer Institute have discovered that substances in pineapples fight cell mutations as shown in laboratory studies.

One-half cup of diced raw pineapples gives you almost a gram of dietary fiber to help protect against colon and breast cancer. There's also a little folate to help keep your cells healthy and less vulnerable to a cancerous attack. Folate may also help reduce your risk of cancer of the cervix, colorectum, lung, and possibly the esophagus. You get some copper to help strengthen your immune system.

Heart disease and stroke. One helping gives you almost 20 percent of the Daily Value of vitamin C. It helps raise levels of the beneficial HDL cholesterol, the stuff that keeps the harmful LDL cholesterol from doing damage. Having a low HDL level may be the most accurate indicator that you're at risk for a heart attack or stroke.

Plums

When you think "plum," you think "purple," right? Not so—colors range from almost green to red to so-purple-they-look-black. And they have great names, such as President, Empress, Tragedy, Freedom, and Elephant Heart, which is mainly used for cooking. Take your pick—they're all plum protection.

Cancer. One medium plum gives you close to 1 gram of insoluble fiber to help fight colon and breast cancer. Vitamin C in plums protects against cancer of the breast, cervix, esophagus, lung, mouth, pancreas, rectum, and stomach. A little vitamin B$_6$ helps round out the anti-cancer forces by boosting your immune system.

Heart disease and stroke. Plums give you

some of the cholesterol-lowering soluble fiber that protects your heart. They're also a source of riboflavin, vitamin B_6, and vitamin C for a cornucopia of heart protection. The result? Higher amounts of protective HDL cholesterol, lower levels of the harmful LDL cholesterol that clogs your arteries, and less risk of blood clots that trigger heart attacks and strokes.

Pollack

Sometimes the imitation is just as good as the original, and even better if it saves you money. Pollack often masquerades as a low-cost imitation crabmeat (often labeled "surimi"). One 3-ounce serving gives you just a bit over 1 gram of fat and 77 milligrams of cholesterol.

Cancer. Pollack provides a healthy helping of vitamin B_6, weighing in at 14 percent of your Daily Value, which helps strengthen the defenses of your immune system. Folate, another B vitamin in pollack, may help lower your risk of cancer of the cervix, colon, rectum, lung, and possibly the esophagus. You need folate to protect DNA's genetic codes and to help cells divide and multiply properly. Damaged cells are attractive targets for cancerous invaders.

Heart disease and stroke. People who eat one serving of fish a week can lower their risk of stroke by about half. A 3½-ounce serving of Atlantic pollack, for example, gives you 421 milligrams of omega-3 fatty acids, along with a little more than 1 gram of fat. In some studies, omega-3 has been shown to fight heart disease. A healthy 77 milligrams of calcium in a serving of pollack contributes close to 7 percent of your Daily Value and may help to lower your levels of hazardous

LDL cholesterol while at the same time helping to drop your blood pressure.

One 3-ounce serving deals out disease protection in the form of 19 percent of the Daily Value of magnesium to help get your blood pressure down. It also helps keep blood from clumping and forming clots that increase your risk of a heart attack or stroke.

Potatoes

Pop quiz: What food makes up the leading source of vitamin C in the American diet?

Yup—potatoes.

Cancer. Eat one medium baked potato with its skin and you will take in more than 43 percent of the Daily Value of vitamin C to help stave off cancer of the breast, cervix, esophagus, lung, mouth, pancreas, rectum, and stomach. There are also substances in potatoes that fight off cell mutation.

Heart disease and stroke. That baked potato also gives you 844 milligrams of potassium to help bring down high blood pressure. (To get the full benefit, eat the skins.) And its vitamin B_6 helps lower your risk of heart disease.

Prunes

Why all the fuss? Prunes are just dried-up plums, right? When water gets removed during processing, nutrients become more concentrated. If foods got Academy Awards for disease protection, prunes would be working on an acceptance speech.

Cancer. One-half cup of these dried delectables contains more than 2 grams of insoluble fiber to help prune your risk of colon and breast cancer.

They are a source of vitamin A and beta-carotene, which may help keep cancers from invading healthy cells. Some studies also suggest that these nutrients help protect against lung cancer. You get 10 percent of the Daily Value of copper to strengthen your immune system.

Heart disease and stroke. In an ounce-per-ounce comparison, prunes contain more fiber than most dried beans, fruits, and vegetables. A lot is soluble, protecting your heart. You get 354 milligrams of potassium, plus an assortment of powerful protectors against heart disease: calcium, folate, magnesium, riboflavin, vitamin A, vitamin B_6, and vitamin C.

Pumpkins

The kind of pumpkin you carve out at Halloween isn't the kind that usually goes into a pie, bread, or soup. Smaller, sweeter (and less stringy) sugar pumpkins get used instead.

Cancer. A variety of nutrients protect: A mug full of pumpkin soup can give you about 1.4 grams of fiber. One-half cup of mashed pumpkin is a source of more than 26 percent of the Daily Value of vitamin A and some beta-carotene, which may reduce your risk of cancer of the esophagus, stomach, colon, breast, cervix, uterus, and lung. You get cancer-fighting, immune-strengthening copper, too. Researchers working with the National Cancer Institute also note that substances in pumpkins keep cells from mutating.

Heart disease and stroke. A 10-year study of 1,795 women heart-attack or angina survivors found that those who ate the highest amounts of beta-carotene, vitamin C, vitamin E, and riboflavin had 71 percent less risk of stroke and a 33 percent reduced risk of a second heart attack. Fortunately, pumpkins contain all these nutrients.

They're one of the few foods that give you even a moderate amount of vitamin E. Several large studies show that vitamin E may reduce the risk of heart disease. It helps prevent the oxidation of cholesterol and helps prevent clumping of platelets in blood vessels. These studies used vitamin E supplements, but foods that contain vitamin E will help, too. One-half cup of canned pumpkin gives you more than 251 milligrams of potassium, along with magnesium, to help keep your blood pressure from going through the roof.

Radishes

What movie features the star brandishing a radish? Here's a clue: "As God is my witness, I'll never be hungry again." Sure, you remember: Vivian Leigh, Scarlett O'Hara, *Gone with the Wind.* And the vegetable that many of us use to garnish salads.

Cancer. Radishes kept Scarlett going, and the substances in them will help your body fight off cancer. Researchers working with the National Cancer Institute have found that eating just a little more than one radish a day may keep tumors from developing and cells from mutating. They're a rich source of vitamin C for protection against cancer.

Heart disease and stroke. Just ½ cup of sliced radishes gives you 22 percent of your Daily Value of vitamin C to raise the levels of the important HDL cholesterol that helps keep your arteries clean. HDL levels are often used as an indicator of whether you're likely to suffer a heart attack—the lower the levels, the greater your risk. Vitamin C also helps lower the dangerous LDL cholesterol that grabs onto artery walls and, over time, leaves them narrow and easily clogged.

Raisins

People have been drying grapes in the sun to make raisins for more than 3,000 years. Talk about wisdom of the ages!

Cancer. A ½-cup serving gives you almost a gram of insoluble fiber to help prevent colon cancer. You get 11 percent of the Daily Value of copper and more than 9 percent of vitamin B_6 to help your immune system.

Heart disease and stroke. Imagine a David and Goliath setup: Little raisins battle big diseases. The winner? The little guys, of course. A ½-cup serving of raisins gives you more than 544 milligrams of potassium to help keep your blood pressure low. You get a bit of heart protection from magnesium. Riboflavin and vitamin B_6, among others, gang up on LDL cholesterol and substances in your body that can damage your heart.

Raspberries

These delicate berries won't keep for long in the refrigerator, so what are you waiting for? Pop them in your mouth for disease protection.

Cancer. Like other berries, raspberries give you a healthy dose of ellagic acid. In the lab it fights cancer of the lung, skin, esophagus, and liver. It may even keep cancerous substances from damaging DNA, the first step in cancer's growth.

One-half cup also gives you a lot of additional cancer protection. You get more than 1 gram of insoluble fiber to help protect against colon and breast cancer. More than a quarter of your Daily Value of vitamin C goes a long way to protect you against cancer of the breast, cervix, esophagus, lung, mouth, pancreas, rectum, and stomach.

Heart disease and stroke. A healthy dose of vitamin C helps protect your heart by raising your HDL cholesterol levels, preventing buildup of plaque in your arteries. It also helps reduce levels of LDL cholesterol and other blood fats that lodge in your arteries. You will also get almost 0.5 gram of soluble fiber to help fight bad cholesterol.

Rhubarb

Talk about a confused plant. Those stalks that look like pink celery protect you from disease—but its leaves are poisonous. Most people don't eat the roots, but they were prized for medicinal use in ancient China.

Cancer. Mmmm, smell that rhubarb pie. And think about how healthy it is. One-half cup of raw rhubarb gives you more than 1 gram of dietary fiber to help protect you from colon cancer.

You get some vitamin C that helps lower your risk of cancer of the breast, cervix, esophagus, lung, mouth, pancreas, rectum, and stomach.

Heart disease and stroke. One-half cup of cooked rhubarb gives you more than 17 percent of your Daily Value of calcium, which may help lower mild blood pressure and reduce harmful LDL cholesterol, which can stick to your artery walls.

Vitamin C takes care of more than one matter of the heart, as it raises your HDL cholesterol and lowers LDL cholesterol and other blood fat.

Rice

The big question: Is there really a difference between white rice and brown rice? The big answer: Yes.

Cancer. Let's do a little math. Copper protects you from cancer because it helps build up your immune system. Eat ½ cup of cooked long-grain brown rice, and you get 5 percent of the Daily Value. If, instead, you go for white rice, you get 3.5 percent. Brown rice gives you almost 2 grams of total dietary fiber, which protects you from colon cancer. The long-grain white stuff gives you 0.4 gram.

Researchers working with the National Cancer Institute have also found that brown rice neutralizes dangerous substances that play havoc with your system and allow cancer to make inroads.

Heart disease and stroke. Eat ½ cup of cooked brown rice and get double protection—vitamin B_6 and magnesium. Both help lower risk of a blood clot, while magnesium also helps lower high blood pressure.

Salmon

As one of the much-touted sources of omega-3 fatty acids, salmon swims against the current of disease.

Cancer. Half of a filet of fresh cooked coho salmon has high levels of vitamin B_6 along with some copper and zinc, which have been shown to heighten cancer-resisting immunity. More than 7 percent of the Daily Value for calcium is available, which may help fight colon cancer.

Heart disease and stroke. Eating fish once a week will cut your risk of stroke in half, researchers say. Make it salmon, and you get plenty of omega-3 fatty acids, which some studies have associated with reduced risk of heart attacks and strokes.

One 3-ounce serving of fresh cooked coho salmon dishes up almost 387 milligrams of potassium, helping to lower your blood pressure. You get almost 63 percent of the Daily Value of vitamin B_{12}, one of the important B vitamins that can help to reduce your risk of heart disease by lowering the amount of homocysteine, a substance that activates the clotting system in the blood. Other B vitamins include riboflavin (more than 8 percent of the Daily Value) and vitamin B_6 (almost 24 percent of the Daily Value). Your body doesn't absorb vitamin B_{12} very well now that you're older, so it's important to make sure that you get a good supply through your diet.

Salmon also gives you magnesium (almost 8 percent of the Daily Value) and a little folate, which, combined with B_{12} and B_6, may lower the homocysteine levels in your blood, to help prevent clogged arteries. Eat salmon and you're going to get calcium, which in some studies has been shown to lower mild high blood pressure. Get extra calcium by eating canned sockeye salmon, which contains edible chunks of bone.

Sardines

When you peel back the lid on a can of sardines, you let out a crowd of disease fighters.

Cancer. That canned cluster of tightly packed fish gives you a healthy dose of zinc and copper to help your immune system function at its peak and to neutralize dangerous invaders. The contents in one can gives you more than 5 percent of your Daily Value of calcium, which may help lower your risk of colon cancer.

Heart disease and stroke. The calcium in sardines also may help keep your blood pressure and levels of harmful LDL cholesterol down. One can, or about 3 ounces, gives you a heart-helping assortment of the B vitamins that cut down your risk of a heart attack or stroke: 137 percent of the Daily Value of vitamin B_{12} and almost 8 percent of the Daily Value of vitamin B_6, to help control blood clots in the blood vessels.

Shallots

Shallots look like a cross between garlic and an onion. So you won't be surprised to find out that they offer just about as much protection as their close relatives.

Cancer. In the lab, substances in shallots block and suppress cancer-causing carcinogens. Shallots also contain beta-carotene and are a source of vitamin A, which may keep cancerous agents from invading healthy cells, stopping cancers before they get started. In one study, beta-carotene is linked to lower rates of lung cancer in nonsmokers. Some scientists believe that they also protect other important organs from cancer invasion.

Heart disease and stroke. The same vitamin A and beta-carotene that may help protect you from cancer might also help your heart. One study found that beta-carotene keeps the harmful LDL cholesterol from oxidizing, the first step in latching onto the walls of your arteries where it can turn into dangerous plaque that increases your risk of heart attack and stroke.

Soybeans

Yes, we're talking about tofu and sprouts. But before you roll your eyes toward the ceiling, consider all of the good things that these products do.

Cancer. Soy products contain genistein, a chemical that attacks cancer the way that Arnold Schwarzenegger goes after bad guys. It blocks the formation of blood vessels around new tumors, stops cancer cells from multiplying, and prevents the absorption of tumor-promoting estrogen. In the lab it keeps breast cancer cells and precancerous prostate cells from growing.

You get protection from other foreign-sounding substances: isoflavones, phytosterols, protease inhibitors, saponins, and phytic acid. The bottom line? They keep cancer-causing substances from getting a grip in your body, stop cancerous cells from reproducing, and slow down tumor growth. One-half cup of boiled soybeans gets you a healthy helping of calcium, 13 percent of the Daily Value, which may help protect you from colon cancer.

Heart disease and stroke. Soybean products give you just about as much protection from heart disease as they do from cancer. Calcium may help lower your blood pressure and reduce the nasty LDL cholesterol that leads to clogged arteries, heart attacks, and strokes. In ½ cup of boiled soybeans, you get almost 14 percent of your Daily Value of magnesium to help keep blood from clotting and gumming up your arteries. Magnesium also helps lower high blood pressure. The beans weigh in with 485 milligrams of potassium to quiet down your blood pressure, too.

Vitamin C in soybeans (more than 25 percent of your Daily Value) helps raise your HDL cholesterol, which keeps fatty deposits from blocking your arteries.

Spinach

Popeye was no fool. Spinach is high on disease prevention and low in calories. Plus, fresh spinach can keep in the refrigerator for 10 to 14 days.

Cancer. Researchers working with the National Cancer Institute note that some of the stuff in spinach keeps cells from mutating. Antioxidants also neutralize the substances that help cancer get started.

One cup of raw spinach (green and tender, not brown and wilted) gives you more than 27 percent of the Daily Value of folate, which protects you against cancer of the cervix, colorectum, lung, and possibly the esophagus. Folate also helps keep cells strong and healthy, so they are better able to fend off a cancerous attack. Some studies show that the consumption of high levels of vitamin E decrease the levels of prostaglandin E_2, a substance that limits the efficiency of the immune system. Although these studies used supplements, dark green leafy vegetables are a known source of vitamin E.

Heart disease and stroke. When Popeye fought Bluto, he may have looked as though his blood pressure was about to go through the roof, but the potassium in spinach probably helped keep it down. Other heart-helping nutrients include vitamin C, magnesium, folate, and vitamin E. Several large studies note that vitamin E can actually slow the development of heart disease by preventing the oxidation of cholesterol and blood clots. Although these studies used vitamin E supplements, foods that contain vitamin E can always help.

Squash

If you just think of winter squash as a decoration for your Thanksgiving table, you're in for a low-calorie, disease-fighting treat. For that matter, summer squash gives you protection, too—just in smaller doses.

Cancer. Winter squash—of any shape and

color—is rich in beta-carotene, an important antioxidant that may help stop cancer before it gets started. One study found that it provides protection against lung cancer. One serving (about ½ cup, cubed) of butternut squash gives you more than 3 milligrams of beta-carotene. The same amount of Hubbard squash dishes out almost 2 milligrams of beta-carotene.

As if that weren't enough, researchers have found that something in squash keeps tumors from developing, although they haven't yet identified the substance with this disease-squashing ability.

Heart disease and stroke. Acorn squash dishes up heart protection, too. A ½-cup serving, baked and cubed, gives you about 18 percent of the Daily Value of vitamin C to maintain high levels of beneficial HDL cholesterol. It also reduces levels of the harmful LDL cholesterol that lodges in your arteries and can lay the groundwork for a heart attack or stroke.

Other nutrients, such as folate, magnesium, and potassium, team up to lower levels of LDL cholesterol, raise levels of protective HDL cholesterol, drop high blood pressure, and keep blood from forming those nasty clots that can lead to heart attacks and strokes.

Strawberries

"Strawberry fields forever," sang the Beatles back in the 1960s. Strawberries will get your immune system humming, too.

Cancer. In one study involving lab animals, researchers found that ellagic acid, found in strawberries, fights cancer of the lung, skin, esophagus, and liver. It also decreases the number of tumors in animals. When applied to the skin of animals, it prevents cancers. Ellagic acid seems to keep carcinogens from damaging the DNA of healthy cells. It's even possible that it eats up substances that carcinogens need to get off the ground.

Glutathione may help boost your cells' ability to divide, thereby launching a strong counterattack against cancer. And the best news for you is that glutathione works best in older folks. You also get 1 gram of insoluble fiber to help protect you from colon and breast cancer.

Heart disease and stroke. One cup of strawberries gives you 247 milligrams of potassium, keeping your blood pressure rosy, and 140 percent of the Daily Value of vitamin C, helping to lower your cholesterol. You also get soluble fiber to help keep cholesterol in check and folate to help keep levels of homocysteine low, preventing blood clots. The magnesium in strawberries helps prevent blood clots and lower blood pressure. Studies show that pantothenic acid, also in strawberries, may lower cholesterol and triglycerides. There is also riboflavin, which lowers your cholesterol.

Sweet Potatoes and Yams

Let's get the confusion cleared up: Sweet potatoes and yams are different critters that belong to different families. And, chances are, you have never seen an actual yam. These giants of the vegetable world hail from Africa and Asia. They can weigh up to 100 pounds. Now, sweet potatoes—that's a whole different story. These vegetables have their roots in the United States and undoubtedly kept more than one family of frontier homesteaders alive. Anytime you go to the grocery store, you're going to come home with sweet potatoes, not yams.

Cancer. One 4-ounce baked sweet potato is a

source of 249 percent of the Daily Value of vitamin A, which may help protect you against cancer of the mouth. And the bright orange color tells you that beta-carotene is on board. So is almost half the Daily Value of vitamin C, which strengthens your defenses against cancer of the breast, cervix, esophagus, lung, mouth, pancreas, rectum, and stomach. And a healthy helping of fiber protects against colon cancer. Researchers working with the National Cancer Institute have also discovered that substances in sweet potatoes actually keep cells from mutating, at least in the laboratory.

Heart disease and stroke. There's plenty of beta-carotene, which may help shut out the harmful LDL cholesterol that leads to plaque buildup and clotting in the arteries. A common misconception about soluble fiber is that some of the best sources are tasteless and often involve oats. It doesn't have to be that way, since sweet potatoes are an excellent source of cholesterol-fighting soluble fiber. Vitamin C in sweet potatoes raises HDLs, which protects you from heart disease. It disarms the harmful LDLs and gets rid of triglycerides. Your blood pressure drops, thanks to a lot of potassium—397 milligrams in one 4-ounce baked sweet potato.

Tangerines

They're a lot like oranges, but easier to eat. You don't get as much vitamin C in a tangerine as in an orange but the amount you do get in a tangerine is nothing to sneeze at.

Cancer. Substances in tangerines keep cells from mutating. Other components strengthen the production of enzymes that make carcinogens more water-soluble so that the body can get rid of them quickly. And others may keep nitrates in the stomach from being converted into dangerous nitrosamines, naturally occurring carcinogens.

In one tangerine you also get more than 43 percent of your Daily Value of vitamin C to help prevent cancer of the breast, cervix, esophagus, lung, mouth, pancreas, rectum, and stomach. Its vitamin B_6 beefs up your immune system, and its fiber lowers your risk of colon cancer.

Heart disease and stroke. Tangerines are a source of vitamin C and vitamin A, which may knock down the levels of the dangerous LDL cholesterol and raise the levels of the good stuff, HDL. Vitamin C also lowers mild high blood pressure, providing an added benefit to tangerines. Potassium in tangerines also helps lower your blood pressure.

Tea

The American colonists started a war by dumping a load of tea into Boston Harbor. If they had known about its disease-preventing properties, they might have selected something else to throw overboard.

Cancer. Whether it's green, black, or decaf, tea protects. Substances in tea help enzymes neutralize cancer-causing agents and may repair damaged DNA. One study showed that tea drinkers have a lower risk of breast and stomach cancer. In other studies, substances in tea block skin cancer.

Heart disease and stroke. Drink tea and cut your risk of heart disease: Black, green, or even decaf varieties are rich in flavonoids, substances that protect your heart and lower your risk of heart disease. In a Dutch study, researchers found that the antioxidant quercetin, found in tea, lowers the risk of stroke by one-third. The effects of tea were reportedly most beneficial to older folks. You get the most benefit from bagged tea because the leaves are more thoroughly crushed.

Tomatoes

Until the 1800s people believed that tomatoes were poisonous. After all, it is a relative of the nightshade family of plants known for poisonous leaves, berries, flowers, and fruit. But researchers found that tomatoes protect, whether on a pizza, in a sauce, or fresh off the vine.

Cancer. Substances in tomatoes fight cell mutation. Tomatoes also arm your defenses with glutathione, which may reduce the risk of oral and throat cancer and makes your immune system work better. And you get the powerful cancer fighter lycopene. Other substances in tomatoes battle nitrosamines, substances produced in our bodies that can lead to cancer.

Heart disease and stroke. One ripe tomato offers a generous 399 milligrams of potassium to lower blood pressure, and 57 percent of the Daily Value of vitamin C, which helps control bad LDL cholesterol. You also get vitamin B_6, which may help reduce the incidence of blood clots.

Trout

Weave all the tales you like about the one that got away. When it comes to trout on your plate, opt for the smaller size—it will contain less fat.

Cancer. Your immune system gets a boost with 17 percent of the Daily Value of vitamin B_6. You also get more than 5 percent of the Daily Value of folate, which is known to reduce the risk of developing cancer of the cervix, colon, rectum, lung, and possibly the esophagus.

Heart disease and stroke. Some researchers

have zeroed in on fish as an easy way to help your heart. In one study people who ate one serving of fatty fish a week lowered their risk of heart attack by 50 percent. Another study reported that people who eat ⅔ ounce of any type of fish a day can cut their risk of stroke in half. In a 3-ounce serving of baked trout, you'll also get heart protection from calcium, folate, magnesium, riboflavin, thiamin, vitamin B_{12}, and vitamin B_6. An impressive 375 milligrams of potassium will help lower mild high blood pressure.

Tuna

Pop quiz: Name the most-consumed fish in America. Yes, tuna. But not all tuna is equal. Look for fresh bluefin or canned albacore.

Cancer. A 3-ounce serving of baked, fresh bluefin tuna is a source of almost 43 percent of the Daily Value of vitamin A, which in some studies has been shown to reduce the risk of cancer. Compare that figure to just over 1 percent of the Daily Value of vitamin A from the same amount of the canned tuna. You also get more than 22 percent of the Daily Value of vitamin B_6 to build up your immunity—that's 4 more milligrams than the canned tuna. Canned tuna contains about 8 milligrams of copper, however, compared to fresh bluefin's 4.

Heart disease and stroke. Bluefin tuna provides a rich source of the omega-3 fatty acids that may help lower your cholesterol and protect you from heart disease. Albacore, or white tuna, also gives you a good helping of protection from omega-3's.

A heart-healthy helping of magnesium lowers your blood's tendency to clot and reduces your risk of a heart attack or stroke. Magnesium also reduces high blood pressure. The assortment of B vitamins in tuna also is a champion in the heart-protection department. Three ounces of fresh baked bluefin tuna provides more than 15 percent of the Daily Value of riboflavin, a B vitamin that helps other heart-saving nutrients work harder and more efficiently. Even better, you get more than 154 percent of the Daily Value for vitamin B_{12}, another important heart protector, and 274 milligrams of potassium to help lower your blood pressure.

Turkey

Ben Franklin had such high regard for the turkey that he wanted to make it the official bird of the United States. But no, we have the eagle on our coins and the turkey on our table, which is good for you, since eating turkey cuts your risk of heart disease, cancer, and stroke.

Cancer. Turkey's a rich old bird—at least in terms of disease protection. A 3-ounce serving is low in fat (2 grams) and cholesterol (30 milligrams); it's the leanest of all meats. And that's important to reduce your risk of cancer. Plus, it gives you more than 8 percent of your Daily Value for zinc, a mineral that's important to your immune system. You also boost your immune system with 9 percent of the Daily Value of vitamin B_6.

Heart disease and stroke. Turkey provides an assortment of heart-protecting B vitamins: pantothenic acid, riboflavin, vitamin B_{12}, and vitamin B_6. Working together, they lower your risk of heart disease. They increase the HDL cholesterol that protects your arteries from plaque buildup and lower the levels of homocysteine. You'll also benefit from potassium, which protects you from deadly high blood pressure.

Walnuts

You could also call them the royal nuts. In ancient Rome, for instance, they were consumed by royalty and dedicated to the god Jupiter. They're good for us commoners, too. Crack some nuts to crack down on your cancer risk.

Cancer. Walnuts are rich in ellagic acid. In lab animals, this substance fights cancer of the lung, skin, esophagus, and liver. The same tests determined that it decreases the number of tumors. When ellagic acid was applied to the skin of mice, it kept cancers from forming.

Researchers at Ohio State University believe that ellagic acid keeps cancerous substances from starting the process of DNA damage. It may also neutralize cancer-causing substances before they do damage. These researchers also believe that ellagic acid may actually beat cancerous substances to the punch—taking in substances they need in order to do their damage.

Heart disease and stroke. Don't like fish but want to get the potential benefits of the omega-3 fatty acids found in fish? Eat English or black walnuts and you may be taking steps to help lower your cholesterol levels and protect your heart. While ⅓ cup of walnuts will load you up with almost 25 grams of fat, the nuts contain no cholesterol. Walnuts also give you other important health helpers: folate and vitamin B_6—B vitamins that lower your risk of heart disease. One-third cup of walnuts gives you 201 milligrams of potassium to help lower high blood pressure.

Watermelon

Isn't it nice—the watermelon that's such a treat on a hot summer day is also great for disease protection? Beyond nutrients, watermelon gives you a lot of—what else?—water, which also is vital to your health.

Cancer. You get a lot of glutathione from watermelon. Researchers at Emory University in Atlanta found that this substance may function as an anticarcinogen to reduce your risk of oral and throat cancer by up to 50 percent. A lab study at Tufts University in Boston found that glutathione helps white blood cells in a test tube fight off invaders—and that means it could possibly make your immune system work as well as that of a much younger person. When you consider that people over age 60 have blood levels of glutathione about 17 percent lower than people under 40, it's easy to see why you should head for foods that provide a lot.

Heart disease. One-half cup of watermelon gives you more than 12 percent of your Daily Value of vitamin C, helping to lower your levels of harmful LDL cholesterol, which can become a permanent and hazardous fixture on your artery walls. You get a healthy helping of vitamin B_6, which helps deactivate your blood's clotting system. Watermelon is also a source of beta-carotene and vitamin A, which some studies show helps fight heart disease.

Wheat Germ

Wheat germ is the part of the wheatberry that is cast off when flour is refined from whole wheat to white. What a waste.

Cancer. Wheat germ gives you vitamin E, which helps your immune system work better by strengthening the T cells that protect you from disease. It also reduces prostaglandin E_2, which interferes with your immune system as you get older. People who get a lot of vitamin E also have a lower risk of stomach cancer.

Heart disease and stroke. Several studies have shown that supplemental vitamin E slows down the progress of heart disease. It helps prevent the oxidation of cholesterol and helps prevent clumping of platelets in blood vessels. These studies used vitamin E supplements, but foods that contain vitamin E are a good bet, too. In people who've had a heart attack, vitamin E reduces the risk of a second attack.

When you eat ¼ cup of toasted wheat germ, you take in 25 percent of the Daily Value of folate. Researchers believe that this nutrient can help prevent heart attacks and strokes because it reduces levels of an amino acid called homocysteine. In a study of 536 men, researchers found that those people with the highest levels of homocysteine had a slightly elevated risk for stroke. Homocysteine injures the walls of your arteries.

Yogurt

It's really just curdled milk mixed with bacteria, all of which sounds pretty awful until you think about how much good yogurt can do for you.

Beyond the nutritional protection it gives, yogurt works as a substitute for less healthy foods. For example, cheese made from low-fat yogurt (basically, yogurt with some of the liquid removed) can substitute for the high-fat kind of cheese and still give you the calcium that you need.

Cancer. An 8-ounce or 1-cup serving of plain low-fat yogurt gives you almost 42 percent of your Daily Value of calcium, which may help guard you against colon cancer. You get folate, which is important to help protect DNA's genetic codes so that they're able to divide and replicate properly, keeping cancer at bay. Folate may also protect against cancer of the cervix, colon, rectum, lung, and possibly the esophagus. Yogurt provides more than 13 percent of your Daily Value of zinc, which helps keep your immune system strong.

Heart disease and stroke. The B vitamins—folate, riboflavin, vitamin B_{12} and vitamin B_6—protect your heart. People who get a lot of folate and vitamins B_6 and B_{12} in their diets may have up to 25 percent lower risk of heart disease. One 8-ounce serving of low-fat yogurt gives you almost 29 percent of your Daily Value of riboflavin, more than 21 percent of vitamin B_{12}, and more than 6 percent of your Daily Value for folate. In addition, its 264 milligrams of potassium helps lower high blood pressure.

Weight Control

Trim Down to Trim Your Disease Risk

When he wasn't acting or directing classic films like *Citizen Kane*, Orson Welles ate. Reportedly, it wasn't uncommon for him to eat four to five large portions of caviar a day, and three huge steaks and mounds of rich desserts for dinner. His lifetime of gluttony weakened his heart and dangerously elevated his blood pressure. Welles died at age 70 of a massive heart attack.

"To my mind, Orson Welles's health was the antithesis of what you want to experience as you get older," says Michael Klaper, M.D., director of the Institute of Nutrition Education and Research in Manhattan Beach, California. "I would rather be a lean older person than an obese one because when it comes to heart disease, stroke, and cancer, it's clear that being overweight puts you at high risk for these diseases."

While most of us certainly don't overindulge as much as Welles did, the pounds do seem to creep up on us and threaten to erode our health as we get older. But it doesn't have to be this way.

"I've seen some people at these ages who have made dramatic turnabouts in their weights," Dr. Klaper says. "If you begin eating a good diet and become leaner and more active, there's a good chance that you'll still be that way when you hit 90 or even 100."

Where Did Those Extra Pounds Come From?

As a person strides toward 60, the amount of muscle in the body naturally drops and fat begins to account for a greater percentage of weight. So even if you didn't gain a pound, you would still have more body fat at 70 than you did at age 30.

At the same time, metabolism—the rate at which your body burns calories—slows down. Many people also get less exercise as they age, yet continue eating the same amount of food as they did when they were younger. The result is more pounds. In fact, many people gain about a pound a year after age 35.

Some increased poundage as you move up the age ladder is normal, which throws those one-size-fits-all height and weight charts out of kilter for folks over 50. As we age, a greater percentage of our body weight is fat, and that is something that most height and weight charts don't make allowances for, says Reubin Andres, M.D., clinical director of the National Institute on Aging Gerontology Research Center in Baltimore.

A more precise measure that weight-control experts turn to is "body mass index," or BMI. This is a calculation that takes into account both your height and weight and has proven to be an excellent predictor of a person's susceptibility to certain diseases like stroke, heart disease, and cancer.

To figure your BMI, multiply your weight in pounds by 700. Divide that number by your height in inches. Then divide by your height again. The result is your BMI. So, for example, if you weigh 150 pounds, multiple that by 700. Then divide that number by your height-let's say 66 inches-twice. The result is 24.

Using that formula, Dr. Andres has found that people older than 60 have lower death rates at slightly higher BMIs than those who are younger. (A healthy BMI for a man or woman over age 60 is below 29, says Jose Morais, M.D., a gerontologist and nutritionist at Royal Victoria Hospital in Montreal.) In other words, even if you are carrying around a few more pounds than you used to, you may still be at a healthy weight for your age.

Still, by age 60, roughly 40 percent of American men and women are overweight. After age 75, the number of people who are overweight dips to 30 percent because many people who were extremely overweight have died. Furthermore, most of us who survive into our eighties naturally begin shedding pounds because of diminished appetites, says Artemis Simopoulos, M.D., president of the

Center for Genetics, Nutrition, and Health in Washington, D.C.

Although excess weight is one of the primary causes of premature death after age 60, how much of an impact being overweight has on your risk of stroke, heart disease, and cancer in these years is a riddle that scientists are just beginning to probe.

"It's a darn good question that we don't fully have an answer for yet," says Edward Saltzman, M.D., a scientist at the U.S. Department of Agriculture Human Nutrition Research Center on Aging at Tufts University in Boston. "In the past, the diseases associated with being extremely overweight would have precluded many people from living into their sixties or seventies. Now that medical technology is getting better at extending life, we're seeing more people who are overweight living longer. So many of the data for these people are relatively new."

The bulk of the emerging evidence suggests that too much body fat—whether it is caused by overeating, a sedentary lifestyle, or the natural reduction of body muscle and buildup of fat as you age—is just as harmful now as it was when you were 40, says Walter Willett, M.D., Dr.P.H., professor of epidemiology and nutrition and chairman of the Department of Nutrition at the Harvard School of Public Health. Researchers believe that excessive body fat at any age increases the production of sex hormones such as estrogen that promote colon, breast, and endometrial cancer. Increased body fat also drives up blood pressure, forces the heart to work harder, and raises low-density lipoproteins (LDLs)—the bad cholesterol that contributes to the clogging of arteries and increases your risk of stroke and heart disease.

Body Fat: Where You Have It Matters

Apples are a food to admire. You just don't want to be shaped like one.

Extra weight around your belly (an apple-shaped body) puts you at greater risk of heart disease, stroke, and cancer than those who are trimmer. With aging, more men and women develop that undesirable shape.

"Body shape—fat distribution—becomes more important as we age because weight, which relects both muscle and fat mass, becomes a less reliable guide," says Walter Willett, M.D., Dr.P.H., professor of epidemiology and nutrition and chairman of the Department of Nutrition at the Harvard School of Public Health.

A pear shape—more fat on your hips and thighs—also means an increased risk of these diseases, but not as much as an apple, says David V. Schapira, M.D., director of the Stanley S. Scott Cancer Center at Louisiana State University Medical Center in New Orleans.

Are you an apple? Measure your waist at its narrowest point and your hips at the widest point (over the buttocks). Divide your waist measurement by the number of inches around your hips. A number greater than 0.75 for women or 1 for men suggests that you are at greater risk of health problems.

The best way to diminish an apple shape is through exercise. Even as little as walking 30 minutes a day, three times a week, can be an important beginning, Dr. Willett says.

It Isn't As Hard As You Think

Fortunately, losing weight after age 50 is easier than you might suspect. In fact, one study has shown that people in their sixties and seventies who enrolled in a weight-control program were twice as successful in their efforts to lose weight and make lifestyle changes than younger men and women, says Eileen Rosendahl, Ph.D., a geriatric psychologist and assistant professor at the Albert Einstein College of Medicine of Yeshiva University in New York City.

That is because you probably have more time to devote to the effort than you did when you were younger, and fat cells on the abdomen, the type that is really harmful, melt away more quickly than fat on the buttocks and thighs, says Lodovico Balducci, M.D., program leader of the senior adult oncology program at the University of South Florida College of Medicine in Tampa.

"You don't have to get down to an ideal body weight to get the benefits of intentional weight loss. I'm starting to believe that losing just a few pounds may be very good for you," says David F. Williamson, Ph.D., a researcher at the Centers for Disease Control and Prevention in Atlanta. One way for an older person to lose those pounds is by improving his level of physical activity, he says.

The Weight of the Evidence

If you're overweight, losing just 10 to 15 pounds (depending on your height) can reduce your risk of life-threatening diseases and improve your overall health. But if you don't make an effort to get your weight under control, you'll be more vulnerable to the big three killers, Dr. Klaper says.

Here's a look at the persuasive arguments that scientists are finding for shedding modest amounts of weight after age 50. Among other things, weight control does the following:

Promotes longevity. In a study of 15,069 overweight women, Dr. Williamson found that those who had lost 20 pounds in the year before the study began were 25 percent less likely to die of heart disease or cancer in the next 12 years than overweight women who didn't lose weight. These women also reduced their overall risk of dying by 20 percent and slashed in half their chances of succumbing to weight-related cancer of the breast, cervix, ovary, and others, as well as reducing their risk of dying with diabetes.

Researchers traced the lives of 19,000 Harvard University alumni men for up to 26 years. Those who weighed 20 percent under the U.S. average for men of similar age and height had the lowest rates of death.

Protects the heart. In the Framingham Heart Study—an ongoing assessment of the health habits of 5,200 people in Massachusetts—researchers showed that men and women in their sixties and seventies who weighed 30 percent more than what is considered a healthy weight were at least twice as likely to develop heart disease.

That's why Robert DiBianco, M.D., associate clinical professor at Georgetown University School of Medicine and a Washington, D.C., cardiologist, urges mature overweight people to lose weight. "Excess weight magnifies the risk factors of hypertension, diabetes, and high cholesterol levels that are associated with heart disease," Dr. DiBianco says. "Developing diabetes, for example, increases cardiac risk by more than 100 percent. But all these

Do You Use Food to Quell Emotions?

Emotions can be savage beasts. Loneliness, frustration, boredom, anger, grief, anxiety, guilt—these are just some of the beastly emotions that challenge us every day. Unfortunately, a lot of people over 50 regularly soothe them with food.

Do you? If so, you may be packing on pounds without really solving the underlying problem.

Here's a simple test, developed by Stephen P. Gullo, Ph.D., author of *Thin Tastes Better*, that will help you analyze how emotions affect your eating habits and determine what to do about it. Rate each of the following statements on a scale of 1 (rarely true) to 5 (always true). Scoring follows.

1. There is no problem that can't be solved by chocolate.
2. I like to treat myself to a nice dinner or some other food treat to celebrate accomplishments.
3. On previous diets I've sometimes cheated because I just felt that I deserved a little treat.
4. When I'm stressed or upset, I feel better after I've eaten.
5. have a favorite restaurant where my friends and I go to celebrate or just get together.
6. I have a particular food that I always crave when I'm under stress.

things are reversible to some extent if you lose those extra pounds."

Slashes stroke risk. In another ongoing phase of the Framingham study, researchers have been tracking the weights and blood pressures of men and women up

7. I always gain weight when I'm under pressure.
8. Whenever I've gone off a diet plan, there was something unpleasant going on in my life.
9. I always overeat when my children or grandchildren visit me.
10. I always overeat after I fight with friends or family.

Now, add up your total.

If you scored 21 or less, you're doing pretty well. You may occasionally turn to food for solace, but it isn't your first line of defense.

If you scored 22 to 36, you may be using food to pacify your emotions, but you're just as likely to use other ways of dealing with feelings—such as talking them out with friends, taking a bath, or exercising—that are less fattening.

If you scored 37 or more, you may be relying too much on food to cope with stress. Before you open the refrigerator, ask yourself if eating is really going to relieve your anger, boredom, depression, or other emotional needs, says Eileen Rosendahl, Ph.D., a geriatric psychologist and assistant professor at the Albert Einstein College of Medicine of Yeshiva University in New York City. Try to find something else to do—take a walk, garden, or visit an ill friend—that will make you feel gratified or happy instead of guilty.

to age 94 for 30 years. Every pound of excess weight, according to William Kannel, M.D., professor of medicine and public health at Boston University Medical Center, causes you to retain more sodium in your bloodstream, increases your risk of diabetes, and drives your systolic blood pressure (the top number in a blood pressure reading) up 4.5 millimeters. Combined, these weight-related risk factors may quadruple your chances of a heart attack or stroke, Dr. Kannel says.

"Weight control is very important for preventing stroke," says Philip Wolf, M.D., professor of neurology at Boston University School of Medicine. "Being overweight doesn't seem to be an independent risk factor for stroke. But if you look at the main risk factors for stroke—high blood pressure, high blood sugar, and high cholesterol levels—losing weight will lower every one of them."

Pounds Add to Your Cancer Risk, Too

Although scientists believe that extra pounds have more impact on heart disease than on cancer risk, slimming down may decrease the possibility that you'll develop some tumors, says Rachel Ballard-Barbash, M.D., an epidemiologist at the National Cancer Institute in Bethesda, Maryland. Specifically, avoiding midlife weight gain can help you:

Stifle breast and endometrial cancer. Dr. Barbash has found that women with more upper-body fat, the so-called apple-shaped bodies, are at 70 to 100 percent greater risk of developing breast cancer than women whose fat is on their lower bodies, the so-called pear shape in which fat clings to the hips and thighs.

Other studies involving women up to age 83 have found that the heaviest women who were apple-shaped have a 5 to 6 times greater risk of breast cancer and had 15 times greater incidence of endometrial cancer than women who were trimmer, says David V. Schapira, M.D., director of the Stanley S. Scott Cancer Center at Louisiana State University Medical Center in New Orleans.

"Theoretically, breast cancer risk can be reduced by 45 percent just by losing 10 to 15 pounds," Dr. Schapira says.

In addition, if a woman who weighs 25 percent or more over her ideal weight develops breast cancer, she is 60 percent more likely to have a recurrence of the disease in the next 10 years than does a woman who has her weight under control at diagnosis.

"Weight control is one of the few modifiable lifestyle behaviors that may reduce a woman's risk of diagnosis and death due to breast cancer," says Ruby Senie, Ph.D., associate attending epidemiologist at Memorial Sloan-Kettering Cancer Center in New York City.

Corral cancer of the esophagus. Men in their sixties who are 20 percent over their recommended healthy weight are at three times greater risk of developing adenocarcenoma, a cancer of the esophagus, than men who tip the scales right on, according to researchers at the National Cancer Institute who studied 174 men who had the disease and 750 who didn't.

Fight off colon cancer. In a six-year follow-up study of 47,723 male dentists, pharmacists, and other health professionals up to age 74, Harvard University researchers found that men who had waist circumferences of 43 inches or more were 2½ times more likely to develop colon cancer than those whose waists were less than 35 inches.

What's Going On?

Doctors suspect that excessive body fat sparks increased production of sex hormones like estrogen and testosterone that are thought to promote breast and endometrial cancer. At the same time high amounts of body fat slash levels of a protein that binds to these sex hormones and deactivates them. The result is a greater risk of developing these cancers, Dr. Schapira says.

Extra weight also triggers gastric reflux, bathing the esophagus with excessive amounts of acid that may promote precancerous growths, says Linda Morris Brown, an epidemiologist at the National Cancer Institute in Bethesda, Maryland.

Researchers are less certain how excess weight contributes to cancer of the esophagus and colon. They do know, however, that some of the same things that cause excess weight—high-fat foods and lack of exercise—also increase the risk of colon cancer. So being overweight may not directly cause colon cancer, but it could be a potent warning that other aspects of your lifestyle are endangering your health, says Tim Byers, M.D., professor of preventive medicine at the University of Colorado School of Medicine in Denver.

You Can Make a Big Difference Now

For many of us, controlling weight has been like trying to catch a live trout with bare hands. But, as discussed, making another effort even after age 50 can have an immense impact on your health and well-being.

"The safety of being thin is huge," says George Blackburn, M.D., Ph.D., associate professor of surgery at Harvard Medical School and chief of the nutrition/metabolism laboratory in the Cancer Research Institute at Beth Israel Deaconess Medical Center West in Boston. "There are 300,000 excess deaths in the non-thin population each year, and we spend $100 billion a year to treat diseases like heart disease, stroke, and cancer that are related to not being thin."

In most cases diet alone won't do the job for you. Your best bet is to use dietary changes as part of a comprehensive effort that includes exercise, Dr. Balducci says.

Remember that the pounds may come off more slowly than in the past, says Sharon Emmons, R.D., a clinical dietitian and geriatric nutrition specialist at the University of South Alabama College of Medicine in Mobile. If you lose a half-pound to a pound a week at this age, you're doing great, she says.

Usually, losing weight at that rate means shaving only 150 calories a day from your menu, Dr. Blackburn says. That's about the equivalent of a slice of cheese pizza, a 12-ounce beer, a ½-cup serving of vanilla ice cream, or five gingersnaps.

Shoot for losing no more than 10 pounds or 5 percent of your body weight (whichever is less) in 12 weeks, Dr. Blackburn says. Then try to maintain that weight loss for three months before attempting to lose more weight. The body, particularly after age 60, is willing to lose weight for about three months, he says. Then it doesn't want to budge for quite a while. If you push yourself too much, you're more likely to start overeating and regain the weight that you have dropped, Dr. Blackburn says. With these goals in mind, here's a look at the nuts and bolts of weight control, beginning with motivation.

Feed Your Head First

Weight control begins in the mind.

"I don't think that you'll seriously be able to get your weight under control without considering what is going on between your ears," says Maurice Larocque, M.D., a Montreal physician and author of *Slim Within*, a 21-day, audiocassette weight-loss program. "The thoughts that you plant in your mind will determine if you succeed or fail."

Here are some ways to help you think more positively about weight control so that you can achieve your goal and permanently reduce your risk of stroke, heart disease, and cancer.

Find new reasons to like yourself. "We know that 80 percent of people who are overweight don't like themselves," Dr. Larocque says. "They can't find any pleasure within themselves that would encourage them to care for their bodies. So you need to learn to love yourself before you can make any progress toward slimness."

Twice a day, take a moment to focus on some aspect of yourself that you like such as your legs, nose, or eyes. As you begin to lose weight, take pride in the features that are improving. Tell yourself, "I'm 60, but look at me. I really like how my belly is trimming down. I'm starting to get back the shape that I had when I was 40."

Write 'em down. Jot down on an index card your three most important motivators for losing weight, such as more stamina, more energy, and lessening your risk of heart disease. Read and think about what those motivators mean to you for 5 minutes when you awaken and just before you go to bed, suggests Peter Miller, Ph.D., executive director of the Hilton Head Health Institute in Hilton Head, South Carolina. Doing that will keep your mind locked on your goal.

Take a picture. Once a month, have a friend or a spouse take pictures of you from front, side, and back views. Focus on the parts of your body where you are making progress, like your shrinking tummy or your strengthening arms and legs. Take a couple of minutes each day to imagine how much better you'll look next month, Dr. Larocque says.

Let go. The more relaxed you are, the more open you'll be to positive thoughts that will help keep your weight under control, Dr. Larocque says. Try the following relaxation exercise twice a day: Get into a comfortable position—either lying or sitting—in a darkened room. Close your eyes and begin breathing very slowly and deeply. Relax the muscles of your forehead and jaw. Part your lips slightly. Now relax the muscles of your mouth, neck, arms, and legs. Now breathe more deeply, inhale slowly. Then push your shoulders upward until it seems as though they are touching your ears. Hold your breath for a count of five, then exhale slowly and drop your shoulders. Push your shoulders up again and repeat the breathing sequence. Sense yourself beginning to feel relaxed. Your arms are very heavy and limp.

Feel the sun's warmth on your arms. They are getting warmer and warmer. Now let your legs go limp and feel the sun's warmth on them. Repeat the sun imagery with your eyelids, jaw, forehead, and finally with your entire body. Feel the sun's energy inside your whole body. See yourself and smile. You are full of energy, and you use it. You appreciate each step that you are taking on your road to weight control. Now count to three, then open your eyes and get on with your day.

Step into the mirror. Like the queen in *Snow White*, you can be the fairest of all. Just use your imagination, says Barbara Morse, an imagery counselor and recreational therapist in San Diego who works with men and women over age 60.

Imagine yourself in a hall of mirrors, each one reflecting a different image of you, Morse says. Try to see as many perspectives in the mirrors as you can. One may make you look short and fat, another tall and skinny. See reflections of yourself as a child, as a person older than you are now, and as you see yourself today. Now look in a mirror and give yourself whatever type of body you would like. Change your hair color or style. Work with the image in the mirror until it reflects you exactly as you would like to be.

Step into that mirror and become that image that you have visualized. When the image fits and you feel comfortable, walk out of the hall of mirrors, taking the magic mirror with you. Ask the mirror what you need to do to maintain this image. Pay attention to the directions and follow them. Wear this new image as if it were an elegant gown or suit perfectly suited for you. Do this visualization twice a day for 5 minutes each, or whenever you feel your motivation to control your weight slipping, Morse says.

Put the scale away. Don't weigh yourself every day, says Maria Simonson, Sc.D., Ph.D., director of the Health, Weight, and Stress Clinic at the Johns Hopkins Medical Institutions in Baltimore. Instead, step onto the scale once a week at the same time of day. It will give a more accurate measure of your progress and be more encouraging than the constant ups and downs of daily weigh-ins.

Lean on others. Sharing your experience with a friend or a support group can help keep you motivated and lessen your temptation to stray. "A lot of people try to lose weight alone and that's difficult," Dr. Rosendahl says. It's even harder as you get older, she says, because the rate of weight loss often is slower than when you were younger, and that can be discouraging.

Discard all-or-nothing thinking. A lot of

10 Quick Low-Calorie Snacks

Here are 10 snacks—all 100 calories or less—that can satisfy your taste buds and still fit into your weight-control effort. This list was developed by Marilyn Cerino, R.D., coordinator of the weight-management and nutrition programs at the Benjamin Franklin Center for Health in Philadelphia.

- 3 chocolate kisses, 75 calories, 4.5 grams of fat
- 24 fresh grapes, 81 calories, 0 gram of fat
- 1 cup fresh strawberries with 1 tablespoon confectioner's sugar, 86 calories, 0 gram of fat
- ½ cup cranberry juice over ice with club soda and an orange slice, 91 calories, 0 gram of fat
- 5 vanilla wafers, 93 calories, 3 grams of fat
- 19 pieces of candy corn, 95 calories, 1.9 grams of fat
- 2 tablespoons low-fat yogurt topped with ½ cup cherries and 2 teaspoons sliced almonds, 96 calories, 3 grams of fat
- 2 cups warm air-popped popcorn tossed with 1 teaspoon melted margarine and 1 teaspoon honey, 97 calories, 3.8 grams of fat
- ½ cup sugar-free instant pudding with skim milk and ½ teaspoon shaved semi-sweet chocolate, 99 calories, 0.6 grams of fat
- 10 (1-inch) cubes of angel food cake topped with ¼ cup frozen raspberries in light syrup, 100 calories, 0 gram of fat

overweight older people are perfectionists, Dr. Larocque says. "They expect to reach 105 percent of their weight goals, and if they only achieve 90 percent of them, they think the whole effort is a failure," he says.

Instead of focusing on your overall goal, set your sights on a modest weight target—like a pound a week—that you can easily achieve. If you don't reach your goal one week, try not to think of it as a failure but as a learning experience. Jot down the things that you did and didn't do that will help you make a better effort in the next seven days.

"You don't have to be perfect, you just have to keep trying," Dr. Larocque says.

Take a day off. "We encourage our patients to take what we call planned holidays," says Patrick M. O'Neil, Ph.D., clinical psychologist and director of the Weight Management Center at the Medical University of South Carolina in Charleston. "It's a time when you decide in advance that you're going to give yourself a rest from weight control and have a do-as-you-choose day."

Doing that about once a month helps you learn how to regain control of your eating habits after a lapse and will boost your self-confidence so that you can get back on track after an unplanned slip, Dr. O'Neil says. A day off will also give you something to look forward to as your weight-control effort progresses.

Squelch the Saboteurs

Although positive motivation can help you overcome your own worst enemy—yourself—there are still plenty of well-intentioned friends and family members who can quickly sabotage your weight-control efforts. The older you get the more important it is to defeat the saboteurs, Dr. Larocque says. "They're one of the major obstacles that you'll face, and one of the main reasons that people in this age group stop losing weight," he says.

Jealousy, guilt, envy, and fear are some of the underlying reasons that provoke saboteurs to derail your efforts, he says. "Often, these people are trying to defend their own reasons for staying fat by attacking you," Dr. Larocque says. "They might tell you, 'Gee, you look so old now that you've lost all that weight. Have you seen your face? It looks like you have a lot of new wrinkles. Are you sure this weight-loss thing is right for you?'"

To overcome these attacks, realize that the saboteur is probably more concerned about his own feelings than your well-being. So ask yourself, why is this person really saying these things or offering me fattening foods that I shouldn't eat? Once you understand what is motivating the saboteur, it will be easier for you to ignore his temptations or criticisms and focus on the compliments of others, Dr. Larocque says.

Many other techniques can help you subdue these saboteurs: Here is a sampling.

Let them in on it. Sit down with your family and close friends and discuss why you want to lose weight and what they can do to help, Dr. Miller says. You could, for example, ask for their compliments and support but discourage them from tempting you with rich desserts.

If friends or relatives ignore your request, politely remind them that you're trying to make important lifestyle changes for your health and happiness. If they persist, be blunt, Dr. Miller says. Make it clear that you, and only you, will decide what you'll eat, when you'll eat it, and why you'll eat it, and you don't appreciate their attempts to undermine your efforts.

(continued on page 286)

How I Did It: An Expert Learns the Hard Way

Unlike some weight-loss experts who have never had to shed a pound in their lives, at age 70-plus, Maria Simonson, Sc.D., Ph.D., knows your struggle all too well.

"I know how you feel," says Dr. Simonson, director of the Health, Weight, and Stress Clinic at the Johns Hopkins Medical Institutions in Baltimore. "I know how easy it is to psychologically pounce onto an excuse so that you have a reason to hold on to that weight."

Why does she know? Well, after a stroke at age 50 temporarily immobilized her, she ballooned up to 348 pounds. "I could've gotten out of my wheelchair after six months, but everyone was feeling sorry for me, and I gloried in it," says Dr. Simonson. "I only got on my feet when the wheelchair got too small."

Then one day when she was preparing to speak about malnutrition to a group of medical interns, she overheard one of them say, "That fat tub is going to lecture about malnutrition? I bet she doesn't even know how to spell it."

That night she took all of her clothes off and stood in front of a mirror, and thought, "My God, I have let myself become this. I won't live another five years if I keep on this way. I made up my mind right then to start anew."

It was a struggle, but success came when she took matters into her own hands. "I decided that if I really wanted to lose weight, I'd have to do it myself," she says. "Reading about it, thinking about it, being told about it were all fine. But it was up to me to follow a program and be consistent."

For weight loss, she cut back on what she ate and began walking. For motivation, Dr. Simonson began noticing other people who were overweight and told herself that although she looked like them now, she wouldn't for much longer. And for inspiration, she prayed.

"It may sound old-fashioned, but I asked God to help me, and it made a difference," she says. "I began to realize that it's not just what you eat but how you feel that is important."

Her early success inspired her to co-found the weight-loss clinic at Johns Hopkins, where she continued losing weight along with her patients. Within two years she lost 190 pounds, and she still maintains 158 pounds on her 5-foot-6 frame.

"Losing that weight gave me a better sense of self-esteem," Dr. Simonson says. "I learned to develop self-discipline and hold on to it."

Dr. Simonson likes a reminder that a friend keeps on her refrigerator, reading: "You deserve the best. That means a long, healthy life with your husband, not a piece of cheesecake."

Says Dr. Simonson, "I think it's one of the most practical and self-motivating pieces of advice to remember. You are worth the effort. Always bear that in mind."

Make a contract. Ask potential saboteurs like your spouse or a close friend to sign a written agreement to support your effort, Dr. Larocque says. In writing, let the person know why you consider being overweight a threat to your health. Point out that any serious attempt to get your weight under control will require changes in habits and attitudes, including those of people close to you. Then list five ways the other person can help you, such as providing cooperation when requested, being attentive and praising even the slightest achievement, not pointing out the occasional slip-up, listening without judgment to your feelings, and providing encouragement to persevere regardless of difficulties. Then ask the person to sign and date two copies. Keep one for yourself and give the other one to the person. Carry your copy with you and, if necessary, pull it out to remind your friend or spouse about your deal.

Help them face their fears. Sometimes friends and loved ones worry that your new weight will ruin your relationship, particularly if their own weight or ailments prevent them from being as active as you are now. Reassure your loved ones that you're still the same inside and that you will always care and be there for them, Dr. Larocque suggests.

Keep binge buddies at bay. Some saboteurs love "eatings" rather than outings. These are the people who ask you out for lunch or dessert all the time. Instead of reluctantly accepting, suggest doing an activity that doesn't involve food, like visiting a museum, says Marilyn Cerino, R.D., coordinator of the weight-management and nutrition programs at the Benjamin Franklin Center for Health in Philadelphia.

Keep playing the same tune. Keep saying no thanks without offering an explanation. Don't say, "I can't because I'm trying to lose weight," because they'll just say, "Gee, I don't think that dieting is good for you." "They will come up with something if you let them," says Susan Olson, Ph.D., a Seattle psychologist and weight-control expert in private practice. "So become a broken record and keep saying no thank you until they get the point."

Move It to Lose It

You can slash calories to the bone and down all the magic pills, instant liquid shakes, grapefruit, cottage cheese, or diet bars you want, but you really won't get your weight under control until you do one critical thing: exercise.

"I know some older people who are very virtuous eaters who are extremely frustrated with their weight," Dr. Rosendahl says. "The trouble is they don't exercise, and unless you exercise, you're not going to lose weight."

In particular, exercise helps you retain muscle and fends off the natural accumulation of body fat as you age, Dr. Blackburn says.

That's important because researchers believe that moderate or mild exercise stimulates the immune system. So if you try to lose weight without exercise, you're going to lose muscle as well as fat. And once weakened this way, your body will sacrifice much of its ability to destroy viruses and abnormal cells that can develop into serious illnesses, says Robert C. Klesges, Ph.D., professor of psychology and preventive medicine at the University of Memphis in Tennessee.

Losing just a few pounds through exercise also may be a beneficial way to reduce your risk of heart disease and stroke, says Robert S. Schwartz, M.D., professor of internal medicine and gerontology at the University of Washington School of Medicine in Seattle.

In his studies of healthy older men up to age 82, Dr.

Schwartz has found that a 5-pound weight loss caused by six months of brisk walking and biking can increase levels of the good high-density lipoprotein cholesterol and lower harmful LDL cholesterol by as much as a 20-pound weight loss caused by calorie reduction alone.

"People are more likely to be successful keeping off weight by exercising," Dr. Schwartz says. "You may not lose as much weight or look very different, but metabolically I think exercise produces tremendous improvement."

Exercise also is a powerful motivator that can help suppress your appetite and keep you on track for weight control. It's an especially powerful lifestyle tool for people over age 50. "After they begin exercising, they often feel an increased sense of well-being and accomplishment and develop better self-esteem and a sense of control over their bodies," says Samuel Klein, M.D., director of the Center for Human Nutrition at Washington University School of Medicine in St. Louis. "All of these things feed into helping them eat better and staying with their effort."

All of the benefits of exercise are discussed in the next chapter, but here are a few specific approaches to help you control your weight and reduce your risk of the big three killers. Be sure to check with your doctor before beginning any exercise routine.

Lift it off. Resistance training will not only strengthen your muscles but also help you increase your metabolism so that you burn extra fat, says Margarita Treuth, Ph.D., assistant professor at Baylor College of Medicine in Houston.

In a pair of small studies involving 15 men up to age 65 and 15 women ages 60 to 77, Dr. Treuth found that those who worked out with resistance-training equipment three times a week for 16 weeks burned an extra 50 calories a day. Over a year, these workouts—one set (12 to 15 repetitions) of several upper-body exercises like biceps curls and two sets of lower-body strengthening exercises like leg presses—can help burn calories, she says.

"At these ages, it appears that resistance exercise can increase resting metabolism and help control weight," Dr. Treuth says.

To do a simple biceps curl, for instance, stand with your back against a wall and grasp a 1-pound food can in each of your hands. Lower your arms so that they are fully extended at your sides. Turn your palms so that they face forward. Then, slowly lift the cans up so that they touch your shoulders. Lower and repeat 10 to 12 times. (If you feel ambitious, after you lift the cans to your shoulder, pause for a count of five, then extend your arms over your head.)

Do that once a day for three weeks, then add a second set of 10 to 12 repetitions to your daily routine, says Mark Bank, an exercise physiologist at Walter O. Boswell Memorial Hospital in Sun City, Arizona, a retirement community near Phoenix.

Walk a mile toward leanness. Just strolling a mile daily burns 110 calories, Dr. Simonson says. That may not seem like much, but if you stick with it, you can lose up to 11 pounds a year even if you don't go fast. "Never overdo it. Keep it safe, even if it means moving slower," she suggests.

Do it a foot at a time. "You don't have to do all your exercising all at once," Dr. Simonson says. "A person over 60 can easily cover a mile a day by doing errands on foot, walking around the house, cleaning up after herself, or parking a few extra spaces away from the mall."

Do what you can. Maybe you can't always play tennis, walk, or lift weights. But you can still move your body, says Dr. Simonson, who lost nearly 200 pounds in two years. Sit in a chair and kick your feet up in the air, bend over and reach for your toes, pretend you're riding a bicycle and pedal your feet up and down, or play classical music on your stereo and flail your arms like a conductor.

"Every bit of exercise will help you burn calories," says Dr. Simonson, who considers herself a senior. "If you don't feel like exercising, just try it for 5 minutes. Even that can make a difference."

Stop Hunger Pangs with Yoga

"Yoga is a good exercise for older people trying to lose weight because it energizes their minds, bodies, and spirits and supplies them with a feeling of satisfaction that can replace any desire to eat," says Morse.

And you don't have to twist yourself into a knot to do it. In fact, you can practice many simple yoga techniques while sitting in a chair. Here are some easy yoga movements that you can do three times a week. Remember to breathe deeply, evenly, and continuously, suggests Carrie Angus, M.D., director of the Center for Health and Healing at the Himalayan International Institute of Yoga Science and Philosophy in Honesdale, Pennsylvania.

Roll your shoulders. Sit tall in a straight-back chair and lift your shoulders up as far as possible toward the back of your neck. Roll your shoulders forward and then relax them down. If you do this correctly, your shoulders should move in a circular motion, Dr. Angus says. Repeat this three to five times.

Bend an elbow. Put your hands on your shoulders and point each elbow out to the side. Slowly rotate your elbows in large circles. Do five rotations forward and five backward.

Reach for the sky. Lift your right arm up as high as possible, make a fist, and look up at your hand. Hold that position for a count of five, then relax. Do that three to five times with each arm.

Make circles. Extend your arms out to the sides, fingertips turned up, and palms away from your body. Slowly rotate your arms forward in circular motions, 5 to 10 times. To determine how wide a circle to make, start small and increase the size until you feel a gentle stretch. Your circles may be as small as 6 inches or as wide as 2 feet. Repeat the motion in the opposite direction.

Do the twist. Sitting slightly forward in the chair, take your right hand and put it on your left knee. Place your left hand behind you on the chair seat. Gently twist to your left so that you're looking over your left shoulder (make sure your feet stay flat on the floor, facing forward). Hold this position, breathing gently for a slow count of 10. Relax and repeat this sequence to the right. Do this three times in each direction.

Fine-Tune Your Eating Habits

After five or more decades, some just don't want to make drastic changes in their diets for any reason. But you don't have to in order to lose weight, says Edith Howard Hogan, R.D., a spokesperson for the American Dietetic Association in Washington, D.C.

"Small changes can add up to big differences in weight," Hogan says. "All it takes is a few little daily adjustments that are so easy that you really shouldn't have any problem incorporating them into a winning weight-control effort." Here's a sampling.

Plan your meals. Take a moment just before

you go to bed or when you wake in the morning to go over your meal strategy for the day, Dr. Miller says. Jot down when you're going to eat, where you're going to eat, what you're going to eat, and try to stick to it. Imagine yourself making the right food choices throughout the day and feeling good about yourself.

Make your kitchen convenient, not cozy. If your kitchen is too comfortable, you'll be tempted to spend more time there nibbling on snacks and other foods. "Some people have a television, a rocking chair, and a desk in their kitchens," Cerino says. "It's the focal point of their homes, and if they have a weight problem, the first thing they need to do is get all of that stuff out of there."

Cancel your membership in the clean plate club. A lot of us in this age group grew up with, "Oh, good for you, you cleaned all the food off your plate," says Barbara Beahm, R.D., a registered dietitian in Great Bend, Kansas, and a spokesperson for the Kansas Dietetic Association. But as we age, that philosophy can make it harder to keep weight down.

"Breaking away from the clean plate club takes some effort," Beahm says. "But one way to do it is to ask yourself, before you eat those last bits of food on your plate, what is more wasteful: to throw something away or to carry unnecessary pounds around on your waist that will add to your risk of stroke, heart disease, cancer, and other medical problems?"

Never say never. "When someone tells me, 'I love cheesecake, but I'm never going to eat it again,' I can guarantee you that she's either going to drop out of our weight-loss group or be one of the few who have gained weight after six weeks," Dr. Klesges says.

So to reach your weight goal, strive for moderation, not denial. "If you don't give in to cravings occasionally, your weight-control effort is headed for failure, because denying yourself too often sets you up for binges," Dr. Simonson says. "Once a month or so, let yourself have a couple of spoonfuls of the foods you love." Remember that even the experts cheat once in a while.

Wait out the wave. Cravings surge and ebb like waves. So instead of dashing for the kitchen, wait 10 minutes, and the craving will probably subside, Dr. Simonson says.

Get naked. "If you're determined to eat something that you shouldn't, take all of your clothes off and sit in front of a mirror as you eat," Dr. Simonson says. "Believe me, you will not be tempted to do it again for a very long time."

Face your tormentor. Schedule a time when you won't be interrupted for 10 to 20 minutes. Then place the food you usually crave in front of you. Look at it, think about why you want it, then eat half of it and throw the rest away, says Dr. Miller. Do that three times a week, eating smaller and smaller portions each time.

Feast on imaginary doughnuts. One simple way to fight off a craving is to imagine yourself giving in to it, says Morse. Visualize a doughnut shop, grocery store, or favorite restaurant that has lots of tempting but fattening foods. Now choose one, two, or as many as you would like. Sit down with your doughnuts and eat them bit by bit, savoring each mouthful. Feel the bites going down your throat and into your stomach. Continue to eat doughnuts until you feel full.

Repeat this visualization whenever you feel a craving for your favorite food. Eventually, you should be able to think "doughnut" and immediately feel full and satisfied without having to eat.

Beware the "comfort" trap. Losing a loved one can lead some to seek comfort in food. "But keep in mind that your loved ones are at peace and watching over you. So please don't let them down," Dr. Simonson says. "They only want what is best for you, and being overweight simply isn't healthy."

Sneak in a nap. When you're tired, emotions can overwhelm you and tempt you to seek comfort from food, says Hogan. Get at least 6 hours of sleep a day. If you feel an urge to eat, lie down, close your eyes for a few minutes, and the emotional tug to chow down should pass.

Become a stove-top eater. Instead of putting foods into serving bowls and placing them on the table, take modest portions—so that they don't overlap on your plate—right from pots and pans in the oven or on the stove, Beahm says. Then quickly wrap up any leftovers and put them away before you eat. You'll be less tempted to go back for seconds, and you'll probably end up with a spare meal in the freezer instead of a spare tire around your belly.

Slow down and chew. Take your time and enjoy eating, Beahm suggests. If you eat too fast, your stomach may be full long before the message to stop chowing down reaches your brain. That is particularly true in later years when your digestive tract reacts more leisurely to food. To prevent overeating, allow at least 20 minutes for every meal.

When you're eating, ask yourself if you really tasted and enjoyed that previous bite of food. If the answer is no, then it's time to slow down the conveyor belt from the plate to your mouth, Beahm says.

Put your fork down between bites and chew

carefully so that you have time to savor the flavors and textures of the food in your mouth, she says. Glance at the clock before you begin eating. If you're finished within 5 minutes, try to stretch that out to 8 minutes during the next meal. Gradually increase the time it takes you to eat until you reach 20 minutes, Beahm says.

Try downsizing. Use salad plates and smaller serving dishes. It will squelch your appetite and shave calories off your meals, Dr. Simonson says.

In restaurants ask for a child's portion or request that the waiter put half of the entrée into a take-home bag before serving you the remaining portion, she says.

Lop off fat. Trimming the visible fats off meats can save you about 60 calories per meal, Hogan says. Over a year, that can add up to 21,000 calories. And that's 6½ pounds less fat that you have to worry about gaining. Slashing other fats including cooking oils from your recipes can make another huge dent in your weight.

Fiber up. Fibrous foods like fruits, vegetables, beans, and grains are good for weight control because they are packed with nutrients and usually have few calories. Fiber also adds bulk to your diet, so you'll feel full faster and eat less, Beahm says.

By the time you're 60, you should be eating 25 to 30 grams of fiber a day (one orange has about 3 grams) for weight control and to prevent heart disease and cancer, Beahm says.

Drink water. Have an 8-ounce glass of water about 10 minutes before you eat, Dr. Simonson says. That way, your stomach will already have something in it, and you won't need to eat as much to feel full.

Munch on carbs first. Kick off meals with a food rich in carbohydrates like an angel hair pasta appetizer or bean or noodle soup, Dr. Blackburn says. That should lessen your fat craving 20 minutes into the meal, and you probably won't yearn for calorie-laden, high-fat desserts.

Eat six a day. If you eat smaller meals more frequently, you'll be less likely to overindulge, Hogan says. After breakfast, have a midmorning snack like yogurt or an apple. Have a hearty lunch entrée like stew, baked chicken breast, or spaghetti. Then have a late-afternoon snack like cheese and crackers, a small dinner, and a light evening snack like a scoop of nonfat frozen yogurt.

Eat breakfast. Skipping meals, especially breakfast, puts your body on a starvation alert. So it is more likely to conserve fat instead of shedding it, Emmons says. Eating such foods as toast, cereal, and leftover pasta early in the morning will get you off on the right caloric track for the rest of the day and help you fend off the afternoon munchies.

If you need another incentive, consider that breakfast skippers—no matter their weight—are three times more prone to develop heart disease and stroke-inducing blood clots than people who stop to taste their oatmeal, according to researchers at Memorial University of Newfoundland in St. Johns.

Brown-bag it. Prepare your lunch the night before, even if you're retired, Dr. Larocque says. If you do it right after dinner, you'll be more thoughtful and probably select lower-calorie foods than you might otherwise choose the next day when you're famished.

Dine light at night. Eat your smallest meal of the day for dinner, especially if you are going to be watching television or doing another sedentary activity in the evening, Hogan says. If you eat most of your calories early in the day when you are most active, you'll have more opportunities to burn them off before they turn into fat, she says. So try a tuna salad or lean turkey breast sandwich and a cup of soup instead of a full-course dinner.

Keep a top 10 list. Write down 10 healthy foods such as carrots or fig bars on an index card and carry it with you, Dr. Miller suggests. Then when you have a craving or are tempted by a high-calorie food, you'll have a handy list of alternatives. Update your list once a week so that you'll always have a few new foods to try.

Alternate yellow and green. To ensure that you're getting plenty of nutrients like vitamins A, B, and C after you begin a weight-control effort, eat fresh, low-calorie yellow or orange vegetables like squash, pumpkin, and carrots one day then switch to green vegetables such as fresh spinach, turnip greens, or dark leafy lettuces the next day, says Virginia Stoner, in her seventies, past president of the Dietary Managers Association and a certified dietary manager from Hampstead, Maryland.

Imbibe cautiously. Alcohol is a double-edged sword. It seems to have a beneficial effect on the heart. But one serving of alcohol contains more than 100 calories, and it hinders your body's ability to burn fat, Hogan says. So if you're trying to lose weight, limit yourself to one serving, Cerino suggests. That's one 12-ounce beer, 6 ounces of wine, or one cocktail containing 1 ounce of liquor a day.

Control it with carbs. "I've found in my weight-management classes that people who avoid eating complex carbohydrates like potatoes and bread in the mistaken belief that these foods are fattening, turn instead to chocolate and sweets in the late afternoon," Beahm says.

And instead of filling you up, sugary sweets can actually stimulate your appetite, Dr. Blackburn says.

Prescription for Prevention

As we age, metabolism slows and fat begins to account for a greater percentage of body weight. Overall, the average person gains about a pound a year after age 35. This extra body fat can increase the production of sex hormones such as estrogen that promote colon, breast, and endometrial cancer.

Greater amounts of body fat also drive up blood pressure, force the heart to work harder, and raise LDL—the bad cholesterol that contributes to the clogging of arteries and increases your risk of stroke and heart disease.

Do:

■ Write down your three most important motivators for losing weight. Read and think for 5 minutes twice a day about what those motivators mean to you.

■ Unwind. Practice a relaxation technique such as guided imagery twice a day. The more relaxed you are, the more open you'll be to positive thoughts that will help keep your weight under control.

■ Exercise regularly. Try walking 30 minutes a day, three times a week.

Eating at least six servings of grains, pastas, and other complex carbohydrates a day can dampen urges for candies, cakes, and other fattening snacks, Beahm says.

Don't touch the finger foods. Most people will eat more with their fingers than they do with a knife and

- Sit down with your family and close friends and discuss why you want to lose weight and what they can do to help.

- Serve yourself directly from the stove and immediately put leftovers away. That will discourage overeating.

- Eat six smaller meals instead of three large ones.

- Use smaller plates and chew slowly.

Don't:

- Weigh yourself daily. Small fluctuations can be discouraging. Step on the scale no more than once a week. The results will seem more dramatic.

- Be pressured into eating something that you don't want. Keep saying no thank you until the person tempting you gives up.

- Make your kitchen too comfortable. You'll be tempted to spend more time there nibbling on snacks and other foods.

- Keep a large stash of nuts, chips, and other snacks in your house. Buy smaller packages and only have one open at a time.

fork. So avoid keeping a large stash of finger foods like nuts, chips, and cookies in your house and stay away from entrées like fried chicken, too. Buy smaller packages and only have one open at a time, Dr. Simonson says.

Pass on the peanuts. A 2-ounce serving of salted peanuts has 328 calories. If you need to nibble on something crunchy, reach for pretzels instead—20 small ones have as little as 80 calories, and most are fat-free.

Just eat one. If you insist on eating high-fat, high-calorie snacks like peanuts or potato chips, don't eat them right out of the package. Instead, divide the chips into individual servings and store them in plastic sandwich bags for later use. That way, when you reach for these snacks, you'll be less tempted to eat more than you should, Emmons says.

Skip the fried shrimp. Boiled shrimp have about 84 calories per 3-ounce serving compared to 206 calories if they're fried, Dr. Simonson says.

Pick pumpkin pies. If you love pie, stick to pumpkin or fruit types. They're lower in calories, Dr. Simonson says. Pecan pie, for instance, has about 430 calories a slice compared to 240 for pumpkin. You cut another 100 calories off if you don't eat the crust, she says.

Back off bacon. An ounce of bacon (slightly more than four medium slices) has 163 calories. A 1-ounce slice of Canadian bacon is leaner and only has about 57 calories, Dr. Simonson says.

Exercise

Protective Programs Designed Just for You

Y ou don't want buns of steel. But you do want to steel your defenses against diseases that kill. And you'd like to do it without stressing the bones, joints, and muscles that need more TLC with each passing year.

Yes, physical activity is good for you. But if you're like most people age 50 and over, you bypass the exercise programs, books, and videos that shout "no pain, no gain." And you've made the smart choice. Research shows that moderate exercise gives you as much—maybe even more—protection from disease as the old grunt-and-groan-and-sweat type of workout.

"Moderate exercise can help you lower your risk of disease and carry on an active lifestyle beyond your eighties," says James M. Rippe, M.D., director of the Center for Clinical and Lifestyle Research at Tufts University School of Medicine in Boston and author of *Fit over Forty*.

Two-Phase Program for Protection

Experts today recommend a two-part exercise program: aerobic exercise (walking or bicycling, for example) to condition your heart and cardiovascular system, and strength-training exercises (calisthenics and high-intensity weight lifting) to build muscle and cut fat. And you need to exercise only two or three times a week.

You can ease into this routine gradually and safely. That's a big plus since "by age 60, just about everyone has some element of osteoarthritis, osteoporosis, joint irritation, or lack of flexibility," says Dr. Rippe. "Light exercise doesn't aggravate these conditions." In fact, exercise usually reduces them.

If you join exercise groups or walking clubs, you reap even more benefits—social activity and new friends. "We like to call this recreation, not exercise," says Gerald Fletcher, M.D., professor of medicine at the Mayo Clinic in Jacksonville, Florida.

Experts note that people who exercise enjoy a better quality of life. "Exercisers are more active in the rest of their lives," says Dr. Rippe. "Many of the age-related declines that we see are tied to the expectation that people become more sedentary and uninterested in things around them as they age. It is true that if you're inactive, your metabolism slows, you gain weight, and you become even more inactive. But it doesn't have to be like that."

Stay Young at Heart

Researchers have found that exercise can give your body's systems the capacity to work as well as someone 20 years younger. So it's not surprising that physically active people—regardless of their biological ages—have lower rates of heart disease and are less vulnerable to strokes.

If you haven't exercised for years, don't be put off: "As soon as you start to exercise, your risk of cardiovascular problems drops by 25 percent," says Dr. Fletcher.

"Studies show that even if you start a regular exercise program in your sixties, you lower your risk of heart disease for the rest of your life," says Dr. Rippe. "If you're 60 years old, you may have another 25 years left, so the quality of life during those years is something to think about."

Don't let a heart attack hold you back. "Exercise has been proven to be a great therapy," says Kenneth H. Cooper, M.D., president and founder of the Cooper Clinic and the Cooper Institute for Aerobics in Dallas, who is also known as the father of aerobics. Studies show that people who become involved in an exercise program after their first heart attacks are 20 to 40 percent more likely to be alive seven years later than those who survived a heart attack and then remained totally sedentary.

Exercise is so important that cardiologists often prescribe (not just recommend or suggest) exercise for patients with heart disease, observes Alan Rozanski, M.D., director of nuclear cardiology and cardiac stress testing at St. Luke's Hospital in New York City.

In one study, researchers followed 68 patients who were on a waiting list for heart transplants and who also participated in an exercise program of graded walking. After three to six months, the hearts of 30 patients had improved to the point that they no longer needed new hearts. Two years later, their hearts were still going strong.

How does aerobic exercise perform these miracles? It makes your heart pump more vigorously to carry extra blood and oxygen to hardworking muscles. Over time, the demands of exercise make your heart physically fit—stronger and more efficient. "The heart becomes a bigger, stronger pump that pumps more blood with each beat," says Bryant Stamford, Ph.D., professor of exercise

Exercise Danger Signals

Exercise intentionally puts an added burden on your cardiovascular system. So if you have any of the following symptoms or medical conditions, stop exercising and see your doctor before you start up again, says Gerald Fletcher, M.D., professor of medicine at the Mayo Clinic in Jacksonville, Florida.

A headache, cramps, or heart palpitations: Or if you feel dizzy, faint, or cool while exercising. With any of these, if you're in the sun, get into the shade or someplace cool.

Discomfort in your upper body, including your chest, arms, neck, or jaw: You might feel aching, burning, tightness, or a sensation of fullness.

Shortness of breath: That includes wheezing or the failure of your breathing to return to normal within 5 minutes.

A cramp in one calf that flares up when you walk and simmers down when you rest: This could be a symptom of intermittent claudication, a condition caused by plaque buildup in the arteries of your leg. If that's the case, you may have similar deposits in your coronary arteries.

An infection: Put off exercise until all symptoms of a cold, flu, bronchitis, or other infection are gone, and until your temperature, white blood cell count, and cultures are back to normal.

physiology and director of the Health Promotion Center at the University of Louisville in Kentucky.

You get practical payoffs: The well-exercised heart doesn't have to beat as fast when you do something demanding. Even though your body is stressed, your heart isn't. When nonexercisers shovel the sidewalk after a snowstorm, for instance, their likelihood of a heart attack jumps to 107 times their normal risk. Someone who exercises five times a week has a risk that rises to only 2.4 times.

Drive High Blood Pressure Down

Heart attacks and strokes don't come out of the blue. Much of the trouble that leads to these killers starts in the arteries, the tubes that carry the blood and allow it to flow to the body's organs. High blood pressure, a condition that becomes more common with advancing years, often sets the stage for all the other problems. Exercise can help get it down.

When you have high blood pressure, the blood circulates too vigorously under too much force. The pressure tears up the artery walls, which allows the harmful low-density lipoprotein (LDL) cholesterol to attach and form plaque. Over time, this turns arteries that used to be as smooth and efficient as the interstate into the equivalent of one-lane gravel roads. "High blood pressure wouldn't be such a serious problem if it didn't do so much damage to artery walls," says Dr. Stamford.

"We think exercise lowers blood pressure because it opens up the small vessels and capillaries and helps blood flow into the working muscles that need the extra nourishment," says Dr. Stamford. An added benefit for the muscles: They become better able to absorb oxygen and glucose (blood sugar). Exercisers with high blood pressure often find that exercise lowers it, which in turn allows their doctors to lower or eliminate their medications.

You reap the benefits of exercise long after your workout, even when you are lolling in a recliner with the newspaper. That's because exercise lowers the resting heart rate, which reduces pressure on the whole cardiovascular system, says Dr. Stamford.

If the blood flow gets blocked completely, which becomes more likely as the arteries narrow, you could have a heart attack (if an artery to the heart gets blocked) or stroke (if the blockage occurs in an artery leading to the brain). This happens when the platelets—the tiny disklike structures that help the blood coagulate—stick to each other and to the artery walls to create a clot. Exercise reduces your risk because it keeps the platelets from clustering excessively and damming the flow.

When you exercise, you also protect your artery walls. Studies in Europe suggest that a combination of diet and exercise decreases the soft plaque that gradually builds up and hardens, narrowing the artery.

The Honolulu Heart Program on Oahu, Hawaii, conducted a 22-year study of 5,362 Japanese-American men ages 55 to 68. The researchers found that nonexercisers were four times more likely to experience one type of stroke and three times more likely to experience another type of stroke when compared to more active men.

Get a Grip with the Good Cholesterol

Any time you exercise, your body ends up with more of the high-density lipoproteins, or HDLs. That's the so-called good cholesterol that grabs the harmful LDL cholesterol and carries it out of the bloodstream before it can attach to artery walls. The biggest predictor of future heart disease is an HDL reading below 35, says Dr. Cooper. (That number is a measure of milligrams per deciliter or mg/dl.)

Warm Up for Comfort

Before you walk or do strength-training exercises, always ease into the effort by stretching your muscles. "Warm-up exercises that stretch your muscles prevent injury," says William J. Evans, Ph.D., professor of applied physiology and nutrition and director of the Noll Physiological Research Center at Pennsylvania State University in University Park.

"I advise older people to go out and walk slowly for the first quarter mile or so, just to warm up their muscles a little, and then stretch," says Kenneth H. Cooper, M.D., president and founder of the Cooper Clinic and the Cooper Institute for Aerobics in Dallas.

Besides walking and stretching, Dr. Evans suggests warming up with an exercise that works the muscles in your lower body. "They're the most important for mobility, so it's important to stretch, limber, and strengthen those muscles," he says.

Step-ups are a good way to do that. You'll need a step stool, roughly 8 to 10 inches high. Stand with both feet on the floor. Slowly raise your right leg and place your foot on the stool. Using the muscles in your right leg, lift yourself to a standing position on the stool. Hold on to something for support if you have balance problems. Now reverse that motion: Step off the stool, again making sure that your right leg does all the work. Repeat 10 to 15 times. Then repeat the exercise with the left leg.

"We used to think that you had to exercise vigorously to raise HDL levels. But now we think that moderate amounts of low-key exercise such as walking can increase HDL levels by about 10 percent," says Dr. Rippe.

Researchers at Stanford University studied men and women ages 50 to 65 who exercised lightly. After two years, an HDL check showed that 52 percent of the exercisers had lowered their risk of heart disease by 10 percent. Another study showed that women who walked a slow 3 miles four or five times a week also upped their HDL levels. And a joint study of postmenopausal women showed that while good cholesterol levels rose with exercise, the amounts of artery-clogging LDL cholesterol dropped.

As you get older, your arteries gradually stiffen, which increases your risk of atherosclerosis, unless you take steps to flex them by exercising your body. Researchers at the Gerontology Research Center in Baltimore evaluated the arteries of 146 older men and women. The arteries of exercisers were up to one-third more flexible than those of couch potatoes.

Build Your Muscles to Block Disease

Strength-training exercises put one of the major risk factors in heart disease, cancer, and stroke into reverse—the otherwise inevitable increase of body fat. We're not talking about weight problems here, just the simple fact that as you age, you lose muscle, and it's replaced by fat.

Even if their weight remains unchanged, nonexercisers will probably greet their eightieth birthdays (assuming they get there) with 30 percent less muscle than they had in their prime.

This alarming ratio makes you older than you have to be. As your muscle decreases, stairs feel like a vertical mountain climb. Hefting that can of beans off the kitchen shelf gets harder and harder. And a common sack of groceries feels like an Olympic barbell in your hands. That's not good for your risk of cancer, heart disease, and stroke—and certainly not good if you want to continue to live independently.

One quick encounter with a tape measure will probably give you all the evidence you need that these changes are taking place. Researchers in England have determined that your body's fat level manifests itself in your girth, not just in your weight. You're at the threshold of increased health risk if your waist measures over 31 inches (for most women) or over 37 inches (for most men).

You can't head off the effects of time with diet alone. Researchers think that the changes in your body are connected to age-related alterations in your metabolism and your oxygen intake.

Exercise is your only defense, and it can go a long way toward reversing the loss that leaves you weak and at risk, observes William J. Evans, Ph.D., professor of applied physiology and nutrition and director of the Noll Physiological Research Center at Pennsylvania State University in University Park.

Just how potent are exercise's effects? Healthy men and women ages 56 to 80 participated in a 12-week strength-training program and on average lost 4 pounds of body fat. Their metabolisms increased by 7 percent, which contributed to their needing 15 percent more calories a day just to maintain their weight.

Regular exercise is associated with lower rates of colon cancer, probably because exercise speeds the passage of substances through the gut, according to Dr. Evans. Researchers at the European Institute of Oncology in Milan concluded that exercise might reduce the risk of colon cancer in men by up to one-third.

Laboratory research gives further support to the importance of exercise as a cancer fighter. In one study exercise was tied to increased killer-cell ability to attack tumors in mice. Some studies also suggest that regular exercisers are less likely to develop prostate and breast cancer.

How Exercise May Jump-Start Your Immune System

Moderate amounts of exercise not only strengthen you but may also muscle up your immune system, some researchers believe. In fact, when you exercise, your blood platelets and white-blood-cell count go up. During moderate exercise, the body manufactures more natural killer cells, which help keep immunity strong and fight free radicals caused by pollutants. With those two factors on your side, your risk of cancer drops.

Experts believe an immune system strengthened by exercise also may help fight some forms of cancer.

A stronger immune system makes life more pleasant on a day-to-day level, too. "We notice fewer colds, coughs, and bronchitis in people who exercise," says Dr. Fletcher.

Researchers aren't sure how exercise effects the immune system, but Dr. Stamford speculates that "when you exercise, you stress all of your body's systems. The immune system reacts like the body's fire department to take care of the stress."

The rest of the body responds to the stress of exercise by becoming stronger and better able to cope with the next round of demands. It's likely that the immune system muscles in on disease, too.

Live Easy with Exercise

You get a lot out of the effort you put into your workouts. Besides lowering your risk for heart disease, stroke, and cancer, exercise helps people over 50 im-

Test Your Rate of Perceived Exertion

The Rate of Perceived Exertion (or Borg) scale lets you decide if you're exercising hard enough—or too hard. It's easy to use.

Just make a mental scale, using 6 to represent the least difficult activity (lying down and doing nothing) and 20 for the most, where you'd be working so hard that you couldn't take another step. So exercise that's very light rates a 7, fairly light gets an 11, and just plain hard a 15.

Until your body gets used to the work, keep your exercise between 11 (fairly light) and 14 (somewhat hard). Within that range, you'll be working at between 50 percent and 85 percent of your peak heart rate, where you get the maximum benefit.

There's no need to move up the scale if you're just trying to maintain your fitness, says Terri Merritt, a clinical exercise physiologist at the Preventive Medicine Research Institute in Sausalito, California. But if you want to improve your fitness, gradually increase your level (no faster than one level every week or two) until you reach 15. At this point you'll begin to get short of breath and feel that you can't go much longer. Don't exercise above 15.

You can vary the intensity and the duration. A long walk at a lower level of activity, perhaps 11, will help as much as a shorter workout at level 14.

Keep in mind that as you become more fit, you'll have to work longer to get the same degree of exertion.

prove their health in lots of other areas. Here's what else exercise can do:

Eases sleep. Without good sleep your body is more likely to catch diseases and less able to fight them off. "If you have a low activity level, it's normally hard to sleep," says Richard P. Allen, Ph.D., assistant professor in the Department of Neurology at the Johns Hopkins University Sleep Disorder Center in Baltimore.

A study conducted through Stanford University looked at 43 people ages 50 to 76. Those who exercised four times a week fell asleep faster, slept better and longer, and felt more rested than those who didn't.

Some studies show that exercise helps improve the quality of slow-wave sleep, the phase of rest that produces the strongest sleep experience.

Cuts the fat. Exercise helps the body get rid of triglycerides, a type of fat in the blood linked to an increased risk of heart attacks, generalized atherosclerosis (hardening of the arteries), and other medical problems. Researchers think that exercise enhances an enzyme in the blood and muscles that plucks triglycerides out of the bloodstream.

Trims the pounds. Extra body weight means extra risk for heart disease, cancer, and stroke. If you don't increase your calorie intake and burn at least 700 calories per week (the amount that you would use if you walked for 20 minutes, three times a week), you'll lose weight. Exercise also seems to help your body use the proteins that it takes in more efficiently.

Reduces stress. "It's not stress that kills, per se," says Dr. Cooper. "Rather, it's the way we handle it. And exercise has been shown to help people handle their stress better and thus should lower their incidence of heart disease and other health problems."

Research also suggests that exercise axes thromboxane, a chemical in the blood that promotes clotting and encourages platelets to stick together, which can trigger heart attacks. Nonexercisers with aggressive type A personalities show the highest levels of the chemical.

Lowers the dose. Because exercise helps the heart work better and may speed weight loss, people with heart disease, high blood pressure, or diabetes may show so much improvement that their doctors can lower the dose of their medicines or drop the pills altogether, notes Kaaren Douglas, M.D., director of the program in geriatric medicine at the University of California, Irvine.

Betters your balance. As you age, your risk of falling increases. Studies show that weight lifting or balance training improves overall balance. In healthy community-dwelling elders, tai chi has been shown to decrease fall rates.

Improves a couple's sex life. Researchers have found that physical impotence often results from poor blood circulation to the penis. Since exercise improves circulation on a system-wide basis, doctors speculate that it will help reduce the problem.

Increases mobility. When you work your heart, more blood goes to all parts of your body, including your brain. Those who exercise, studies show, perform better on mental tests and respond faster to stimuli.

Makes more muscle. Strength training also produces larger, stronger muscles. The stress of exercise probably creates microscopic tears in the muscle fibers, according to Dr. Evans. In between exercise sessions, the muscles repair and strengthen the fibers and learn to synthesize and use proteins more efficiently. The brain gets into the act, too, putting more muscle cells to work to meet the extra demands.

Improves your mood. "There is no question that exercise has been shown to improve mood and relieve anxiety and depression, although the reasons why are hard to prove in a laboratory setting," says Robert S. Brown, Sr., M.D., Ph.D., clinical professor of psychiatric medicine at the University of Virginia in Charlottesville and a longtime researcher on exercise and its effect on mental health. "I've never treated a physically fit person with a major depression."

Exercise also produces physiological changes that may elevate mood. "My theory is that exercise—at least to the point of sweating—raises body temperature, which speeds up the metabolism," Dr. Brown says. "That results in more oxygen going to the brain, optimizing essential chemical reactions." Exercise also releases endorphins, the so-called pleasure chemicals in the brain that can block pain and invoke feelings of well-being—or even euphoria like the much-ballyhooed runner's high experienced by long-distance runners and other athletes.

Controls diabetes. Exercise helps your body produce the insulin that it needs to process glucose (blood sugar) and get it out of the blood and into the cells. "Millions of people are insulin-resistant," Dr. Stamford says. Glucose stays in the blood, which creates real problems because it crystallizes. A sugar crystal looks like a medieval mace, a weapon consisting of a ball with spikes on it. It tears up the lining in small blood vessels, which sets the stage for harmful cholesterol to attach to the artery walls and balloon into atherosclerosis, or hardening of the arteries. Exercise can help prevent that.

Strengthens bone. Exercise strengthens bones weakened by osteoporosis because it increases blood flow and helps cells create new, healthier bone. A study at Tufts University in Boston followed 39 women ages 50 to 70 and found that bone mass, muscle mass, strength, and balance all improved with exercise.

Eases joint pain. Because exercise develops the

Give Yourself a Lift

Ever want to feel like a kid again? Well, maybe you remember calisthenics from grade school, those exercises that use the body's own weight to build and tone muscles. They're not complicated, and they require no special equipment. The following three exercises are recommended by William J. Evans, Ph.D., professor of applied physiology and nutrition and director of the Noll Physiological Research Center at Pennsylvania State University in University Park.

Bent-knee pushups: Lie on the floor facedown, feet together, knees and palms against the floor. Keeping your knees against the floor, push your body up with your arms. Keep your back as flat as possible. Return to starting position.

Calf raises: Use a chair or wall for support, if necessary. Stand with the balls of your feet on a 2-inch-thick book or board, your heels off the edge. Push yourself up onto your toes, then slowly lower your heels as far as you can.

Modified squats: Stand behind a chair, holding the back of the chair for support. With your feet flat on the floor, point your toes outward. Bend your knees slightly while keeping your back straight and feet on the floor. Return to starting position.

muscles that support your joints, says Dr. Evans, it usually eases the pain of arthritis and other joint ailments.

Get Off to a Good Start

Here are the guidelines that you'll need to get your total exercise program of aerobic and strength-training exercise off the ground safely.

Get a physical. Exercise works because it stresses your body, which grows stronger as a result. It's important to make sure that your body's systems can handle the extra work, so you'll want to schedule a checkup with your doctor, says Dr. Stamford.

Checking with your doctor before you begin an exercise program is even more of a must if you have more than two risk factors for heart disease, Dr. Fletcher says. These risk factors are high cholesterol levels, high blood pressure, diabetes, a smoking habit, or a family history of heart disease.

If you're at risk for heart problems, your doctor probably will want to do an exercise tolerance test to check for cardiovascular disease, custom-design an exercise program to ease you into the swing of things, and monitor your progress.

Warm up. Experts recommend 10 to 15 minutes of warm-up activity, which can include stretches, light calisthenics, or slow walking.

As you get older, your body needs to ease into exercise more gradually, according to Richard Birrer, M.D., vice chairman of family medicine at the Catholic Medical Center in New York City. That's because by ages 65 to 70 most physiological systems are down by about a third and take longer to warm up and cool down, notes Dr. Birrer. For example, the pulse rate goes down, he adds.

Break it up . . . or don't. Exercising more than

30 minutes at a time helps you lose weight, if you exercise three to five times a week and follow an appropriate diet, experts say. If you don't need to lose weight, three 10-minute exercise sessions per day will be just as beneficial for disease protection, Dr. Stamford says.

Start slowly. Most people don't realize how out of shape they are. "It's not unusual for someone to get halfway around the block and feel winded," says Terri Merritt, a clinical exercise physiologist at the Preventive Medicine Research Institute in Sausalito, California, who works closely with Dean Ornish, M.D., president and director of the institute, whose regimen for reversing heart disease is known the world over. "You have to start exercising gradually."

Keep the faith. "If you haven't walked in 25,000 years, you're going to be winded after a block or two," says comedian Sid Caesar, who started exercising at age 57 to get his life moving toward good health. "But if you keep walking, in another week or two, you won't be."

Says fitness guru and author Jack LaLanne, "Any time you exercise, it's like putting money in the bank. If you can only start with a nickel, that's okay. Eventually, it'll add up. Any exercise is better than no exercise."

Keep setting goals. On your first walk or exercise session, you may decide to walk for 10 to 15 minutes and do three repetitions of each exercise. Even that may be hard at first, but when you can easily meet your goal, up your efforts. Lengthen your walks or vary the terrain to make the work harder. Increase the number of repetitions for each exercise or add weights to make the exercise more difficult. Don't get carried away, though. Even as you increase the workload, the effort should never be too taxing, says Merritt.

Time it right. Experts say that you'll be able to

Stay Clear of Cramps

You can avoid those painful cramps by stretching and strengthening your leg muscles with these three exercises recommended by Gary Gordon, D.P.M., director of the Running and Walking Clinic at the Joseph Torg Sports Medicine Center at Allegheny University of the Health Sciences in Philadelphia.

Leg lifts: Lie on the floor. Tighten one leg's thigh muscles and lift it 12 inches off the ground without bending your knee. Hold it there for 10 seconds. Then lower the leg and repeat with the opposite leg. Repeat the exercise, alternating legs. Work up to the point where you can do 30 lifts with each leg. When this becomes easy, strap on leg weights to add 1 to 2 pounds to your ankles and work your way up to 30 lifts again.

Calf stretches: Stand with heels apart and toes pointing in, your arms straight out in front of you, palms touching a wall. Keep your back straight and bend your arms, then move your chest toward the wall. You should feel a stretch through the backs of your calves. If you don't, move farther away from the wall and try again. If your calves hurt too much, move closer to the wall. Hold the stretch for 10 to 30 seconds. Repeat 5 to 10 times.

Knee and ankle bends: Stand with your feet about 6 inches apart. With your back straight and your feet on the ground, bend your ankles and knees, lowering your body as far as is comfortable. Keep your hands on your thighs for support. The movement should be coming from your knees, not your back, Dr. Gordon says. Hold for 10 to 30 seconds. Repeat 5 to 10 times.

stay with your program better if you exercise at the same time each day.

Wake up first. If you're a morning person, exercise after you have been up and about for at least 10 minutes. While you sleep, fluids sometimes pool throughout your body, even in such important places as the disks in the spinal column, in ligaments, and in muscles, Dr. Birrer says. If you get up suddenly and begin to exercise, the accumulated fluids can cause major injuries, such as a herniated disk.

Avoid internal conflicts. Exercising right after eating causes problems because both your intestinal tract and your muscles will need extra blood. The conflicting needs of each system may leave you with cramps or a feeling of nausea or faintness. Give your body 2 hours to complete its digestive chores.

Choose your shots. If you have diabetes, avoid injecting insulin into a muscle that will soon be used for exercise. Working muscles process insulin differently than do nonworking muscles.

Play it safe. Find a place where you can do the walking phase of your program safely. "Your neighborhood isn't safe if you don't feel safe," Dr. Douglas says. "If that's the case, look for other locations. Drive to another neighborhood or a public area where you feel comfortable."

Mall-walking programs, often operated by hospitals or health centers, provide a haven where you can walk regardless of the weather. Call local malls to find out about programs, suggests Dr. Douglas. She recalls a trip to the Midwest, where "they opened up the mall at 7:00 A.M. just for walkers, and the place was mobbed with people doing laps. There were so many people, they practically knocked me over."

(continued on page 322)

Give Your Cancer Defenses a Lift

Sure, Arnold Schwarzenegger's over 50 now too. But you don't have to work out like he does. Even a little weight lifting provides women and men a mighty defense against cancer.

You'll need some weights for the weight-lifting exercises that follow. You can either buy free weights—dumbbells or barbells—or use plastic bottles or milk jugs filled with water or sand. You'll probably want to buy inexpensive weights that you can attach to your ankles.

Finding the best weight for you takes trial and error, says William J. Evans, Ph.D., director of the Noll Physiological Research Center at Pennsylvania State University in University Park. The weights should be heavy enough that your muscles benefit, but not so heavy that your muscles can't handle the stress. Find the heaviest weight that you can lift five times and work with that weight. The goal is to do three sets of five repetitions of each exercise. Choose two or three for your upper body and two or three for your lower body, he recommends. Dr. Evans suggests the following exercises.

Military presses: Use a barbell or secure a weighted milk jug on each end of a broomstick. Hold the bar behind your head, arms bent. Slowly raise your arms until they are straight. Return to starting position.

Shoulder raises: Sit in a chair with your feet flat on the floor. Hold a weight in one hand, resting at your side, palm facing in. Keep your elbow straight but not locked as you slowly bring your arm forward and up, until it is fully extended above your head. Return to starting position. Repeat for one set, then switch to the opposite side.

Triceps extensions: Sit in a straight-back chair, feet flat on the floor, parallel but not touching. Hold a weight in each hand and raise both arms over your head. Bend your elbow and lower one hand behind your head, then raise it back overhead. Repeat with the opposite arm.

Biceps curls: Sit in a chair with your legs apart, feet flat on the floor, and one hand on your thigh. Holding a weight in your other hand, extend that arm straight down, while resting your elbow against your inner thigh. Flex your arm and slowly curl the weight to shoulder level. Return to original position. Repeat for one set, then switch arms.

Knee extensions: Sit on a chair, with a weight strapped to the ankle of one leg, foot on the floor. Slowly straighten the leg. (Don't point your toe— keep your foot at about a 90-degree angle to your leg.) Then lower the leg to the starting position. Repeat for one set, then switch sides.

Knee flexions: Strap a weight to the ankle of one leg. Stand and hold on to the back of a chair for support. Slowly lift your heel toward your buttock. Lower your leg to the starting position. Repeat for one set, then switch sides.

Dress for comfort. Your body has to get rid of the heat produced by exercise, so wear loose-fitting cotton or high-tech fabrics, such as Gore-Tex, that breathe. Use layers of clothing to stay warm and simultaneously dispel perspiration and heat. Use sweat suits only in cold weather when you need to stay warm. In hot weather and in direct sunlight, wear light-colored clothing and a cap to avoid sunburn or overheating, says Merritt.

Wear athletic socks designed to wick perspiration away from your body like acrylic or other breathable materials.

Check the water supply. It's easy to become dehydrated as you exercise. Drink water or juice beforehand to make sure that your system doesn't run dry, especially if the temperature is above 70°F. Bring liquids with you as well. Some experts advise that you take a drink of water every 20 minutes. Avoid excessive coffee, alcohol, and other diuretics that will contribute to dehydration, says Dr. Fletcher.

Cool down. End your session by walking very slowly for 5 minutes or by doing stretching exercises, advises Dr. Fletcher. Don't sit down immediately after exercise; slow movement will help your body cool properly. It will reduce the likelihood of muscle cramps and help the blood circulate. Massaging muscles after your cooldown will also help keep the blood moving, according to the American Medical Association.

In hot weather, wearing sweaty clothes after exercise will help your body cool. In cold weather, change wet clothes to help keep warm. Hot showers slow the cooling process, so wait about 45 minutes until your body temperature has returned to normal before you indulge.

Keep tabs on medication. Some medications,

even common over-the-counter medicines such as decongestants, raise your heart rate and blood pressure. Dr. Fletcher suggests that you decrease exercise if you're on medication.

One word of caution: We haven't suggested that you take your pulse because, if you're on medication, your readings may not accurately reflect the stress of exercise to your system. To keep from overdoing it, make a habit of methodically estimating your level of exertion. If you want to take your pulse anyway, don't take it by pressing on the artery in your neck. That can cause a stroke. You can safely take your pulse by pressing your wrist, says Dr. Fletcher.

Listen to Your Body

Most exercise-related injuries happen because people try to do more than their bodies can handle. If you're overloading your system, your body will let you know. Listen to it. After exercising, you should be:

Very energetic. Exercise should give you additional energy. "If you're exhausted when you finish exercising, you've overdone it," LaLanne says. "You should finish a session feeling exhilarated, yet relaxed. That way, you won't do too much and get hurt." If exercise leaves you languid, shorten your walk or lighten your strength-training weights.

If you still haven't recuperated a half-hour after stopping exercise, check with your doctor, Dr. Fletcher says.

Clearheaded. A feeling of nausea or faintness lets you know that your efforts are too intense for your body, although these symptoms can also mean that you're not spending enough time on your cooldown exercises. Review your routine. Add or lengthen the cooldown exercises. If that doesn't make a difference, shorten your walk and reduce your weights, says Dr. Fletcher.

Breathing easily. While your breathing rate will increase when you exercise, you should still be able to carry on a conversation. If you can't talk and walk or talk and lift at the same time, your work pace is too intense. Slow down and lighten your weight load, recommends Dr. Fletcher.

Pain-free. Exercise isn't supposed to hurt or leave you feeling stiff (although you may feel some soreness when you begin to exercise). Devote more time to warm-up and cooldown exercises, because they provide maximum protection against aches and pains, Merritt advises. If problems persist, see your doctor or a fitness expert to rule out underlying problems and to make sure that you are doing exercises correctly.

If you're overweight, your knees may not be strong enough to support you. If they hurt, shorten (or eliminate) your walks and concentrate on strength-training sessions to build up muscles and tendons to take some of the load off the joints, Dr. Evans recommends.

You may experience lower back pain when you start to exercise. That's because, if you have spent a lot of time sitting, your hamstring muscles have shortened. When you walk or exercise, these muscles pull on the buttock muscles which, in turn, yank on the lower back muscles. If your abdominal muscles aren't strong enough to help support the lower back, you'll feel it. Include abdominal-strengthening exercises with your warm-up and cooldown stretches says Merritt.

Remember that warm-up and cooldown exercises protect muscles and tendons as well as the cardiovas-

How I Did It: Life Begins at 78

Al Markstein started exercising at age 78, spurred on by his high school buddy and World War II Navy roommate Jack LaLanne, the fitness guru. (They also share the same birthday.)

"Jack kept telling me I had to exercise. I made excuses," says the Orinda, California, resident, now in his eighties. Then one day LaLanne simply signed up his friend for an exercise program at a nearby gym. LaLanne also checked up on Markstein every two weeks. "If he hadn't, I probably would have dropped out," Markstein recalls. "When I started, I could barely pick up a 5-pound barbell. Now I'm doing 27 pounds."

Going to a gym can seem intimidating to older men and women, but Markstein likes the mix of ages at his. "Some people are older than I am," he says. "You meet all kinds of people."

Of his pre-exercise life, he says, "When I owned my own company, I was always the first person there and the last to leave. But after I retired, I used to just sit down and be ready to fall asleep. People would ask me to play a game of golf or go to a ball game. I'd make arrangements, but when the day arrived, I'd find an excuse not to go."

But now, when asked about an average day, Markstein replies, "Today, I exercised for 2 hours. I'm about to participate in a charity golf tournament. I'll stay at the club for dinner and a raffle. You name it, I'm ready to do it."

cular system. Don't try to shorten your workout by omitting them.

Walk toward Longevity

Ideally, half of your exercise program should consist of aerobic exercise. And to many experts, walking is the aerobic exercise of choice, especially if you're 60 or over. That's because when you walk, the pressure on your joints never rises above 1.5 times your body weight. Jogging or dance or step aerobic exercise can put a lot more pressure—4 times your weight or more—on your bones.

Start slowly and gradually increase the length and difficulty of your walks, says Dr. Rippe. Here's how to strengthen your heart without overtaxing your system.

Try airport aerobics. To get the most benefit, walk briskly. Imagine that you're walking through the airport to catch a plane, suggests Dr. Stamford. But don't overdo it. Start your walking program with a goal of 10 to 15 minutes, advises Dr. Douglas.

If you're really out of shape and concerned that you may get too tired to make it back home, wear a watch. Check the time when you start to walk and keep walking around the block until you get a little tired. Glance at your watch to see how long you have walked. That's the length that your walks should be for the next week or two, Dr. Douglas says.

"If you get tired on the way home, stop, rest, then walk some more," advises Dr. Douglas. Some days you may tire more easily or the work may seem too much. Just shorten your session.

Once you're comfortable, you can gradually increase the length of your walks by about 10 percent every two weeks, according to Dr. Fletcher.

How I Did It: A Comeback from Heart Attack

In 1991 Alice Ann Hamilton began attending exercise classes at Emory University in Atlanta at age 60. "I started two months after my heart attack," she says. "I had never done any organized exercise."

Hamilton, a retired assistant superintendent for personnel in the DeKalb County, Georgia, school system, found it hard to accept that she really had suffered a heart attack. "You never believe that anything like a heart attack is going to happen to you," she says.

Now she reflects that there were warning signals: "Not long before my heart attack, I went on a trip to New York with some friends and was surprised at how tired I got after a day of walking around."

Once she made the commitment to a comeback, she worried about measuring up. The heart attack had left her energy level set on low. But she started out with stretching exercises. She then walked a quarter mile on the track and rode on the stationary bicycle for a few minutes.

The program gradually became more demanding. "I had to walk faster around the track and do more exercises," Hamilton says. Now, she has graduated to a high-powered step aerobics program.

Hamilton's effort has given her the energy to do volunteer work in her community. She even found an unexpected bonus in getting out to exercise: "I met people who live right around the corner, but I had never known them." Her evaluation of her new life? "I feel great," she says.

Keep it constant. Try to maintain the same level of exertion for your entire walk. That way, you'll ask your heart to work hard (but not too hard) for your entire session. Your heart gets the biggest benefit from a sustained workout.

You may want to use walking as part of your warm-up. If that's the case, make this phase of your routine slower and more relaxed, says Dr. Fletcher.

Slow for hills. If you come to a hill, forget the heroics. Slow your pace to maintain the same level of exertion that you had on level ground.

Track the temperature. Your work will seem harder if it's hot or humid. Adjust your speed and intensity so that you stay at the right exertion level. If the temperature soars—say, over 95°F with 80 percent humidity—don't exercise outside for more than 30 to 45 minutes, advises Dr. Fletcher. If you have heart problems, reduce your time in the heat by at least 25 percent.

Get More Health from Your Walks

Once you get into a regular walking program and can keep up a set pace, vary it. "If you do the same thing over and over, your muscles aren't challenged and they don't respond as well—and you can get bored," says LaLanne. "I change my program every three to four weeks."

Here are ways to keep a little pep in your step.

Step lively. Take a tip from racewalkers. They take short steps and get their speed by packing a lot of steps into each minute, says Dr. Stamford.

Weigh it down. Weighted belts are popular. If your condition permits it, the belt will add extra resistance, according to Dr. Evans. Or you can load a knap-sack with plastic jars full of water or sand, starting at 2 to 3 pounds and then gradually working up to heavier weights. (Weigh yourself on a bathroom scale—with and without the containers—so that you'll know how heavy your homemade weights are.) When you walk with weight on your back, you'll expend more effort, he adds.

Walk with a swing. The more you move around, the more intense your workout. Swing your arms vigorously. Raise them and punch at the sky, first with one arm and then with the other. "You can get a great cardiovascular workout in 12 to 17 minutes if your exercise is vigorous," says LaLanne.

Beef Up Your Muscles to Pummel Disease

Toning your muscles isn't just an exercise in vanity. When you build muscle, the ratio of body muscle to body fat tips a little more in your favor. This lowers your risk of cancer, heart disease, and stroke.

Calisthenics use your body's own weight to work your muscles. You'll need to work some muscle groups with light weight-lifting exercises using weights that you make or buy. As you get started in a calisthenics program, use these basic guidelines from Dr. Evans to get the most out of all your exercises.

Keep it slow. Perform all exercises slowly. Unless otherwise noted, spend 2 seconds in the lifting phase of the exercise and 4 to 6 seconds in the lowering part. If you move too quickly, you won't get the muscle-strengthening benefits and you could hurt yourself.

Everyday Exercise

A regular exercise program will benefit everyone. But Bryant Stamford, Ph.D., professor of exercise physiology and director of the Health Promotion Center at the University of Louisville, suggests that some people over 50 may be happier—and more willing to exercise—if they simply do more of the things they enjoy.

"If you like to garden, figure out a way to turn that into 30 minutes a day of vigorous activity," Dr. Stamford advises. "It'll help you ward off lethal diseases."

According to a report issued by The Centers for Disease Control and Prevention and the American College of Sports Medicine, your risk of coronary heart disease increases as your level of activity goes down. Those two groups suggest a number of everyday activities to get that activity level up, including:

- Taking the stairs (not the elevator)
- Walking instead of driving short distances
- Doing housework
- Raking leaves
- Dancing

Another suggestion from Dr. Stamford: "Make things more difficult, not easier. Usually, if you have trouble getting up the stairs, everyone suggests that you move into a one-story house. But in reality the stairs give you trouble because you have become weaker. If you stop doing stairs, soon you won't be able to get up them at all. Do more of what's difficult, not less."

Remember the ins and outs. Always inhale before you lift, exhale as you lift, and inhale as you lower the weight for maximum benefit.

Pick and choose. Pick several exercises for your upper body and several for your lower body from the resistance and weight-lifting categories. You can switch to different exercises anytime you feel like it.

Up the ante. Unless otherwise noted, work up to the point where you can do three sets of exercises. In each set do 5 to 15 repetitions of the exercise. (Don't rest within the sets. You can rest briefly between each set.) When the work becomes easy, add weights or increase the amount you do.

Get rhythm. If you have trouble establishing a rhythm to your exercise routine so that you perform each repetition within a set with the same gusto, Dr. Evans suggests that you listen to triumphal march music as you exercise.

Be Sweet to Your Feet

Exercise in shoes that are designed for the job—otherwise, you're issuing an open invitation to aches, pains, and even stress fractures in your feet and legs.

"A lot of people just put on any old shoe—and they get hurt," notes Gary Gordon, D.P.M., director of the Running and Walking Clinic at the Joseph Torg Sports Medicine Center at Allegheny University of the Health Sciences in Philadelphia. Walking or running shoes absorb the shock of your stride, thanks to a slightly elevated heel that also helps prevent injuries to the legs' muscles and tendons.

Other types of athletic shoes, such as tennis shoes, take the impact of sideways movement and quick turns. Women who normally wear high heels should avoid flat tennis-type shoes because the sudden shift in foot position may cause a strain, says Dr. Gordon.

While shoes may last for years, their shock absorption lasts for only a few months. If you walk fewer than 25 miles a week, Dr. Gordon suggests that you get a new pair every four to six months. If you walk more than 25 miles a week, replace shoes every two to three months. Use the castoffs for work around the house.

If you already have a pair of shoes made for walking or running, examine the tread. Get a new pair if the bottom tread has worn off, which means there has been enough wear to interfere with shock absorption.

If you need new shoes, follow this advice when shopping for a replacement pair.

Examine the patterns. Bring a well-worn pair of everyday shoes with you when you shop for walking shoes. Your wear patterns, particularly in the heels, may help the salesperson pick out the best pair for your feet, advises Merritt.

Help it fit. To get the best fit while fitting new athletic shoes, wear the same kind of socks that you'll exercise in. Shop in the afternoon in case your feet swell during the day. Plan to try on lots of shoes to identify the ones that are most comfortable.

Thumbnail the toe. There's enough toe room if, when you stand, you can fit your thumbnail (about a half-inch) in the space between the end of your big toe and the end of the shoe, says Dr. Gordon. If you have a long thumbnail, of course, stick to the half-inch rule, he advises.

Check the width. A shoe is too wide if the eyelets meet when you lace them up. Your foot will slip around inside the shoe, and you won't get enough support. You may end up with blisters, says Dr. Gordon. A too-narrow shoe will be hard to tie because the eyelets are too far apart.

Some people think they need a wide shoe because their little toe flares out. Ask for a normal-width, curve-lasted model that won't give your little toe a pinched-in feeling, advises Jim Stewart, a registered professional shoe fitter and owner of the Finish Line Running Store, a store specializing in athletic footwear in Allentown, Pennsylvania.

Keep an upright heel. Put the shoe on and have someone look at it from behind, says Stewart. The heel counter, the extra-firm section of the shoe that cradles your heel, should be perpendicular to the ground. If it isn't, you're not getting the heel support that you need from the shoe.

Get enough stiffness. In some shoe models, the shock-absorbing layer of sole is rigid; in others it is more pliable. If you weigh more than 190 pounds, you need the rigid model just to get enough shock absorption, says Dr. Gordon. If you weigh 100 pounds or less, the rigid construction may make your foot work too hard, straining the arch or calf muscles. If you are between 100 and 190 pounds, you may wear a shoe with either a rigid or pliable sole. Unfortunately, you can't easily tell the difference. Ask salespeople at quality athletic shoe stores for recommendations.

Add an insert. You can get additional shock absorption through over-the-counter shoe inserts such as Spenco (which also prevents friction and blisters). This won't help your shoes last longer but will increase your shock absorption protection, says Dr. Gordon.

Leave Inactivity Behind

The exercise clothes are ready to go. The new pair of shoes wait by the door. Weights, present and accounted for. But, if you're like most people, it is still hard to take that final step and, as they say in the ad, "just do it."

Odds are, this isn't the first time that you've tried to set up an exercise routine, and you know how important it is to silence that little voice from within that says, "I'll 'just do it'—tomorrow." Here's how to get on the fast track to disease prevention.

Share the load. "Get someone to go with you," advises Merritt. "You may not want to walk or do strength-training exercises because it's too cold or you just feel lazy. When you depend on someone and they depend on you, it makes it easier for both of you."

In fact, a study conducted by the University of Southern California showed that people who exercise with friends at a health club and socialize with them outside the club work out more frequently and enjoy it more.

Adds LaLanne, "When people work out together, they encourage each other and make sure that they are doing the exercises correctly. They also get competitive and, as a result, they both get a more intense workout than they'd get if they worked alone."

Plug in for pleasure. Some experts recommend using the beat of the music to energize your workouts. Try picking something with a faster tempo for your actual workout and then something slower for your warm-up and cooldown. Choose a rhythm that's comfortable for you, Merritt advises. Listen to your body, not the music, to lessen the chances of overexertion.

Keep a record. If you measure your progress,

Prescription for Prevention

A two-part exercise program protects women and men over 50 from cancer, heart disease, and stroke: Aerobic exercise (walking or bicycling, for example) conditions your heart and cardiovascular system; strength-training exercises (calisthenics and weight lifting) build muscle and cut fat to reduce your cancer risk.

Do:

■ Warm up with stretches, light calisthenics, or slow walking before you exercise.

■ Exercise for more than 30 minutes per session if you want to lose weight. Otherwise, three 10-minute sessions per day will protect against disease.

■ Wear loose-fitting clothing that breathes. Use layers of clothing to stay warm and, simultaneously, dispel perspiration and heat. Wear athletic socks designed to wick perspiration away from your feet. Make sure your shoes fit and support your feet.

■ Cool down by slow walking or stretches.

Don't:

■ Become dehydrated.

■ Drink coffee, alcohol, or other diuretics before or while you exercise.

■ Exercise so vigorously that you can't talk and exercise at the same time.

you'll find it easier to stay motivated. Write down in a calendar or a notebook the number of minutes you walk and the number of exercises you do. You'll be surprised at how quickly you're able to do more.

Smoking

It's Never Too Late to Snuff Out This Major Risk

L ong before all of the illusions about tobacco evaporated like a stale smoke ring, lighting up was the thing to do. Betty Grable, who would eventually die of lung cancer, was a wildly popular World War II pinup girl and cigarette smoker. In the 1950s a cigarette dangling from James Dean's lips defined coolness for an entire generation.

Not only was smoking considered hip, manufacturers even claimed it was healthy. It steadied nerves, increased energy, and suppressed appetite, they said.

In fact, for several years one tobacco company proclaimed that more doctors smoked its brand than any other. Attractive young women from tobacco firms regularly visited doctors' offices to replenish the supply of free cigarettes available in waiting rooms for patients.

So when you were enticed to begin puffing—along

with a lot of other unsuspecting men and women—the powerfully addictive nature of smoking and its devastating effects on the body were virtually unknown.

But now that you know better, can quitting after even decades of smoking really make a difference? You bet. The evidence is unimpeachable: Stamping out your last cigarette at 50 or even 80 can halt many of the worst effects of smoking.

"Quitting will significantly reduce your risk of stroke, heart disease, and cancer regardless of your age and improve your quality of life," says Thomas Brandon, Ph.D., associate professor of psychology at the State University of New York at Binghamton and a smoking-cessation expert.

Who Is the Older Smoker?

A typical male smoker in his sixties or seventies began at age 17 and has smoked about 27 cigarettes a day for 51 years. If you are a woman in the same age range, you probably first lit up at about age 24 and have been smoking 20 cigarettes a day for 45 years.

And like about 80 percent of the people who smoke, you have probably tried to quit at least once. But 46 percent of older smokers doubt that smoking is very harmful or that the benefits of quitting are really worthwhile.

If you're one of those doubters, ponder these facts: Within 8 hours of quitting, your pulse rate and blood pressure drop, and oxygen levels in your body rise. Within 24 hours your risk of a heart attack dips. At around a month your circulation improves, your energy levels surge, and your lung function expands by up to 30 percent. By 1 year, your risk of heart disease is half that of someone who

What Are You Really Smoking?

When tobacco giant Philip Morris announced an unprecedented recall of 8 billion defective cigarettes several years ago, a young woman smoking in New York told a newspaper reporter, "At least it's not cyanide."

Wrong.

Not only does tobacco smoke contain hydrogen cyanide—a deadly poison used in prison gas chambers—it also harbors 4,700 other chemicals and toxins, including at least 43 cancer-causing substances. Here's just a sampling of what a typical smoker inhales with each puff, with a description of the chemical or its uses in parentheses.

Acetone (paint stripper)
Ammonia (floor cleaner)
Arsenic (ant poison)
Butane (lighter fluid)
Cadmium (car battery component)
Carbon monoxide (car exhaust)
Formaldehyde (morgue preservative)
Methanol (antifreeze)
Naphthalene (mothballs)
Nicotine (insecticide)
Polonium 210 (radioactive substance)
Toluene (industrial solvent)

continues to smoke. In 5 years, your stroke risk begins to slide; and in 10 years, your chances of getting lung cancer are the same as that of someone who has never smoked.

"I've had 75-year-old patients tell me that the day they quit smoking, in their thirties and forties, was the greatest day of their lives." says Alan Blum, M.D., assistant professor of family medicine at Baylor College of Medicine in Houston. "The feeling of finding something that you had thought you had lost—your health—is better than if you had never lost it at all. And to know that your risk of sudden death from smoking-related heart disease has dramatically decreased is tremendous."

Each Puff Is Harmful

With each puff a smoker inhales more than 4,700 chemicals that have a wide-reaching effect throughout the body.

Some of the milder effects include accelerated wrinkling of the skin, yellowing of the teeth and fingers, and slow wound-healing. Smoking also increases the risk of osteoporosis, hip fractures, cataracts, diabetes, tooth loss, and emphysema.

Then there is smoking's real downside. Every day, 1,147 Americans die of smoking-related causes. That adds up to more than 418,000 lives annually, making smoking the most preventable cause of death in the United States. Nearly 80 percent of those deaths are caused by cardiovascular disease and cancer. Specifically, 29 percent of all smoking-related deaths are attributed to lung cancer.

Switching to low-tar, low-nicotine cigarettes won't reduce the peril much. "Light" and "ultra-light" cigarettes still contain dangerous amounts of nicotine, carbon monoxide, and tar—the gaseous residues of those 4,700 chemicals.

"Smoking a low-tar cigarette is like jumping off a 20-story building instead of a 30-story one," Dr. Blum says. "There simply is no such thing as a safe, safer, or safest cigarette."

Here's a quick look at how smoking magnifies the impact of certain diseases and how quitting can slash your risk of developing them.

Smoking Breaks Your Heart

The chemicals in tobacco smoke, including nicotine and carbon monoxide (the same gas found in automobile exhaust) raise blood pressure, constrict blood vessels, and starve the heart of oxygen, forcing it to work harder. At the same time, smoking increases the stickiness of blood platelets so that they are more likely to form dangerous blood clots. It also raises total and low-density lipoprotein (the so-called bad cholesterol), lowers levels of high-density lipoprotein (the good cholesterol), and accelerates the accumulation of plaque in arteries causing atherosclerosis, also known as hardening of the arteries.

People age 64 and over who smoke have arteries clogged with about the same levels of plaque as people a decade older who have never smoked, according to researchers at Bowman Gray School of Medicine of Wake Forest University in Winston-Salem, North Carolina.

The bottom line is that a person who smokes is three times more likely to develop heart disease and has four times the risk of having a stroke as a nonsmoker. In addition, one in every four deaths is linked to smoking.

If you quit, your risk of a heart attack is sliced by 50 percent in one year, and after about five years your chances of having a stroke can be slashed to virtually the same risk as someone who never smoked.

Cancer: Smoking Tops the List

Smoking is linked to one in three cancer deaths and nearly 90 percent of all lung cancers. Smoking is associated with

How We Did It: A Couple Douses Their Deadly Habit

Tracy Gibson, a two-pack-a-day smoker since his teens, had just lit a cigarette after a July 21, 1993, swim at Rehoboth Beach, Delaware. Seconds later, his heart stopped. Paramedics and, later, emergency room staff administered repeated electroshocks to his heart to keep it beating. Tracy doesn't recall much of those events, but he knows why they happened.

"My heart failure was caused by hardening of the arteries due to smoking and a fast-food diet," says the former gas station owner, who is now in his sixties. "Having something like that happen was like going through a very advanced stop-smoking clinic. I've never really had a desire for a cigarette again."

But quitting was harder for his wife Bernice, who ditched her own two-pack-a-day habit after watching her husband's near-death experience. "My toughest times were after dinner or after I ate because I was used to having a cigarette then," says Bernice, also in her sixties. Her solution? She changed her routine.

"I sat in a different spot at the table than I normally would," she says. "After I was finished eating, I would get right up and start doing the dishes."

Three years later, the couple was walking three miles a day, eating a low-fat, high-fiber diet, and never lighting up.

cancer of the mouth, throat, esophagus, bladder, pancreas, kidneys, and 30 percent of cervical cancer.

"If it weren't for smoking, these cancers would barely exist," says Andrea LaCroix, Ph.D., associate professor of epidemiology at the University of Washington School of Public Health and Community Medicine in Seattle.

Tobacco smoke contains at least 43 cancer-causing substances that can scramble a cell's genetic code, causing it to reproduce abnormally. Constant exposure to the toxic compounds in smoke can cause these abnormal cells to gradually transform into cancer.

But if you quit—even at age 65—your risk of developing lung cancer by age 75 is less than half that of someone who continues to smoke, according to researchers at the University of Michigan. The risk of developing many other cancers—including those affecting the mouth, kidney, and pancreas—begins to diminish within 10 years of quitting.

"The time to quit smoking is when you still feel fine, because by the time you develop cancer and it is detected, it may be too late to cure it," says Teresa Hayes, M.D., an oncologist at Baylor College of Medicine in Houston. "If you quit smoking, not only will you stop adding to your risk, but if you do develop cancer, your chances of survival will be better because your body will be in better shape and you'll be able to tolerate whatever therapy is needed better than someone who continues to smoke."

Quitting Is Easier Than You Think

Like four of every five smokers, you may have tried to quit several times only to be lured back to tobacco. But don't blame yourself. It's not a sign of weakness, smoking-cessation experts say. Nicotine, the prime ingredient in tobacco, is one of the most addictive drugs known. Once you're in its grasp, it takes a determined effort to break free, particularly

Outsmarting Your Favorite Smoke of the Day

If you smoke, there are probably special moments when lighting up gives you the greatest pleasure. "For most smokers, the after-dinner cigarette seems to be almost irresistible," says Murray Jarvik, M.D., professor of psychiatry at the University of California, Los Angeles, School of Medicine.

Why? Eating a big meal like dinner slightly reduces the amount of nicotine in the blood, and that may trigger physical cravings. You also can develop a strong psychological urge to smoke if you associate finishing a meal with lighting up an after-dinner cigarette.

Other typical "special smokes," according to researchers at Stanford University and the West Los Angeles Veterans Affairs Hospital, are the first in the morning, the last of the day, and any with an alcoholic beverage.

A key part of quitting smoking is getting past those moments. How? Change your routine, says Michael Cummings, Ph.D., director of the smoking cessation clinic at Roswell Park Cancer Institute in Buffalo, New York. After a meal, go for a walk or do the dishes. Have a low-fat dessert in a room where you normally don't eat. Avoid food or drinks that make you crave tobacco.

If you enjoy a smoke first thing in the morning, get up and go straight to the shower, dress, eat breakfast, and then plunge right into your daily activities. Dr. Cummings even suggests that you make early appointments and let yourself sleep late so you'll have to rush and won't have time to smoke.

if you have been smoking for many years. But you can do it.

"Many older people have smoked for so long that they don't think they can overcome it," says Gary DeNelsky, Ph.D., director of the smoking-cessation program at the Cleveland Clinic. "But I've helped people who have smoked for 50 years quit successfully. Quitting isn't easy, but it isn't like climbing Mount Everest either."

In fact, of the people over age 65 who have ever smoked, 77 percent have stopped, according to the Office of Smoking and Health at the Centers for Disease Control and Prevention in Atlanta. That still adds up to nearly 16 million people who continue to smoke after age 65, let alone age 50.

How to Become Smoke-Free

About 1.3 million Americans break free of tobacco's hold each year and become nonsmokers. Most quit on their own using a variety of techniques ranging from Nicotine Anonymous to nutrition.

Remember that the first 7 to 10 days of any effort to quit smoking are the toughest because you'll go through withdrawal symptoms—such as upset stomach, difficulty concentrating, drowsiness, insomnia, and irritability—as your body adjusts to the lack of nicotine, Dr. Brandon says.

Once nicotine is flushed out of your body, your cravings should gradually subside. But you still may be tempted to smoke for months or even years afterward. (Eleven years after he quit, President Dwight Eisenhower scribbled, "God, I wish I had a cigarette," on a memo pad during a tense meeting with Soviet Premier Nikita Khrushchev.) But the longer you go without smoking, the more likely you will be able to resist the urge.

"Everybody needs to find his own way to quit. That's the key. You have to be motivated to quit and be creative in finding ways not to smoke," says Mitchell Nides, Ph.D., a psychologist at the University of California, Los Angeles.

But no matter how you choose to quit, smoking-cessation experts say there are a few fundamentals to keep in mind.

Set a quit date. People who designate a definite day to quit and stick to it are more likely to stop smoking than those who don't, Dr. Brandon says. Avoid picking stressful holidays like Thanksgiving, and don't select a date that's weeks or months away. Chances are that your resolve to quit will melt away by then. Instead, once you decide to stop, choose a day that falls within the next two weeks.

Go cold turkey. President Eisenhower began smoking when he was a cadet at West Point. By World War II Ike was up to four packs a day. In 1949 doctors advised him to cut back on his smoking. He tried it for a few days then decided that rationing his cigarettes was worse than not smoking at all. So he quit cold turkey and never had another cigarette in his life, says Stephen Ambrose, Ph.D., author of *Eisenhower: Soldier and President*.

All he did was put smoking out of his mind and developed "a scornful attitude toward those weaklings who did not have the willpower to break their enslavement to nicotine," Dr. Ambrose says.

It worked for Ike, and it can work for you. "If you quit cold turkey, you'll probably have a week to 10 days of withdrawal, but then you'll be almost over it," Dr. Brandon says. "Most people find it a lot easier to quit cold turkey than to gradually reduce their smoking."

Toss 'em overboard. On your quit date, throw out all of your tobacco products. That includes lighters, matches, and ashtrays. Don't hold back. If

345

you have any cigarettes hidden in places like sweaters, pockets, and glove compartments, toss those as well, says C. Tracy Orleans, Ph.D., director of Tobacco Control Research at Fox Chase Cancer Center in Philadelphia.

Banish the booze. Alcohol dissolves your resolve and makes it easier for you to light up again, says Thomas Cooper, D.D.S., a nicotine dependency researcher and professor of oral health sciences at the University of Kentucky College of Dentistry in Lexington. Avoid drinking for at least a month after you quit.

Yield not to temptation. Nicotine is a lifelong addiction, so smoking just one cigarette—even after years of abstinence—can lead to another and another. "Smoking one won't hurt me," has probably been the downfall of more smokers who are trying to quit than any other single thing, says Dr. Cooper, who smoked for 36 years before quitting in 1984.

Psychologically, smoking just one often makes people who have quit feel bad about themselves. And to cope with those bad feelings, they will smoke more cigarettes and quickly tumble back into the habit, Dr. Nides says. So if you're severely tempted, get away from the situation that's tempting you, or call a supportive friend who can help talk you out of it, Dr. Nides suggests.

Behavior Modification: Change Is Good

When you wake up, you smoke. Take out the garbage, you smoke. Go bowling, you smoke.

The urge to have a cigarette is often triggered by

everyday tasks and routines. But if you change your behavior, you can become a nonsmoker, doctors say. These self-help techniques, used alone or in combination, will help.

Write an instruction book. Every time you smoke, jot down the time of day and what you were doing. Then describe the step-by-step process of lighting up. A description of an after-dinner cigarette, for example, might read: "I push my chair back from the table. I take a deep breath. I reach into my pocket and grab the package. I tap the package on the table. I slip out a cigarette and twiddle it in my right hand. I put the cigarette in my mouth and reach for my lighter. I light the cigarette and take my first puff."

This record keeping is an important starting point for later changes, because it helps you become aware of your smoking patterns and the complex rituals that you have created for lighting up, says Dennis Gersten, M.D., a San Diego psychiatrist in private practice and publisher of *Atlantis: The Imagery Newsletter*.

Switch hands. Once you are aware of your smoking rituals, try to break up that routine somehow. "You can try to break the pattern any way you want, but I find that switching hands makes people very uncomfortable, which turns out to be a good thing," Dr. Gersten says. "I had a patient who had been smoking for 40 years. He simply switched from smoking with his right hand to his left, and that was the end of his smoking. It broke the pattern right on the spot."

Short-circuit stress. A lot of people smoke to cope with stress. "So when you quit, you have to come up with some new coping devices," says Michael Cummings, Ph.D., senior research scientist and director of the smoking-cessation clinic at Roswell Park Cancer Institute in Buffalo, New York. For starters, try deep breathing, meditation, squeezing a rubber ball, or pushing your tongue into the roof of your mouth for 10 to 15 seconds.

Quit early in the week. "We suggest that our patients try to quit on a Monday or a Tuesday of a busy week," Dr. Cooper says. "You don't want to quit smoking when you have a lot of time on your hands to think about it."

Dive into the smoke-free world. Plan out your day so that you'll be less tempted to smoke. Browse in a smoke-free shopping mall, eat in a smoke-free restaurant, or go to a movie or museum where smoking is prohibited, suggests Dr. Nides.

Give yourself daily pep talks. Every morning and at bedtime, write down all the reasons why you want to quit. It will reinforce your resolve to stop smoking. "It's easy to forget why you're trying to quit when you're going through nicotine withdrawal," Dr. Brandon says. "So reminders are an important way to keep yourself on track."

You also might try jotting down something you did that day—like walking a mile—that you weren't able to do when you smoked, Dr. Nides says.

Reward and punish. Sign a contract with yourself, Dr. Brandon suggests. Every day that you go without a cigarette, reward yourself—buy a magazine, sleep in for an extra 30 minutes, or take a long stroll.

If you smoke, punish yourself with an activity you detest, like cleaning out the refrigerator or washing out the gutters, Dr. Brandon says.

Give to the bad guys. In the first two weeks after you quit, every time you give in to the urge to smoke, pledge a dollar to an organization that you absolutely despise, Dr. Brandon says. It should be such a detestable group that it will make you think twice before lighting up. At the end of each day, give the money to a friend or spouse and insist that they send it off.

"Some people have told me that this particular technique helped stop them from smoking for those critical first few days," Dr. Brandon says.

Save those dollars. Put the money that you would normally spend on cigarettes into a clear container so that you can see it add up. After six months, use that money for a big reward, like a dream vacation, Dr. Brandon suggests.

Stall for time. When an urge hits, if you can delay lighting up for just a minute or two it may pass, Dr. Cummings says. Carry a picture of your grandchildren or other loved ones and pull it out every time an urge strikes. Write down the reasons why you want to quit and keep the list handy for these moments, too.

Nutrition: Eat Well, Stay Smoke-Free

If you start eating like a nonsmoker eats, you may even become one, says William McCarthy, Ph.D., director of science at the Pritikin Longevity Center in Santa Monica, California.

In fact, dietary changes when used in conjunction with other smoking-cessation methods can be a potent ally in your effort to quit, Dr. McCarthy says.

"Dietary changes are a way of moving away from the smoker lifestyle," Dr. McCarthy says. "If you simply extinguish the cigarette and do nothing else about your lifestyle habits, you will still be acting and living like a typical smoker."

How do typical smokers act and live? In terms

of diet, they tend to eat more meat, drink more coffee and alcohol, eat fewer fruits and vegetables, and consume fewer cereals and grains. They're more likely than nonsmokers to be deficient in vitamins A, C, E, and minerals like calcium, selenium, and zinc.

Smokers who begin eating a typical nonsmoker's diet are more likely to be smoke-free a year later than those who attempt to quit without dietary changes, Dr. McCarthy says.

What's more, dietary changes—particularly cutting fats and adding fruits and vegetables like oranges, apricots, carrots, and sweet potatoes, which are loaded with antioxidants—can help offset some of the ill effects of smoking and reduce your risk of stroke, heart disease, and cancer, says James Scala, Ph.D., a nutritional biochemist and author of *If You Can't/Won't Stop Smoking*. Antioxidants like vitamin C help block or reverse some of the harm done by free radicals, which are unstable molecules that damage cells and tissues.

"Research indicates that it is sensible to take up to 1,000 milligrams of vitamin C daily and about 400 international units of vitamin E to reverse some of the bad influences of smoking," says Dr. Scala.

A good diet also will help you cope with some of the challenges of quitting, such as weight gain, Dr. Scala says. That's an important benefit, because fear of gaining weight is an imposing barrier for many smokers who are trying to quit.

In a survey of 1,234 people who smoked, ages 50 to 74, nearly half believed that gaining 20 pounds is more harmful than smoking. "Actually, you would probably have to gain at least 100 pounds to equal the health risks of continued smoking," says Robert C.

Klesges, Ph.D., professor of psychology and preventive medicine at the University of Memphis in Tennessee.

In reality, about half of all people who quit smoking don't gain weight, and those who do put on about 10 pounds. The weight gain only occurs shortly after you quit smoking, and you do not continue to gain weight any faster than someone who had never smoked.

The following dietary changes may help prevent excessive weight gain after you quit. But Dr. McCarthy suggests that you alter your diet long before you stop smoking, because waiting until the day you quit may make it too difficult to make major changes in your diet at the same time that you have to cope with nicotine withdrawal. So adjust your diet first. Then, when you feel comfortable with your new eating habits, quit smoking.

Balance the pyramid. If you follow the basic U.S. Department of Agriculture food pyramid guidelines, you'll be eating more like a nonsmoker and may be less tempted to light up again, Dr. McCarthy says. That means 2 to 4 servings of fruits and 3 to 5 servings of vegetables a day; 2 to 3 servings of dairy products like milk and cheese; 6 to 11 servings of breads, rice, and cereals; and no more than one 3-ounce serving of meat, poultry, or fish or 2 to 3 servings of beans, egg whites, and nuts.

Sip on OJ. Tobacco smoke destroys vitamin C. Replenish your supply by drinking two 8-ounce glasses of orange juice daily, particularly in the first few days after you quit, Dr. Scala says.

Orange juice will also help flush nicotine out of your body and help you become nicotine-free faster, Dr. Cooper says. Avoid orange juice, however, if you're using the nicotine patch or gum, because you want that nicotine to stay in your body to help avoid withdrawal symptoms.

Cap the caffeine. Laying off tobacco increases the stimulating effects of caffeine. So if you drink coffee, you may feel more jittery and might start craving a smoke, Dr. Brandon says. Switch to decaffeinated coffee and drink no more than two 8-ounce cups a day, he suggests.

Stay fluid. Carry a squeeze bottle of water around with you. Whenever you feel the urge for a smoke, take a swig of water instead, Dr. Cummings says. Water helps flush nicotine and other tobacco toxins out of the body and speeds withdrawal. In addition to the normal amount that you drink, he recommends having another six to eight glasses daily when you're trying to quit.

Eat breakfast. People who smoke often use a cigarette to elevate blood sugars and suppress appetite, Dr. Cooper says. It's important to replace your early-morning smoke with an energizing low-fat breakfast like a low-fat bran muffin and a glass of apple juice.

Be Johnny Appleseed. Snacking on an apple twice daily for the first 90 days after you quit will help get you past the midmorning and midafternoon slumps without reaching for a cigarette, Dr. Cooper says.

Try new foods. Avoid eating or drinking any foods that you link with smoking, Dr. Brandon says. So if you have always had a cup of coffee and a muffin for breakfast followed by a cigarette, try a glass of milk and a piece of raisin toast instead. The change can dampen your urge to smoke.

Make food work for you. In the first few days after quitting, keep low-fat foods like breadsticks, crackers, carrots, celery, and popcorn handy to toss into your mouth whenever you feel the urge to smoke. If you need something to do with your hands, try eating foods that require peeling, such as oranges, sunflower seeds, tangerines, nuts in the shell, or arti-

A Medical Advance to Ease Quitting

It's only a few inches around and doesn't look like much, but the transdermal nicotine patch is a formidable weapon in the struggle to quit smoking. And it's rapidly gaining in popularity.

When worn on the skin, the patch releases tiny amounts of nicotine into the bloodstream for up to 24 hours. That eases withdrawal symptoms and makes it easier to quit. Over several weeks, the dosage of the patch is gradually reduced to wean you off the drug.

In a survery of 1,070 male and female patch users ages 65 to 74, nearly 30 percent were still smoke-free six months later, says C. Tracy Orleans, Ph.D., director of Tobacco Control Research at Fox Chase Cancer Center in Philadelphia. Most of those who had tried to quit before said that the patch made quitting easier.

"The patch is the state of the art," Dr. Orleans says. "It increases quit rates two to three times. We're recommending it for anyone who has had trouble dealing with withdrawal symptoms in the past."

Nicotine gum, another form of nicotine replacement, also has helped many people quit. Both the patch and gum are readily available over the counter, but be sure to check with your doctor to see if either is appropriate for you.

chokes, suggests C. Barr Taylor, M.D., professor of psychiatry at Stanford University School of Medicine and author of *The Facts about Smoking*.

Indulge your sweet tooth. If eating a sweet will prevent you from smoking, do it, Dr. Taylor says. If possible, avoid high-fat sweets like cake, ice cream, and chocolate. Instead, pick alternatives that are lower in fat like jelly beans, sherbets, hard candies, or fruits like grapes, bananas, or dates.

Meditation:
A Single Thought Can Banish Urges

The average person has about 15,000 thoughts a day. If you're trying to quit, it can seem like every one of those thoughts is the same: Smoke!

But meditation can help you dampen that mental noise and help you become a nonsmoker, says Dr. Gersten.

Meditation is a form of concentration that allows you to focus your mind internally and step back from your thoughts and feelings, Dr. Gersten says. In its simpler forms, meditation uses pictures, words (mantras), objects (such as a candle flame), or sensations (such as breathing) to focus the mind. If your mind begins to drift, you refocus your attention on your chosen image or word.

Studies have shown that meditation can help reduce the severity of many medical conditions, including anxiety, asthma, migraines, high blood pressure, and chronic pain. And it can help you quit smoking, Dr. Gersten says. Every time you feel an urge to smoke, try this meditation. Each time you inhale, say the word "peace," and as you exhale, say "love." If your mind begins to wander, refocus it on the words. Do that for five minutes,

Nicotine Anonymous: No Names, Lots of Support

Here's another possible aid in your quest to quit smoking: Nicotine Anonymous is a 12-step program similar to Alcoholics Anonymous that offers support to those who want to become and remain nicotine-free.

The organization, founded in 1982, has about 500 chapters worldwide. Members acknowledge that nicotine is an addictive drug and that they can't control their use of it. The only requirement for membership is the desire to abstain from nicotine.

No formal studies of its effectiveness have been conducted, but those who attend Nicotine Anonymous meetings often credit the mutual support they find there for helping them stay smoke-free.

"I heard things in meetings from others who had quit before me, and I thought, 'Oh my God, I'm going through that, too,'" says Lynn H., a Chicago woman who smoked for 34 years before quitting in her sixties. "I just realized that what I was experiencing was normal. There is a lot of caring, friendship, and support. I still go to remind myself what it was like because it's so easy to forget. And I know that if I forget and decide I can smoke socially, I'll end up right back where I started."

For more information, write to: Nicotine Anonymous World Service Office, Department R, P. O. Box 591777, San Francisco, CA 94159-1777. Be sure to enclose a stamped, self-addressed envelope.

and by then the urge to smoke may have passed or sub-sided to the point that you can resist it, Dr. Gersten says.

"This meditation will help you deal with the craving," Dr. Gersten says. "You're not saying that the urge to smoke isn't there. You're acknowledging that the urge exists, but you don't have to do anything about it. You just turn your mind back to your mantra."

Nicotine Fading: Letting Go Slowly

Although going cold turkey is your best bet, there is a gradual alternative that works for some people, says Dr. Orleans.

The process is known as nicotine fading, and Dr. Orleans calls it a form of "cool turkey" because it pre-pares you both physically and psychologically for the day when you finally quit altogether.

"Quitting abruptly on a target date is the best way to go," Dr. Orleans says. "But nothing says that you shouldn't prepare yourself for your quit date. Nicotine fading is one of the ways you can do that."

By making small weekly drops in nicotine, you avoid strong withdrawal symptoms when you quit, par-ticularly if you smoke a high- or medium-nicotine brand.

High-nicotine brands include unfiltered cigarettes and any filtered brand that isn't labeled with the words "mild," "light," or "ultra-light." Medium-nicotine brands are labeled "mild" or "light." Low-nicotine cigarettes bear words like "extra mild," "ultra," and "ultra-light."

The program allows two weeks to complete the nicotine fading process if you smoke a high-nicotine brand, and one week for medium- or low-nicotine brands.

Let it fade. Fading is fairly simple, Dr. Orleans says. If you smoke a high-nicotine brand, switch to a medium for one week and then to a low brand for another week before you quit. That way you will cut your dose of nicotine by one-third each week. If you smoke mediums, switch to lows for a week, and if you smoke lows, try an ultra-low brand for a week.

Don't jump off too fast. Avoid going directly from a high-nicotine brand to a low one, Dr. Orleans says. If the nicotine in your body drops too rapidly, it can cause cravings and withdrawal symptoms, which will defeat the purpose of fading.

Be cautious. The way you smoke affects how much nicotine you take in, so keep your cigarette use on an even keel. Dr. Orleans warns that if you switch to lower-nicotine cigarettes but smoke more of them, you risk getting the same dose of nicotine that you were getting before. Also, avoid inhaling more often or deeply than you have in the past and try not to cover the tiny airholes near the bottom of the filter with your fingers or lips.

PART 4

Defeating Disease

Anemia

Ironclad Solutions

Karen was a dynamo, juggling family outings, work assignments, and out-of-town trips with seemingly boundless energy. But then she started noticing that her get-up-and-go had gotten up and gone. She even slipped away from work sometimes to grab a quick nap at home. "I was afraid of getting caught, but I couldn't help it," she says.

Finally, fearing the worst, Karen dragged herself to the doctor, who took a blood sample and gave her some good news. "You have a touch of iron-deficiency anemia," the doctor said, "and a little boost of iron should do the trick."

Low Oxygen, Low Energy

People with anemia have a shortage of red blood cells and hemoglobin, the protein that carries oxygen to cells throughout the body, says Allan Jacob Erslev, M.D., professor of medicine at Thomas Jefferson University Hospital in Philadelphia. In other words, the body doesn't have enough oxygen to work at peak efficiency. The result can be fatigue, mood changes, headaches, and heart palpitations.

Lots of disorders can cause anemia, but too little iron in the blood is the most common. This kind of anemia often comes on so slowly that people get used to it and don't even know something's wrong. "But when I give them iron, they suddenly discover they feel so much better," Dr. Erslev says. "The difference can be quite striking."

Are you at risk for iron-poor blood? Well, most women over 50 (and all men) will escape the most common causes—overmenstruation and pregnancy. "In women, iron-deficiency anemia almost always is due to excessive menstrual flow," Dr. Erslev says. Menstruating women typically lose twice as much iron as either men or nonmenstruating women do. And during the nine months of pregnancy, when a baby is growing and sharing the mother's nutrients, they can lose even more.

There are, however, other routes to iron-deficiency anemia. Gastrointestinal bleeding caused by ulcers, parasites, or cancer, for example, can very quickly deplete iron stores. In such cases, doctors naturally tend to be more concerned about those underlying causes than about the anemia itself.

It's also possible to become anemic by not eating enough iron-rich foods. Rapidly growing children, particularly fussy eaters, may have difficulty meeting their body's needs. And since the type of iron found in fruit and vegetables is not as readily absorbed as the iron in meat, strict vegetarians who don't take supplements may be slightly more prone to iron deficiency anemia than meat-eaters.

In rare cases, iron-deficiency anemia may lead to bizarre food cravings. How bizarre? Well, people with this condition, called pica, can crave such unsavory (and not at all iron-rich) substances as laundry starch, clay, cigarette ashes, or dirt. Pica isn't always caused by iron deficiency, Dr. Erslev says, but when it is, it's easily treated. Once people with pica are given supplemental iron, the cravings will usually disappear, often within 24 hours.

Iron isn't the only key to avoiding anemia. To have healthy blood cells, you also need vitamin B_{12}, a nutrient found in meats, eggs, and dairy products. It doesn't take much: Most people need only 2 micrograms (a microgram is one-millionth of a gram) a day. But those who abstain from eggs and dairy products may be deficient in this essential nutrient and are susceptible to a condition called pernicious anemia, which doctors estimate affects approximately 1 percent of people over 65.

Pernicious anemia isn't as pernicious as it used to be. "It's one of the most treatable things we have," says Michael L. Freedman, M.D., professor of internal medicine and director of geriatrics at New York University Medical School. There is a protein in your stomach called intrinsic factor (IF) that transports vitamin B_{12} from your stomach to the lining of the small intestine, where the vitamin gets absorbed into your bloodstream. As people age, they begin producing less IF. For people who don't produce IF, supplemental doses of B_{12}, usually given by injection, will "cure" the disease. Vegetarians can protect themselves merely by taking B_{12} supplements.

Animal and Vegetable Know-How

Iron deficiency is the most common cause of anemia, but not all iron is created equal. Meats contain a type of iron called heme (pronounced heem) that's easily absorbed by the body. For that reason, doctors used to recommend liver—a veritable iron mine—as a quick-acting answer to low iron stores. But liver is also loaded with cholesterol, an unwelcome addition at today's heart-conscious tables.

Fortunately, there are healthier sources for heme iron than liver and hamburgers, says Elaine McDonnell, staff nutritionist at Pennsylvania State University's Nutrition Center. Lean meats such as chicken, turkey, and top round steak (trimmed of fat) all can help you boost your iron stores without contributing unhealthy amounts of fat and cholesterol to your diet.

The second type of iron is nonheme iron, found primarily in plant foods. It isn't as easily absorbed as heme iron. Generally you can expect to absorb 23 percent of heme iron but only 2 to 10 percent of nonheme iron.

However, there's a trick to boosting your absorption of nonheme iron, McDonnell says. "When you eat foods that have only nonheme iron, try to eat another food at the same meal that's high in vitamin C," she suggests. Vitamin C has been shown to help enhance absorption of nonheme iron. In fact, meat also improves the absorption of nonheme iron, so combining meat and vegetables at mealtimes is an excellent way to put extra iron in the bank.

As you might expect, there are also foods that can block iron absorption. The best examples are tea and coffee. Does this mean you have to give up your favorite brew if you have iron-deficiency anemia? Not necessarily, McDonnell says. Just avoid them within 1 hour after a meal.

Iron Out Anemia

Anybody over 50 who's worried about anemia should keep one thing above all in mind: Too much iron can cause as many problems as too little. Feeling a little tired is no reason so start pumping up your iron intake or loading up on iron supplements. Anemia is not self-diagnosable. If you suspect something's wrong, your doctor can tell you how much or how little iron you really need.

But if blood tests do indeed reveal that you're low in iron, there's a good chance you have the medicine you need right in your kitchen. To stay healthy, men and post-menopausal women need to consume approximately 10 milligrams of iron a day. Here are some ways to make sure you get enough iron and save some up for a rainy day.

Lean on red meat. It really is a good source of heme iron. Still, you don't want the fat and cholesterol that sometimes go with it. To get the benefits of red meat without the risks, shop for *lean* meats. A lean shoulder-cut pork chop, for example, contains 1.3 milligrams of iron. A 3-ounce serving of chicken breast or turkey breast (without the skin) has about 1 milligram of iron.

Pop a potato in the oven. Remember, the heme iron in meats can boost the absorption of the nonheme iron in cereals, salads, and vegetables. So while you're preparing that chicken breast, bake a potato too. One tasty, high-iron spud with the skin contains almost 3 milligrams of iron.

Don't forget the beans. "Beans are a great source of iron," McDonnell says. One serving of navy beans contains 2.3 milligrams of iron, while lentils pack an iron punch of 3.3 milligrams.

Try some chard. This leafy green contains 2 milligrams of iron per ½-cup serving. Or for an iron whammy, have some spinach (3.2 milligrams) or beet greens (1.4 milligrams).

Cook it in iron. Those trusty cast-iron pots are more than just versatile kitchen tools. Foods that are cooked in cast-iron pans actually absorb some of the iron, passing it along to you, McDonnell says.

Fill up on cereals. They're quick to prepare, great to eat, and usually pack iron. Some 85 percent of ready-to-eat breakfast cereals are enriched with added

(continued on page 368)

Iron: Going to the Source

Here are the best sources of both heme and nonheme iron.

Food	Portion	Total Iron (mg)
Heme Iron Sources		
Clams, cooked, moist heat	1 doz.	15.10
Oysters, cooked, moist heat	6 med.	5.63
Deer, game meat, roasted	3 oz	3.80
Tuna, light, canned in water	3 oz	2.72
Shrimp, cooked, moist heat	3 oz	2.62
Top round, lean, broiled	3 oz	2.34
Lamb loin, lean, roasted	3 oz	2.07
Ground beef, extra lean, broiled	3 oz	2.00
Chicken leg, roasted	3 oz	1.31
Pork tenderloin, lean, roasted	3 oz	1.31
Skinless turkey, light meat, roasted	3 oz	1.31
Haddock, cooked, moist heat	3 oz	1.14
Chicken breast, roasted	3 oz	1.04
Veal loin, roasted	3 oz	0.73
Salmon, sockeye, cooked, dry heat	3 oz	0.47

Food	Portion	Total Iron (mg)
Nonheme Iron Sources		
Tofu, raw, regular	½ cup	6.65
Blackstrap molasses	1 Tbsp	5.05
Potato, baked with skin	1	2.75
Kidney beans, cooked	½ cup	2.58
Lima beans, cooked	½ cup	2.08
Spaghetti, enriched, cooked	1 cup	1.96
Hummus	½ cup	1.94
Artichoke, cooked	1 med.	1.62
Oatmeal, cooked	1 cup	1.59
Edible-podded peas, cooked	½ cup	1.58
Kidney beans, canned	½ cup	1.57
Figs, dried	3	1.25
Pearled barley, cooked	½ cup	1.05
Prunes, dried	5	1.04
Whole-wheat bread	1 slice	1.00
Raisins	¼ cup	0.93
Broccoli, cooked	½ cup	0.89
Apricots, dried	5	0.83
Romaine lettuce, shredded	1 cup	0.62
Brown rice, medium grain, cooked	½ cup	0.52

nutrients. So while a cup of regular oatmeal contains 1.6 milligrams of iron, a cup of fortified instant oatmeal contains 8.3 milligrams. Other fortified cereals contain anywhere from 1.8 to 18 milligrams of iron per serving.

Enjoy dried fruit. Dried apricots, figs, prunes, and raisins contain healthy amounts of blood-building nonheme iron.

Wash them down with OJ. Taking vitamin C along with your meals can boost your absorption of nonheme iron, McDonnell says. So have some orange juice with your breakfast cereal, or slice a ripe tomato to garnish a leafy lunchtime salad.

Consider supplements. "When your iron stores get depleted, it can be very difficult to build them up just with a good diet," Dr. Erslev says. Consequently, your doctor may recommend iron supplements along with your high-iron diet. While iron supplements are most effective when taken on an empty stomach, they occasionally cause stomach irritation, so your doctor may suggest you take your supplement with meals.

It's worth repeating: Taking too much iron can be dangerous. In very large doses, it can cause vomiting, diarrhea, even convulsions. In addition, as many as 1 in 300 people suffers from hemochromatosis, a genetic defect that can lead to iron overload. So, again, don't take iron supplements without checking with your doctor first.

Back Problems

How to Put Them Behind You

Do you know 10 people? Chances are, at least eight of them will eventually have back problems.

Make that *expensive* back problems. With lost wages, doctors' fees, and other expenses, the nation's bad backs cost an estimated $16 billion each year. But the good news, according to Augustus A. White III, M.D., professor of orthopedic surgery at Harvard Medical School and chief of the Spine Surgery Division at Boston's Beth Israel Hospital, is that serious back problems such as ruptured disks are quite rare. Sure, backaches hurt, but surgery and long-term pain rarely belong in the picture.

"For the most part, back problems are caused by some type of sprain in the muscles or tendons," says Dr. White, author of *Your Aching Back: A Doctor's Guide to Relief.* "It may hurt like crazy for two or three days. Then it hurts moderately for maybe two weeks. Then after four or five weeks, you'll probably be more or less normal."

For back-pain sufferers, this probably sounds only partially reassuring. Serious or not, that weeks-long journey from "ouch!" to "more or less normal" is nothing to sneeze at. (Indeed, back pain veterans will tell you that sneezes, as well as coughs, momentarily double the pain.)

Worse, folks over 50 aren't likely to avoid the situation, as that 8-in-10 statistic indicates. It doesn't take six rounds with a heavyweight to wrack your back. Just sleeping wrong can do it, or taking out the trash, or bending over to pick up a paper clip. In fact, backache is second only to sore throats as the most common condition doctors treat.

Spinal Architecture

Reach behind and feel your spine, imagining it as a tall, curved stack of doughnuts. (The hole in the middle is for the spinal cord.) Your spine may feel solid, but it's eminently flexible. Every time you nod your head, brush your teeth, or lumber through the limbo, your spine's muscles, ligaments, and vertebrae bend along with you.

But anything that moves can also *stop* moving, including stressed muscles. But instead of merely relaxing while off-duty, they might bunch themselves into powerful, painful contractions called spasms. Those muscle spasms are rarely the *cause* of back problems, Dr. White says. Rather, they're simply a response to other things, such as strained ligaments or too much hard work.

Malfunctioning facet joints can also cause back pain, Dr. White says. The facet joints are the gliding surfaces between vertebrae. Partially coated with slick cartilage, they allow you to twist your hips when you dance the twist. That is, until they get sore. Then your twist gets twisted, and you sit out the next 10.

Perhaps the most infamous back problems are caused by faulty spinal disks. Terms like ruptured disks, slipped disks, or herniated disks all mean pretty much the same thing: trouble! A quick look at what spinal disks are all about will give you a good idea of why that's true.

How I Did It: A Successful Surgery

One Sunday afternoon, Patricia Ambrosini, of Helmetta, New Jersey, lost her balance behind some boxes at the retail store where she worked. "It felt like somebody shot me in the back," she remembers. "Everything locked up from my shoulders right down to my hips. It was a horrible feeling."

She told herself that she'd just strained her back. But by that night, she wasn't so sure. "I started getting numbness in my fingers and radiating pains down my arms," she says. "My legs felt like they weren't there, and my feet were tingling."

Painkillers, inflammation-fighting drugs, and orders to take it easy yielded no improvement. Daily physical therapy sessions seemed to do the trick at first. But after she returned to work, the pain returned, worse than before.

Tests indicated that two herniated disks were putting pressure on her spinal nerves. Recommendation: back surgery to remove the pressure. Not without fear, she agreed.

As it turned out, Ambrosini's problem was not ruptured disks but damaged ligaments, which her surgeon removed. "When I woke up after the surgery, I didn't have that pain," Ambrosini says. "I knew I was better."

One thing still hurts, though. "Until I actually had the surgery, a lot of people seemed to think that this whole thing was in my mind," she says. "I just felt awful, because people didn't have any idea what I was going through."

You may not think about it much, but every time you jump out of bed, run to the store or pirouette past the petunias, your back takes a heck of a lot of pounding. That's why your vertebrae have their very own shock absorbers, the spinal disks. Remember the doughnuts we stacked up earlier? Well, your disks really are like jelly doughnuts: flexible outsides wrapped around a soft, gelatinous middle. When you squeeze a doughnut (or a disk), it absorbs the pressure; release the pressure, it springs right back.

But aging does to your disks what it does to doughnuts—makes them dry and brittle. Now, disks often dry out without causing problems, but in some cases, the flexible outside will crack open (herniate), allowing the soft middle to ooze right out. That means the spine loses the use of one of its shock absorbers.

Even that's not always a big problem, Dr. White says. There are plenty of healthy, pain-free people walking around with moderately herniated disks. In most cases, they don't even know anything happened. But if the disk begins to push against nearby nerves, the "pinched" nerve can send shooting pains into both arms and legs. It can cause muscle weakness or even paralysis. In some cases, it can cause loss of bladder control.

Watch Your Back

None of the above means back pain is inevitable once you climb into your fifties and sixties. Even when disks rupture, the pain often goes away on its own. On the other hand, a bush-league backache can still cause major-league pain. It's always better to prevent a backache, Dr. White says, than to wait for it to go away.

As you might expect, much of the advice doctors give for avoiding back pain begins with "don't." Don't lift too much. Don't work too hard. And so on. But there are also plenty of "do's."

Work on your trunk. Think of your back as a building. When the foundation is strong, it stands up; take away the foundation, and the only way it can go is down. That's why doctors agree that strong trunk muscles can help keep backs feeling good. The most important ones to strengthen are your *psoas* (which connect the lower back to the inside of the hips) and the *erector spinae* (running parallel to the spine).

Swimming is an excellent way to strengthen these muscles, doctors say. And because swimming, in effect, reduces gravity, it's an ideal exercise if you have arthritis or other joint problems. Don't know how to swim? No problem: Walking in waist-high water also does the trick.

Put on your walking shoes. Or your running shoes, aerobics shoes, or any-exercise-you-want shoes. (If you're a swimmer, lose the shoes.) Aerobic exercise lessens your chances for spending painful weekends inspecting ceiling tiles, says Richard Plummer, D.C., director of Springfield Chiropractic Services in Inman, South Carolina. By improving circulation, it helps keep your spinal disks supple, he says.

"For most people, walking is the simplest, easiest exercise, and all you need is a pair of sneakers," Dr. Plummer says. "People can walk every day of the week in their neighborhood, up and down stairs, or inside shopping malls when the weather's bad. Walking, when you're upright and your arms are swinging, is one of the best exercises for your lower back."

Plan more strenuous workouts for later in the day, Dr. Plummer advises. Your disks take on extra fluid at night and, like most tipplers, are a bit unruly in the mornings. So let them wake up before dragging them to the gym.

Hug your garbage. Try to hold things close to your body when you pick them up, doctors advise. When you lift a bag stuffed with garbage, the temptation is to hold it at arm's length. But what's good for your nose isn't always good for your spine.

Take a stretch. You're looking for trouble when you let your pants wear fastest at the seat. Long-term sitting is extremely hard on your spine, not to mention more southerly parts of your anatomy. Sitting puts about 50 percent more stress on your spine than standing does. All that extra pressure, Dr. White says, may irritate structures in the spine, including the disks. So give your back (and your bottom) a break. "When you feel tightness or tension in your back or neck, get up and move around a little bit, even if it's only for 30 seconds," Dr. Plummer says.

Pull those shoulders back. You probably argued when Mom told you to stand up straight. Now it's time to apologize to her. Even though good posture doesn't guarantee healthy backs, people who slump (when they sit, stand or talk on the telephone) are asking for trouble.

Smooth the sway. When you look in the mirror, you'll see that your back naturally has some curve to it. But if you stand around flat-footed for long periods, a little curve can feel like a sharp hook right into your lower back. Standing with one foot up on a step or stool will reduce the curve, doctors say, and that eases the strain. No matter where you are, there's probably a step somewhere. At the store, for example, rest your foot on the shopping cart.

Drop some weight. Your back has enough to do just carrying you and your clothes around all day, every day. Aside from all the other health problems being overweight can cause, adding extra pounds makes your back bend with the extra weight, Dr. White says. So give your back a break and put that spare tire back in the car where it belongs.

Ease into exercise. One of the worst things you can do to your back, Dr. Plummer says, is push it into action on a moment's notice. Going straight from eight sedentary hours at work into your tennis game is not the way to do it. Warm up first. You don't have to stretch for hours, Dr. Plummer says, but limber up before you boogie down.

Lower the vibes. It's not really road bumps that bash bad backs, Dr. White says, but car vibrations. Most cars vibrate at frequencies between 4 and 5 cycles per second—precisely the frequencies that can put your spine in park. Limit your driving time to 2 hours a day, he advises. If you have to drive more than that, consider buying a car that vibrates at different and safer frequencies.

Snuff the butts. One more reason to quit: "Smoking is a vasoconstrictor, which means it limits the supply of blood to some parts of your body," Dr. White says. "When you interfere with the nutrition of the disks, that can cause problems."

Saving Your Back

Even if you do good things for your back and avoid all the dangers, you could still get hurt, Dr. White says. In fact, back injuries are so common that few people never experience a back problem. Fortunately, doctors agree that there are things you can do to beat the pain and to hasten your recovery.

The word *cure*, says Alan S. Bensman, M.D., medical director of the Minnesota Center for Health and Rehabilitation in Minneapolis, really doesn't belong in conversations about back pain. "The word *rehabilitation* is more accurate," Dr. Bensman insists. "Rehabilitation doesn't mean your problems have gone away. It means you've learned to do the very best with the body you've got." So whether you've had back pain all your life or you just pulled a muscle in the garden, some of the following probably can help.

Get comfy. Everyone with back problems has at least one posture or position that puts the least strain on the back. Some people might be most comfortable when they stand with their back bent slightly forward; others will feel better when they're ramrod straight. Find yours.

But there's a catch, Dr. Bensman says. Your favorite position has to be functional as well as comfortable. "I have people who come in here all bent over like pretzels, and they say, 'It's comfortable for me,'" he says. "Well, it might be comfortable, but it's not functional."

Put it to bed. Doctors agree that lying in bed can take painful pressure off that sensitive spine. People who have ruptured disks often feel better after two or three days of bed rest. "Most back injuries will resolve when the pressure is removed," Dr. Bensman says.

In the past, doctors advised people with acute back pain to spend at least 20 hours a day—for up to 10 days—between the sheets. But studies suggest that two days are probably enough for most people. Now, that doesn't mean you should hoist refrigerators on the third day. Give yourself a few weeks to recover.

Catch some Zzzs. Since you're in bed anyway, you may as well get some relaxing, healing sleep. "Deep sleep has been identified as a time when muscle healing occurs," Dr. Bensman says. When

Precision without Incision

Back surgery's tough stuff. To get a good view, surgeons have always preferred large incisions 4 or even 5 painful inches right up the middle of your back.

But the cuts are getting smaller, says Oheneba Boachie-Adjei, M.D., associate medical director of the Southern California Complex Spine and Scoliosis Center in Whittier. That's because surgeons are learning to use magnification to perform complicated surgery with minute instruments.

In fact, a still-evolving technique called percutaneous diskectomy may someday revolutionize back surgery, Dr. Boachie-Adjei says.

Instead of making incisions, the surgeon inserts a hollow tube about one-half the diameter of a pencil into a small hole in the back. Into this tube go even smaller instruments. To see, the surgeon uses a fluoroscope, a type of x-ray machine. "If it can be proven to be as successful as conventional surgery, the advantages will be tremendous," Dr. Boachie-Adjei says.

Some surgeons are skeptical, though. For example, they ask, how is a surgeon to remove disk fragments that are bigger than the tiny incision?

These concerns are valid, Dr. Boachie-Adjei says, but surgeons can still use the technique. "Then if they encounter large disk fragments, all they have to do is perform traditional surgery," Dr. Boachie-Adjei says. "They've left their options open."

you're not sleeping, he adds, find positions in bed that don't hurt your back. Most people find that lying on their stomach is out because it puts too much pressure on the spine. Lying on your back with your knees slightly bent may be the best position. If you usually sleep on your side, curl up and tuck a pillow between your knees.

Open the medicine chest. For most people, aspirin is the drug of choice for fighting pain and inflammation, Dr. White says. If you can't take aspirin, other over-the-counter nonsteroidal anti-inflammatory drugs such as acetaminophen or ibuprofen can help. (However, acetaminophen only fights pain; it does not attack inflammation.)

Or ask your doctor about prescription drugs. They sometimes work when over-the-counter remedies don't. If your pain is really ferocious, your doctor might recommend stronger prescription drugs, such as codeine or other narcotics. But these drugs can delay recovery, so they're rarely recommended for long-term use.

Finally, your doctor may suggest another kind of prescription if he thinks that a lack of deep sleep might be hindering your body's ability to heal itself. "Amitriptyline (Elavil), an antidepressant with sedative effects, taken in low doses (10 to 15 milligrams) 1 to 2 hours before bedtime, may be useful for just this reason," says Dr. Bensman.

Ice it. Like aspirin, ice cubes are a simple (and inexpensive) way to relieve muscle strains and ligament pains, Dr. Bensman says. Because cold reduces the swelling and helps the muscle relax, it can help reduce painful inflammation. Before you lay on the ice, wrap it in pillowcases or washcloths, Dr. Bensman advises. You want to chill your back, not freeze it solid.

Get hot. After a few days of ice, go ahead and

warm things up for a change. Heating your back with a heating pad and a hot bath (not at the same time) can help relax muscle spasms, Dr. Bensman says. Follow treatment with some light stretching. Remember, however, that applying heat soon after an injury can increase pain and inflammation.

Rub it out. After a few days of chilly compresses, reward yourself with a long, leisurely, luxurious massage. It won't cure your backache, Dr. Plummer says, but it should make you feel better—and not only on the outside. "Massage stimulates the circulatory system and the lymphatic system, and that helps bring fluid and nutrients into the muscles," he says. "It also helps remove the lactic acid, a painful by-product of damaged tissue."

Hit the switch. Transcutaneous electrical nerve stimulation, or TENS, is a new therapy for back pain. Small electrodes are placed on the skin near the injury, and electrical currents are shot into the body. Researchers believe these currents interrupt the passage of pain signals from your hurt back to your brain. TENS may also raise the body's production of painkilling endorphins.

Some doctors, however, aren't convinced. A study published in the *New England Journal of Medicine*, for example, found that people treated with TENS units improved about as much as those treated with placebo (inactive) machines. So if TENS doesn't seem to help, Dr. White says to stop using it.

Take a deep breath. But first close your mouth. "When you take a slow, deep breath through your nose, you're helping yourself relax, and you're stimulating the production of endorphins, your body's natural pain reducers," Dr. Bensman says. (If you have a stuffy nose, this technique isn't for you!)

Stretch it out. Stretching is one of the best

things you can do for a bad back, Dr. Bensman says. You don't need a fancy program, and you don't have to spend a dime. In fact, you can do your morning stretches before your feet even hit the floor. Just stretch your legs, your arms, your neck, and your back. Do this for a few minutes every morning, he says, and you'll be more mobile and less prone to back pain. Abdominal exercises, such as sit-ups, also help strengthen the back.

Stay with it. The secret to a pain-free back, Dr. Bensman says, is daily care—whether your back's hurting or not. "You can't stop taking care of your back just because you're feeling better," he warns. "The biggest mistake people make is to think their back problems are just going to end. They are not."

Cancer

Beating the Big C

While the war on cancer rages in hospitals and laboratories, health-conscious men and women of any age have opened up a front closer to home—in their own home, kitchens, and dining rooms.

"Each and every one of us needs to start taking more personal responsibility for the disease," says John Laszlo, M.D., the American Cancer Society's (ACS) senior vice president for research and the author of *Understanding Cancer*. "We're going to have to stop waiting for scientists to cure what may be easier to prevent."

Experts now feel that as much as 70 percent of all cancers may be due to factors within our control. "More than 80 percent of people who get lung cancer, for example, are smokers," Dr. Laszlo says. "And more and more, we're seeing how the effects of dietary fat, alcohol abuse, obesity, and excessive exposure to the sun can increase cancer risks."

In short, we need to start thinking of the Big C as standing for *Control*. "If we did everything possible to prevent cancer and also followed the latest recommendations for early detection, we might be able to reduce cancer deaths substantially over the next generation," says Clark Heath, M.D., ACS vice president of epidemiology and statistics.

Getting Cancer Before It Gets You

How much of a commitment does it take? Really, moderation and common sense are all that's needed, says Dr. Laszlo. A survey of leading cancer experts has even come up with a Top 10 list of strategies to ward off cancer. These are everyday things you can start doing *right now* to give you control over this largely preventable disease.

Break the tobacco habit. Besides lung cancer, the habit increases risks of cancers of the mouth, pharynx, larynx, esophagus, pancreas, uterus, cervix, kidney, and bladder. "The list of chemicals in tobacco includes some of the most potent cancer causers known," says Dr. Laszlo. Bottom line: Smoking is thought to be responsible for about 30 percent of cancer deaths overall.

So, if you've got a pack of cigarettes in your hand right now, drop it. Your cancer risk will drop with it. "The odds of getting lung cancer drop steadily and dramatically when people quit," says Dr. Laszlo. "Natural repair of the cells that line the air passages begins almost immediately. In many cases, precancerous changes that have been caused by smoking can be totally reversed."

Avoid passive smoking. Some studies suggest that "sidestream" or "passive" smoke may be worse than smoke directly inhaled, because the tar content hasn't traveled through the cigarette's filter. "Living with a smoker may increase a nonsmoker's risks of cancer by as much as 50 percent," says William Shingleton, M.D., former director of the Cancer Center at the Duke University Medical School. Working in a smoky environment for 8 hours a day also can substantially elevate your risk. If your spouse smokes, it's time for a talk. If your workplace is smoke-filled, stand up for your rights.

Stay out of the sun. If there's anything good to say about skin cancer, it's that it can easily be prevented, says Dr. Laszlo. Nearly all of the 600,000 cases of skin cancer diagnosed each year are thought to be sun related. So prevention is as easy as avoiding prolonged exposure to direct sunlight between the hours of 10:00 A.M. and 3:00 P.M., wearing protective clothing when out in the sun, and applying sunscreen.

Be especially careful to protect yourself from the sun's rays at high altitudes and in areas near the equator, Dr. Laszlo says. And don't think that getting a suntan at a tanning parlor is without hazard. Despite advertising claims that may tell you otherwise, rays from a bulb that tan you are just as much of a risk for cancer (and wrinkles) as rays from the sun.

Go easy on alcohol. Studies leave little doubt that as the drinks go down, the cancer risks go up. One study found that heavy drinkers have a 2- to 6-fold greater-than-average risk of cancers of the throat and mouth. Some studies (but not all) suggest that the risk of breast cancer may double for women who drink. Even bigger trouble appears to be in store for heavy drinkers who also smoke: Risks of throat and mouth cancer skyrocket to 15-fold, and risks of esophageal cancer may increase by as much as 25-fold, when cigarettes and alcohol are combined.

Why this is true is still a matter of guesswork. Perhaps by overburdening the liver, heavy drinking may compromise that vital organ's ability to detoxify potentially cancer-causing substances, especially those resulting from smoking. Heavy drinking of hard liquor particularly may irritate tissues of the mouth, throat, and esophagus in a way that makes them more susceptible to cancer. Or certain drinks, particularly darker liquors such as rum, bourbon, and scotch, may produce cancer-causing by-products in the distillation process.

Whatever the biological mechanisms involved, the statistics don't lie. More than a few drinks a day increases your risks of cancer of the mouth, throat, pancreas, esophagus and liver. And according to some studies, heavy drinking may also boost your risks of cancer of the breast, stomach, and rectum. "If you're going to drink, you should keep your intake to no more than two or three drinks a day," says Dr. Laszlo. "And avoid drinking the hard stuff straight." The less diluted the drink, the more irritating to the gullet, and the greater the risk of cancer to the upper gastrointestinal tract, he says.

Cut down on fat. A diet high in fat seems to increase risks of cancers of the breast and colon, and perhaps of the prostate and ovary. Scientists still aren't certain if it does that by activating cancer-causing hormones, inciting cancer-causing digestive enzymes, or feeding cancer cells directly. But dietary fat seems to be what scientists call a cancer "promoter," a substance that does not initiate cancerous changes in cells but does encourage continuation of already existing changes by providing a favorable environment.

In the case of breast cancer, for example, a diet high in fat seems to elevate levels of the hormone estrogen, which is suspected of feeding tumor growth. With colon cancer, a high-fat diet may do its harm by causing the excessive release of bile acids, which in large amounts act as promoters on the lining of the intestine.

Regardless of what the mechanics may be, it makes sense to reduce the amount of fat in your diet. "In countries where less fat is consumed, we find fewer cancers," says the ACS statistics expert Dr. Heath. That being the case, the American Health Foundation recommends that total fat in the diet not comprise more than 20 to 25 percent of total calories. If you're an average American, that means you should be eating about half the fat you eat now. A good way to start cutting back is to add more fruits and vegetables to your diet and to go easy on animal products, such as meat and cheese.

Bulk up on fiber. Fiber's your body's scrub brush. Rather than getting digested, it passes right through you, often escorting potential carcinogens along with it. For example, fiber is thought to remove bile acids that could promote colon cancer. In the case of breast cancer, some fiber may reduce levels of cancer-promoting excess estrogen.

The Department of Health and Human Services

says that if Americans would eat more fiber and less fat, colon cancer could be reduced by 30 percent. Researchers from the National Cancer Institute say that a daily intake of 20 to 30 grams of fiber could cut colon-cancer rates in half.

Insoluble fiber from wheat bran, whole-grain cereals and breads, vegetables and fruit seems to speed things through the intestines best. But soluble fibers—prevalent in oat bran and beans—also seem to have cancer-fighting effects. Authorities agree that it's probably best to get a good mix of both types. Here's a sample combination that will get you 20 grams of fiber before dinner: for breakfast, one bowl of wheat bran cereal with a tablespoon of raisins and an apple; for lunch, a bowl of baked beans with a large salad and a slice of pumpernickel bread.

Splurge on fruits and vegetables. Your goal should be to consume at least two servings of vegetables and two of fruit each day. Help them do their work by eating them fresh, cooking them minimally, and leaving on the skins and peels. "Population studies leave little doubt that a varied diet containing plenty of fruits and vegetables can reduce risks for a wide range of cancers," says Dr. Heath.

Fruits and vegetables fight cancer in lots of ways. Most are full of fiber and extremely low in fat. They're rich in cancer-fighting nutrients such as vitamins A and C, beta-carotene, and bioflavonoids, which guard cells from cancer-encouraging free radicals. And the pulpy portions of citrus fruits contain nutrients that enhance the anticancer activity of your body's own enzymes. A similar enzyme boost may also be exerted by cruciferous vegetables (broccoli, Brussels sprouts, cauliflower, and cabbage) in a way that helps the liver break down and eliminate potential carcinogens from the body.

Stay slim. It doesn't matter if the fat is on your plate or on your waist. Get rid of it and you reduce your risk of cancer. Start by pinning this information to your refrigerator door: An ACS study found that obesity (measured as being 40 percent or more above your ideal weight) increases cancer deaths in women by 55 percent and in men by 33 percent. Overweight women have higher death rates from cancer of the endometrium, uterus, gallbladder, cervix, ovaries, and breast. Overweight men have higher death rates from colon, rectal, and prostate cancer.

What's the connection? It could be that extra calories mean extra metabolism, hence more frequent cell division. Also, points out Dr. Heath, the type of diet that tends to promote obesity—that is, one high in fat and low in fiber—may itself be a factor.

Avoid environmental hazards. "Allow for plenty of ventilation when painting, varnishing, or using any chemical product indoors," says John Vena, Ph.D., a professor with the Department of Social and Preventive Medicine at the State University of New York at Buffalo. Also be careful with pesticides and herbicides around the home. Read the labels carefully. Wash fruits and vegetables before eating to remove any chemical residue. And have your house checked for high levels of radon, a naturally occurring gas that has been linked to lung cancer.

What about carcinogens in the workplace? "There are certain work-related substances some people may need to worry about, such as nickel, chromates, asbestos, and vinyl chloride," Dr. Vena says. "But most industries now control these substances fairly well. It

Superfoods to the Rescue

Doctors have been saying it for years: Eating fruits and vegetables decreases the risk of certain cancers. Now the National Cancer Institute (NCI) is poised to go one step better. Its Designer Foods Research Project aims to hunt down nutrients known as phytochemicals in common foods and find some way to concentrate them in "superfoods" with super cancer-fighting potential.

The Designer Foods Research Project is still in the diaper stage, but it's looking to a future in which even desserts might be cancer-fighters. "There's an awful lot of research that has to be done, but the future certainly looks bright," says Herbert F. Pierson, Ph.D., a toxicologist at the Diet and Cancer Branch of the NCI. Looking ahead, he says that someday with the right addition of phytochemicals and subtraction of fat it may be possible that even potato chips and other "junk" foods will be manufactured so as to be good for our health!

The cancer-fighting nutrients targeted in this program would be engineered into their purest and most powerful form. "Studies say that about half of all chronic diseases like cancer may be linked to diet," says Dr. Pierson. "If that's true, then making foods healthier, by taking advantage of what Mother Nature has already given us to work with, may lead to a significant reduction in cancer."

would still be a good idea to learn about the substances you are working with. Also for anyone who has had a history of working with chemicals or dusts, it's important to let their doctor know, so that any complications could be detected as early as possible."

As for recent speculations on the cancer risks posed by electromagnetic fields, the research is still very preliminary, according to Dr. Vena. "It does make sense to update certain appliances that could be showing wear—things like electric blankets or hair dryers that involve very close contact," he says. "This would offer as much protection against fire and electrocution as against cancer."

Get regular exercise. Cancer seems to have a tougher time hitting a moving target. So try to get at least 30 minutes of some sort of physical activity at least three times a week, even if it's as moderate as a brisk walk, washing windows, or weeding the garden. That may be all it takes to keep cancer defenses in good shape. Dr. Vena's own research has found risks of colon cancer to be twice as high in sedentary people as in those who are physically active. "Exercise might be underrated as a cancer-fighting strategy," Dr. Vena says.

The reason for exercise's protective effect is still a matter of speculation. It combats obesity, of course, but there's probably more to it. "Stress reduction could be a factor, as could improved bowel regularity," Dr. Vena says. "It's also possible that people who exercise regularly tend to eat more healthfully and take better care of themselves generally."

The Importance of Early Detection

Say someone agreed to give you just a penny this year, but two next year. Then four the year after, eight the next, and so on, doubling the sum every year for 30 years. Would it be worth the bother?

Only if you could use an extra $5,368,709.12, which is how much a penny doubled every year for 30 years would produce. Unfortunately, the same surprising arithmetic lies behind the importance of early detection of most types of cancer. And that arithmetic becomes a required subject when your years accumulate beyond 50.

"There are mitigating circumstances, such as the strength of a person's immune system, but most tumors will do their best to grow in what's known as an exponential fashion," says Michael Bookman, M.D., of the department of medical oncology at the Fox Chase Cancer Center in Philadelphia. "This means that one cell becomes two, two becomes four, four becomes eight, and so on. As with the example of the pennies, it doesn't take long for the numbers to become huge."

Hence the importance of catching and arresting the spread of most cancers as early as possible. Not only is treatment of the initial tumor more likely to be successful if it's done early on, there's less chance that it will have metastasized—that is, spread to other sites.

That's why regular screening (as outlined in Medical Testing on page 55) is essential, especially if you're over 50. The checkup can usually be done by your family physician.

Tried-and-True Treatments

So prevention is job one in the fight against cancer, and early detection is job two. Job three, should it be necessary, is getting the best and most appropriate treatment should a cancer be found. Many experts recommend getting at least two professional opinions before deciding on a course of treatment. You want to be as informed as possible, because the first shot at curing cancer is always the best shot. Recurring cancers become progressively more difficult to treat.

Here's a brief description of the major types of treatment being used today. Sometimes these treatments are used by themselves, but more often in combination.

Surgery to remove the cancerous growth, or as much as possible, is the oldest form of treatment for cancer, dating back to the Middle Ages. It's often used in conjunction with other therapies in cases where all of a tumor is not removed or if the cancer is thought to have spread.

Radiation is sometimes an alternative to surgery and works by finding cancer cells through exposure to high doses of x-rays. Since cancer cells exist around and among normal cells, however, a drawback to radiation therapy is that it can't always spare healthy tissue. This can make the therapy inadvisable for treating certain cancers involving major organs. On the plus side, however, radiation therapy is painless. Treatments take only a few minutes daily and are usually done on an outpatient basis.

Chemotherapy introduces drugs, usually through injection, that kill cancer cells by interfering with the way they reproduce. It often takes a variety of drugs to combat the uncanny ability of cancer cells to adapt to and resist chemotherapy's effects. But if the right combination is used, results can be dramatic. Also dramatic, however, can be chemotherapy's side effects: nausea, vomiting, hair loss, sores in the mouth, diarrhea, and increased susceptibility to infection. Fortunately, new drugs are bringing some of these side effects under control.

Antihormone therapy, using drugs to keep troublemaking hormones under control, has been quite successful in the treatment of breast and prostate

How I Did It: June Adler Beat Breast Cancer

June Adler, age 44, was devastated. The discovery: A lump the size of a grape in her right breast. The diagnosis: cancer. The recommended treatment: radical mastectomy (complete removal of the breast).

"That's when I called the self-help group Y-Me," she says. "I wanted to know all my options, and they were extremely helpful." At the group's suggestion, Adler sought second and third opinions about treatment and discovered she was a good candidate for a lumpectomy—a surgery that removes the lump without removing the entire breast.

The lumpectomy was followed by 11 months of radiation and chemotherapy treatments. "The cancer had spread to my lymph nodes, so they wanted to be sure they got it all," Adler says.

But they didn't. A small tumor was discovered on her left lung. "That's when I really had to gather my strength," she says. "I was just beginning to feel my ordeal was over. But I wasn't going to give up. After the surgery, I enrolled in a course that taught me how to use visualization to combat cancer. I was going to fight my disease in every way possible."

Today, thanks to continued follow-up care and a fighting spirit, June is cancer-free. She's gone on to direct one of Y-Me's regional offices in Northbrook, Illinois. "Their help was invaluable to me," she says. "They helped me make decisions that helped me save not just my breast but my life."

cancer. Tamoxifen, the antihormone drug most commonly used to treat breast cancer, has few side effects. Those drugs used for prostate cancer, however, may cause troublesome nausea and breast tenderness.

Immunotherapy boosts the body's own abilities to fight cancer naturally. Interferon has been the most publicized of the drugs used in immunotherapy. "Interferon has been highly successful in treating one rare type of leukemia but has been considerably less effective against more common forms of cancer such as lung, colon, and breast," Dr. Laszlo says. "The area of immunotherapy remains a highly promising one, however, and much encouraging work continues to be done."

Depression

Beating Back the Blues

Depression can be a minor funk or a major clinical problem. Big or small, it's the nature of depression to hide hope under a black cloud. But there's actually every reason for hope, says psychiatrist Michael Gitlin, M.D., associate clinical professor of psychiatry and biobehavioral sciences at the Neuropsychiatric Institute and Hospital of the University of California, Los Angeles. "Depression is more treatable now than it has ever been," he says.

In fact, unless you're suffering from a serious case

of clinical depression, there's a lot you can do on your own to pull yourself out of it. Here are ways to get a handle on the run-of-the-mill blues.

Get busy. Some people let themselves slowly withdraw from the world as they work their way through their fifties and sixties. That's bad anti-depression strategy, says psychologist William Leber, Ph.D., associate professor of psychiatry and behavioral sciences at the University of Oklahoma Medical School and director of clinical neuropsychology at the Veterans Administration Medical Center in Oklahoma City. Instead, he recommends making an extra effort to get involved with life.

One way to get busy is to get moving. "Revving up the body to a higher speed tends to have a counteractive effect on depression," he says. "Add exercising and socializing on to the end of your day, before you let yourself get close to your bed. Or you might get up earlier and exercise or play before you go to work."

Talk it out. Hey, what are friends and family for? Just make sure you don't overdo it to the point where people hide when they see you coming. "It's good to talk to people who are close to you," Dr. Leber says. "But it's not good to dump on everybody you come in contact with."

Change your routine. A change of pace brings sunshine into your life, psychologically speaking. "It could be something as simple as going out for lunch more often instead of eating at your desk or at home," Dr. Leber says.

Redirect your thoughts. As you grow older, there's a tendency to dwell on the way things "should"be. Get more flexible, Dr. Leber says. Think positively about how you can adapt to reality and make the most of it.

Limit the cocktails. Alcohol is one of the most powerful depressants known. The more you drink, the more you risk making your problems worse.

A Deeper Shade of Blue

For depressions that go deeper than the blahs, professional help may work best. Clinical depression—the serious kind—seems to be on the rise, although this may be due to better recognition and reporting of the problem. But at any one time, 2.5 million Americans have clinical depression.

You may already know that the go-go-go type A personality weighs heavy on the heart. But depression is actually worse, says Robert Carney, Ph.D., professor of medical psychology at Washington University School of Medicine in St. Louis. "Depression appears to be a risk factor for heart disease," he says. "It's more important than a type A personality, but probably not as significant as high blood pressure and cholesterol."

Still, he notes that depression is often treated long before patients show signs of heart disease. All the same, depressed people may have higher risk for heart trouble not because of their emotional states alone but because they're more likely to smoke and ignore doctors' recommendations.

You don't necessarily have to feel overtly sad to be clinically depressed. Changes in basic drives such as eating, sleeping, energy, and sex may be the only signs you have. Experts at the National Institute for Mental Health say that if you have at least four of the following symptoms most of every day for at least two weeks, you probably have clinical depression:

♦ You don't feel like eating and you start losing weight. Or you start eating more than usual and packing on the pounds.

♦ You can't sleep. Or all you do is sleep.

♦ You slump through the day as if you're Jacob Marley dragging his chains around Ebenezer Scrooge's bedroom. Or you're so hyper that you're up all night polishing the silver and scrubbing the floor.

♦ Your sex drive doesn't shift out of low gear.

♦ You tell yourself that you're worthless, punish yourself for things you think you said or did, and blame yourself for everything that goes wrong.

♦ You can't concentrate on what you're doing; you can't even decide what to have for dinner. You feel as if you can't figure out the simplest matters.

♦ You keep having thoughts and images of killing yourself. Or you wish you were dead. Or you actually try to commit suicide.

Once you decide therapy's for you, you'll find you have lots of choices. Problem solving in four to six months is the goal of many of the newer forms of therapy. "The hot thing in psychotherapy these days is brief therapy," Dr. Leber says. "It focuses on immediate problems as opposed to life history, and the therapist is both active and interventionist."

Cognitive therapy is probably the most popular of the new styles, Dr. Leber says. "It helps you examine your thought patterns and how those patterns keep your depression going," he says. "The therapist helps

Psychotherapy Enters the Computer Age

Morton doesn't look like any therapist you've ever seen. Morton is a computer program.

What does Morton do? During a first session, it might flash on the screen something like, "Hello, Jane, my name is Morton. I hear you've been feeling depressed lately. Is that true?" You answer by choosing one of several possible responses, using the keyboard.

"Some people can relate to the computer as if it were a person," says Morton's designer, Paulette M. Selmi, Ph.D., a psychologist in private practice and director of psychology at Desert Vista Hospital in Mesa, Arizona. "There's a sense that the computer has really listened to them."

A hunk of hardware that listens is interesting. But does it work? Well, Dr. Selmi conducted a study that provided some subjects with six cognitive behavioral therapy sessions with a flesh-and-bones therapist, and others an equal number of Morton-led sessions. Morton proved "as effective in the treatment of mild to moderately depressed outpatients as a therapist," concluded Dr. Selmi and her associates.

Dr. Selmi predicts that many therapists may soon be using computers for depression. "I don't see the computer as a replacement for human beings," she says. "I see it as a tool that may assist the therapist and reduce costs for the patient."

you discover some fallacy in the way you see yourself and the world."

Another major form of brief therapy is interpersonal therapy. "It focuses on the relationships in your life, and it uses relationships to help you gain insights into why you're depressed," says Dr. Leber. Interpersonal therapy also examines the transitions you go through from one stage of life to another—marriage, parenthood, divorce, changing jobs, retirement, death.

Traditional psychoanalysis is still an avenue for some. "After you've dealt with your immediate problems and you're feeling better, you may want to go into a longer-term therapy that deals with your major life issues," says Dr. Leber. "It depends on you; some people are better off with one kind of therapy over another."

Mulling the Medications

The more severe your depression, the more likely it is that medication is warranted, says Dr. Gitlin. The so-called tricyclic antidepressants (imipramine, amitriptyline, nortriptyline) have fewer side effects than the monoamine oxidase (MAO) inhibitors (pargyline, phenelzine, isocarboxazid). But newer drugs such as bupropion (Wellbutrim) and fluoxetine (Prozac) have the least side effects of all.

Prozac quickly became America's antidepressant of choice after its introduction in 1987. Its popularity, says Dr. Gitlin, was due to a resounding success rate and apparent safety. But several years later, the drug became embroiled in controversy, where it remains today. Some people have reported reacting badly to Prozac, even to the point of attempting suicide. Since suicidal thoughts are often a part of depression, it's hard to tell if the drug actually causes them, Dr. Gitlin says. If it does, this occurs in only a very small percentage of the people who take it. "Prozac has probably saved a lot of lives," he says, "and more people can tolerate it than other antidepressants."

The argument over Prozac clearly illustrates why you and your doctor have to discuss your symptoms and your drug reactions thoroughly. What works for someone else may not work for you.

Diabetes

Avoid Getting Type-Cast

While 50-plussers naturally concentrate their health efforts at preventing heart disease, stroke, and cancer, you might make room in your consciousness for another common killer—type 2 diabetes.

First off, it helps to know that your body's a sugar junkie, whether you have diabetes or not. No, we're not talking about the white stuff you sprinkle on cereal. We're talking about glucose, the simple sugar your body extracts from fruits, vegetables, and many other foods. Every single cell of your body uses glucose for fuel. Your red blood cells consume more than 1 ounce every day; your central nervous system gobbles about 5 ounces.

If you're healthy, your body extracts from your diet exactly the right amount of glucose, then stores the rest.

But if you have adult-onset (type 2) diabetes, much of the glucose isn't used or stored. Instead, it remains in the blood, where it creates all kinds of problems.

Diabetes seriously increases your risk of developing cardiovascular disease. According to the American Heart Association, approximately 80 percent of people with diabetes die of some type of heart or blood vessel disease. This is because diabetes increases triglyceride levels and lowers helpful HDL cholesterol levels.

Diabetes is also the leading cause of blindness, kidney failure, and nerve damage.

A Sweet Poison

You can picture how your body makes use of sugars by imagining a counter stacked high with glucose entrees, glucose salads, and glucose desserts. Every cell in your body is ready to feast on all that glucose, but where's that waiter when you need him? Enter insulin, a hormone produced by your pancreas. Basically, insulin makes it possible for glucose to move from your bloodstream (where it accumulates after you eat) into your hungry cells.

People with adult-onset diabetes do produce insulin, but it doesn't work efficiently. The glucose can't get into cells in the normal manner, and so it accumulates in the blood. This condition is called hyperglycemia. "You may be eating tons of food, but if your body can't use it, you're starving," says Priscilla Hollander, M.D., vice president for adult diabetes and special studies at Park Nicollet Medical Center in Minneapolis.

So you're often tired and run-down. You probably drink and urinate a lot, this being your body's futile attempt to eliminate surplus glucose. What's more, glucose at high concentrations can damage nerves, blood vessels, and even the arteries leading to your heart.

But even though you can't entirely prevent this hereditary disease, you can slow its progress or, occasionally, even reverse it. "Some people have a predisposition for diabetes," says John Ivy, Ph.D., a professor of kinesiology at the University of Texas at Austin and director of the school's Exercise Science Laboratories. "But it can be prevented and often even reversed if people eat properly and exercise."

The Best Treatment— Pound for Pound

Doctors aren't sure why, but as your pounds add up, your insulin efficiency goes down. In fact, at least 80 percent of people with adult-onset diabetes are overweight. You can't change your genes, but you may be able to control the disease by keeping your weight in check. Here's how to let your diet help you avoid problems:

Cut the calories. "For many people, the day they cut the calories down is the day they see an effect on their blood sugar," says Linda M. Delahanty, a clinical and research dietitian at Massachusetts General Hospital in Boston. "There's an immediate response." And you don't have to be model-thin to experience long-term benefits. Some people can significantly lower their blood sugar by losing as little as 10 pounds.

Trim the fat. It doesn't take long for high-fat foods to contribute to a high-fat you. Not only will extra weight make your insulin work less efficiently, it can also raise your cholesterol—bad news for people with diabetes, who are already at risk for heart disease. The American Diabetes Association recommends consuming less than 30 percent of your calories from fat.

Load up on complex carbs. Grains, potatoes,

and other complex carbohydrates are packed with glucose, but they won't substantially raise your blood sugar because they slowly release glucose over a long period of time, Dr. Hollander says. That makes them a much better food choice than fats.

Say sayonara to sweets. Pure sugar is pure trouble. Unlike complex carbohydrates, it's dumped into your bloodstream all at once. Your insulin won't have a chance to catch up. If you must have a sweet, eat one that has other things in it too. Accompanying proteins and complex carbohydrates—even fats—will help slow the absorption of the sugar. In other words, you're going to be better off with a slice of cake or a bowl of ice milk than with a handful of jelly beans or a tangle of cotton candy.

Nosh between meals. If you eat a lot at one sitting, your body will be hard-pressed to meet the increased demand for insulin and you can get sudden rises in blood glucose levels. "Distribute your food throughout the day, so that any one meal isn't so large that it overwhelms the pancreas," Delahanty suggests.

Fill up on fiber. Besides lowering cholesterol, beans, oat bran, and other high-fiber foods put the brakes on glucose as it enters your bloodstream. That may lower your need for insulin.

Work It Out

Older adults with diabetes—or at risk for it—have added incentives to exercise. It helps you lose weight, which is so important in controlling diabetes. It lowers blood pressure and cholesterol levels, reducing the risk of heart disease that diabetes itself raises. Finally, exercise can help make your insulin work more efficiently. "Exercise may help by increasing the number of insulin receptors in the body, as well as the number of glucose transporters," Dr. Ivy says. His suggestions:

Start walking. "People can benefit greatly just by doing some good, brisk walking," Dr. Ivy says. But if you have diabetic neuropathy, a nervous system disorder that causes pain, tingling, or numbness in the feet and legs, walking may make you uncomfortable. If so, read on.

Get the upper hand. How? By working your upper body. Exercises such as rowing, pullups, or lifting weights are great for people over 50 because they can keep you in tip-top shape without straining your feet and legs.

Push the pedals. Bicycling is an excellent way to work your legs without overworking your feet, Dr. Ivy says.

Take the plunge. Swimming exercises just about every muscle in your body without putting pressure on your joints or limbs. If you can't swim, walk through the water, Dr. Ivy suggests.

Do it daily. You don't have to join a health club to stay in shape, Dr. Ivy insists. The trick is to look for opportunities to be active. Push that lawn mower. Take the steps instead of the elevator. Walk, don't drive, to the corner store.

Times That Try Men's (and Women's) Soles

Diabetic neuropathy can be the most uncomfortable aspect of this generally uncomfortable disease, says Richard A. Guthrie, M.D., professor of pediatrics at the University of Kansas School of Medicine, president of the Mid-America Diabetes Association, and co-author

A Cure on the Horizon?

It's virtually impossible to duplicate with drugs your body's ideal balance of blood sugar and insulin, says Richard A. Guthrie, M.D., professor of pediatrics at the University of Kansas School of Medicine, president of the Mid-America Diabetes Association, and co-author of *The Diabetes Sourcebook*. So researchers are investigating new technologies to help your body help itself.

One is an implantable sensor that can sense your blood sugar level and broadcast that information to a receiver, perhaps your wristwatch. "You can look down periodically and see what your blood sugar is," Dr. Guthrie says.

The next step will be a surgically implanted sensor, pump, and reservoir. The sensor would sense changes in blood sugar, then signal the pump to release exactly the right amount of insulin from the reservoir. Essentially this "closed-loop system" would be an artificial pancreas, Dr. Guthrie says.

Researchers also hope to grow healthy cells in the laboratory that could be transplanted into a misfunctioning pancreas. If the technical difficulties can be overcome, Dr. Guthrie says, cell transplantation could actually be a cure for diabetes.

Finally, with advances in genetics, doctors may learn to diagnose and treat diabetes long before it becomes a problem. "We will probably screen the cord blood of all newborn infants for it, just like we screen them now for thyroid dysfunctions," Dr. Guthrie says.

of *The Diabetes Sourcebook*. Caused by the nerve damage resulting from high levels of blood sugar, neuropathy can cause tingling, pain, and finally numbness in the feet and legs. "When you lose all sensation, that nerve is dead," Dr. Guthrie says.

To keep your heels on an even keel, try the following.

Peek at your feet. It's not uncommon for people with diabetes to injure their feet without even knowing it. Worse, they're particularly prone to infections. This means that little injuries can turn into big problems: Among diabetics, about 20,000 toes, feet, and legs are amputated every year. Stay on the lookout for blisters or cuts, Dr. Guthrie says. If you have a cut that won't heal or a rash that won't go away, call your doctor.

Keep your shoes on. Even if your idea of paradise is walking barefoot through the park on a hot summer day, don't take chances. Protect your feet from sharp objects by wearing shoes whenever you leave the house.

Soap those soles. You don't want to give bacteria opportunities to cause trouble. Clean your feet every day. Keep your toenails trimmed and free of ragged edges. Can't reach your feet? Ask a friend to help. Better yet, get a pedicure. Once you quit giggling, you may be hooked!

Wear soft socks. Socks made from rayon or other absorbent materials feel good and can wick away rash-causing moisture. Check your shoes, too. Shoes that don't fit can rub you the wrong way.

When Self-Care Isn't Enough

Diabetics have a pancreas that's not working at full steam and tends to slow down over time. So just about everyone with adult-onset diabetes will eventually need either synthetic insulin or drugs that make their natural insulin work more efficiently, Dr. Hollander says.

If your insulin/blood sugar balance isn't dangerously skewed, your doctor may prescribe drugs, taken orally, that will help your pancreas churn out more insulin. Called sulfonylureas, they not only boost your insulin supplies but also increase the number of insulin receptors. This makes the insulin you produce work even more efficiently.

In more advanced cases, people often need regular injections of synthetic insulin to augment their natural supplies, Dr. Hollander says. Their pancreas may recover after a few weeks or months of injections. More often, they'll need insulin injections—sometimes a little, sometimes a lot—for life.

Synthetic insulin isn't without side effects, Dr. Hollander says. For starters, it can stimulate the appetite—the last thing a diabetic wants. It may also encourage the formation of artery-clogging plaque. Finally, there's the risk of hypoglycemia, in which your supply of glucose precipitously falls, sometimes to dangerously low levels. Ask your doctor how to manage this powerful, lifesaving drug.

According to Dr. Hollander, researchers are investigating a third type of drug, alpha glycosides inhibitors, that may help slow the passage of glucose from the intestines into the bloodstream. This would give the insulin more time to prevent your blood sugar from rising to unmanageable levels. But even if alpha glycosides inhibitors don't pan out, additional drugs for diabetes clearly are needed. "Right now, we only have the oral drugs and insulin," Dr. Hollander says. "They're very good, but they can't do everything."

Emphysema

Breathe Easy Again

Emphysema is the disease that teaches you to never take your breathing for granted. It also teaches—the hard way—that smoking is about the worst thing you can do to your body.

Emphysema is caused by the body's own white blood cells chewing up the lungs. White blood cells are the shock troops of the body's immune system. When they sense "invading" smoke particles entering the lungs, they descend to gobble them up. "The problem is that white blood cells are sloppy eaters," says Robert Sandhaus, M.D., Ph.D., assistant professor of medicine at the University of Colorado Medical Center in Denver and director of the intensive care unit at Littleton Hospital in Littleton.

As these sloppy eaters do their work, they accidentally do serious and permanent damage to the lung's air sacs. Called alveoli, these sacs look like bunches of grapes. As the alveoli are destroyed, breathing gets tougher. Eventually, those with emphysema may run out of breath just walking across a room.

Love Your Lungs

Emphysema is almost totally preventable. Can you guess the number one prevention measure?

Stop smoking now. Smoking tobacco is the

cause of emphysema. So stop before it's too late. "Of people with emphysema, 99.99 percent are current or former smokers," says Dr. Sandhaus.

Stay away from smoke, period. Breathing others' smoke doesn't do your lungs any good, either. You're perfectly justified in asking smokers to light up far away from you.

Avoid air pollution. The typical pollutants from cars and factories are also irritants to your lungs, says Dr. Sandhaus. Generally, air pollution isn't as dangerous as inhaling cigarette smoke, but you'd certainly be doing your lungs a favor to dodge areas of thick pollution.

Take antioxidants. If you're at risk for emphysema, consider supplements of vitamins C and E. They're antioxidants, which may help protect a protein in the blood that can shield your lungs from the damage of sloppy-eating white blood cells. "We don't have good, solid scientific evidence that antioxidants help, but the rationale is solid, and these vitamins won't hurt you," Dr. Sandhaus says. "We usually recommend 500 milligrams twice a day of C and 800 units twice a day of E."

Consult with your doctor if you take supplements of vitamin E, because it has potential side effects, especially if you're taking blood-thinning drugs.

Living with Bad News

Exerting yourself can be a real challenge when you have emphysema. So can breathing. But challenges are made to be met. Consult your doctor, stop smoking if you haven't already, keep following the prevention measures above, and use the tips below. They'll help you feel better and enjoy the maximum possible independence.

Avoid cold air. "Cold is a trigger that can make the airways spasm shut," says Dr. Sandhaus.

Exercise moderately. And work up to the moderate level gradually. Exercise can trigger airway spasms, but moderate exercise is essential to strengthen your heart and breathing muscles. The stronger they get, the more work they can do with less oxygen. Walking is probably the best exercise. Mild calisthenics are also good. Work with your doctor on developing a safe exercise program.

Eat properly. Emphysema can make eating difficult, but don't let it prevent you from doing it right. You've got to keep up your interest in food to keep up your strength.

Drink up. Liquids keep your lung fluids thin and easy to cough up. Check with your doctor before increasing your fluid intake, though. Alcohol, by the way, shouldn't be one of those liquids. It's a central nervous system depressant that can slow breathing.

Avoid sick people. Stay away from people with colds or the flu. A lung infection will hurt you a lot more than it hurts them.

Get organized. Arrange your chores to make the best use of your energy. Think of your energy as money that you have to invest wisely. Spread big jobs around throughout the day. For example, if bathing and dressing give you the vapors, bathe before breakfast and dress afterward.

Breathe deeply. That is, breathe so that your belly, not your chest, expands with each inhalation. (Check yourself with your hand.) And wait a full second after each exhalation before inhaling again. This will help force stale air out of your lungs, so that you can breathe in fresh air.

How Your Doctor Can Help

There are treatments that can help you breathe easier and prevent complications. One such complication for many with emphysema is airflow obstruction from asthma. "The asthma part of emphysema is reversible with a bronchodilator," Dr. Sandhaus says.

Lung infections really complicate things for emphysema sufferers. "Upper respiratory tract infections make the airways spasm, and they also call white blood cells into the lungs, where they do more damage," Dr. Sandhaus says. "We make sure our patients have a stock of antibiotics at home, so that they can start them at the first sign of a lung infection."

Other medical options might include a flu shot, nasal and oral steroid sprays to reduce swelling in the airways, and diuretics to get rid of extra fluid. Supplements of the mineral potassium may also be prescribed to replace the potassium lost because of the diuretics. In the very worst cases, a portable oxygen tank may be needed.

More optimistically, a laser developed by lung specialist Akio Wakabayashi, M.D., associate professor of surgery at the University of California, Irvine, Medical Center, allows surgeons to remove the cysts that fill the lungs at the final stages of the disease. By threading the tiny laser into the lungs through a device called a thoracoscope, the cysts can be shrunk and dissolved under the pinpoint heat. Dr. Wakabayashi cites end-stage patients who, instead of dying, no longer need to be on oxygen tanks after the laser treatment.

And work has been done on ways to stop emphysema from forming in the first place. "It won't reverse the destruction that has already taken place, but it will prevent additional destruction," Dr. Sandhaus says.

Fatigue

Energy-Boosting Strategies

Even after five or six decades on this planet, nobody wants to feel tired all the time. If you do, your spouse may say it's all in your head, even though you're tired down to your toes. Your doctor may say it's not chronic fatigue syndrome, not anemia, not anxiety disorder—not any of fatigue's usual suspects. So what's causing you to feel like you're walking through life underwater?

It could be lots of things. Lack of exercise, poor sleep, or boredom can cause long-term fatigue. Many diseases and medical conditions can cause chronic tiredness (a good reason not to ignore fatigue as a symptom). But for ordinary, run-of-the-mill fatigue—the kind you might get from burning the candle at both ends, so to speak—there are things you can try to get your engine started again.

Moving and Shaking

You sit behind a desk all day. You go to bed by nine. You never overexert yourself. Yet you're always tired. How can that be?

Experts agree that not being active can make you feel lethargic and fatigued. "It's common sense," says D. W. Edington, Ph.D., director of the Fitness Research Center at the University of Michigan in Ann Arbor. "The body at rest tends to remain at rest."

Regular exercise, on the other hand, can make you more energetic, not only in the long run but on the spot. What's more, the benefits can last for hours, says Robert Thayer, Ph.D., psychology professor at California State University in Long Beach. So if you're fatigued at 50 (or 70), use the following tips to get moving. (If you've been inactive up until now, consult your doctor before jumping into any exercise program.)

Ease into it. The "no pain, no gain" theory has no place for older adults already pained by fatigue. Start out slowly and advance gradually, says Dr. Thayer. A brisk walk, for example, is a good beginning energy booster.

Choose the right workout. Vigorous aerobic exercise such as a 30-minute session at an aerobics class will eventually be a great fatigue-fighter when done regularly, but that kind of exercise wears you out right after you do it. That's another reason those brisk walks are so good for beginners—you feel more energetic right away.

Make a date. Exercise works best when it's regular, and it's much easier to exercise regularly if you have a set schedule for doing it. To help you stick to your exercise program, set aside a specific 30 minutes several times a week.

Don't overdo it. How hard should you push yourself? As a guide, try the "talk test." If you can't talk comfortably while you're exercising, you're probably working too hard. Any kind of pain—either while exercising or the day after—means you're probably pushing yourself too hard. And, of course, if you experience chest pains or dizziness, it's time to get off the track and into your doctor's office.

Beware the midnight oil. Sure, some people can exercise at any hour and still get plenty of sleep. But for most, late-night workouts turn into all-night insomnia. Avoid vigorous exercise before bedtime, doctors say.

Rude Awakenings

Early to bed and early to rise is a good fatigue-beating policy. But if the quality of your sleep is poor, you're coming out behind.

An often undetected cause of fatigue is called obstructive sleep apnea, which is most common for those in their fifties, expecially men. If you suffer from sleep apnea, your throat tissue "collapses" during sleep, causing your breathing to stop for 20 to 40 seconds at a time. Each episode is accompanied by a brief awakening. Multiply this by hundreds of times a night, and you can see why some people with apnea feel so tired all the time.

If you suspect you have sleep apnea (loud snoring might be a sign), see your doctor. He may refer you to a specialist in sleep disorders, who may recommend drugs or surgery to correct the problem. Meanwhile, lose weight if you need to, because extra tissue in the neck and throat, combined with poor muscle tone, can restrict the movement of air through the upper airway. And remember that alcohol's depressant effect increases muscle relaxation and enhances airway blockage. Skipping alcohol can improve your overall sleep quality, boosting the next day's energy levels.

Another sleep problem that affects at least 15 percent of Americans over 50 (compared to 8 percent of the overall population) is what doctors call periodic leg movements, or nocturnal myoclonus. These nighttime leg movements can be anything from a toe flex to a full-fledged kick—sure to catch a bed partner's attention.

Sleep disorder experts aren't sure what causes

Breathe Away Fatigue

Tired? Maybe it's your breathing.

Doctors suggest that many fatigued patients may have a condition called hyperventilation syndrome, in which shallow, rapid breaths cause excessive carbon dioxide loss and insufficient oxygen flow through the body. In other words, you breathe quickly, but you get less air.

Lots of things can cause hyperventilation syndrome, including anemia, diabetes, heart and kidney disease, and stress. Another possible culprit is good posture. That's right—*good* posture. According to Robert Fried, Ph.D., director of the Institute for Rational Emotive Therapy in New York City and author of *The Breath Connection*, people who keep their stomach firmly tucked in when they stand up straight may be tensing the diaphragm muscles, making it difficult to take in a full breath.

How's your breathing? Put one hand on your chest and the other on your abdomen. If your hands don't rise with each breath, you may be hyperventilating. You can "relearn" proper breathing techniques, says Dr. Fried, simply by relaxing your tummy and keeping your mouth closed. When you breathe through the nose, it's virtually impossible to hyperventilate because the nasal passages are too narrow. So you're breathing easier, and recouping some of that lost energy as well.

these involuntary movements. Some suspect lower back injuries, while others suspect central nervous system problems. What they do know is that these movements, which can occur hundreds of times a night, may cause fatigue. So if you suspect your legs are doing laps while the rest of you is sound asleep, see your doctor. Periodic leg movements can't always be eliminated, but taking medication can help reduce the number of awakenings during the night, thus reducing fatigue.

Not Enough Stress?

Sure, stress can cause fatigue. But so can a lack of stress, in the form of what we might call "excitement." "It's sort of like the tension on a violin string," explains Paul J. Rosch, M.D., president of the American Institute of Stress. "If you have too much tension, the string is going to break. If you don't have enough tension, it's not going to make any music."

Here's how to get yourself in tune.

Restress. "You have to find out what works for you," says Dr. Rosch. "Some people leave everything to the last minute, so they can get that little surge of adrenaline."

Get involved. A lack of creative engagement can be more taxing than doing too much, says Dennis T. Jaffe, Ph.D., author of *Take This Job and Love It*. Try getting involved in more things, he suggests. Brush up on your Shakespeare. Give a speech at Toastmasters. Take up swimming or tennis.

Help somebody else. "I used to write prescriptions for becoming a volunteer," says John Renner, M.D., president of the Consumer Health Information Research Institute in Kansas City, Missouri. "I recommend that you get into something where you are needed. Work with children, or work with an agency that needs your help." Getting interested in others' lives, he says, can add oomph to your own.

Lose It Right

Being overweight is fatiguing, but so is eating poorly. Weight-loss diets and being too rushed to eat properly are open invitations to fatigue. You're not taking in enough calories to sustain your body's normal functions.

So what happens? "The body starts to live off itself," says Manfred Kroger, Ph.D., professor of food science at Pennsylvania State University in University Park. "This whole process is abnormal and very stressful to the body, and one of the many symptoms of this type of stress is fatigue."

By all means, lose the weight if you need to. But lose it without losing energy. Here are two keys for doing that:

Forgo the fat. Calories from fat in foods are more easily turned into body fat than those from proteins or carbohydrates. Plus, fats contain more calories per gram of food. Replace fatty foods with high-carbohydrate foods like fruits, vegetables, grains, and pasta. That will give you an edge in losing weight without reducing energy.

Lose in moderation. It's reasonable to lose 1 or 2 pounds a week. Any more than that is getting risky. Drastic weight loss, doctors say, only increases your chances for feeling fatigued.

Hearing Loss

Our Deafening Society

Hearing loss is mainly about noise, not age. The roar of modern life is making us deaf before our time.

In fact, in the best of all worlds, such a time would never come. A study of Bedouin tribespeople in northern Africa showed that people well into their eighties could hear as well as ten-year-old children. That's because they don't have to listen to much beyond sheep bleating and camels grunting and children playing, not the jackhammers and power drills and 18-wheelers and amplified music we live with.

Yes, collecting years helps hearing loss along, but it still amounts to only a fraction of the damage caused by noise, says John S. Turner, Jr., M.D., head of otolaryngology at Emory University in Atlanta and chief of otolaryngology–head and neck surgery at the Emory Clinic.

"It's to be expected that as you age, you'll have physical changes in your ears, nerves, and brain that will begin to impair your hearing," Dr. Turner says. "It's unusual to reach your late seventies without some degree of hearing impairment, but most of the impairment should be minor, usually at the high-frequency end of the hearing spectrum. That means trouble communicating with women and children, who have higher pitched voices."

Another way your 50-plus years contribute to

hearing loss is simply the cumulative effect of all that noise. "Noise damage is additive," Dr. Turner says. "It builds up over the years, gradually destroying your sense of hearing. We often see hunters who have lost much of their hearing by age 50 because of the noise of shotguns."

Noise over 90 decibels stimulates the cells in your inner ears that conduct sound to the auditory nerve. "It exhausts the chemicals in the cells," Dr. Turner says. "If it's just a brief exposure, the cells can recover. But if the noise lasts a few hours, the damage is permanent. The cells are destroyed; they've done so much work they burn themselves out."

What's "over 90 decibels"? Well, a screaming child can hit 115, and a jackhammer 120. A firing gun blasts out 140 decibels, and a firecracker 160.

The Big Turnoff

Hearing loss is preventable, Dr. Turner says. Since noise is the top cause, it makes sense that turning down the volume can save your hearing. Here are the best things you can do to protect your ears from deafening noise.

Wear ear protection. Earplugs and earmuffs have become standard equipment in many noisy jobs. But if you're exposed to loud noise for long periods of time off the job—by using a power mower, weed whacker, or chain saw, for example—make ear protectors a habit. Don't worry that you won't hear what you have to: Ear protectors can sometimes improve hearing in a noisy environment by filtering out extraneous noise.

Protect your head. Head injuries from car, motorcycle, and bicycle accidents are a common cause of hearing loss. "The impact compresses the inner ear fluid, which then squeezes against the hair cells so strongly it damages them," Dr. Turner says. So wear your seat belt and helmets.

Turn it down. Long hours listening to music at high volume can definitely damage your hearing, Dr. Turner says. Problem is, members of the first rock and roll generation now working their way through their fifties may have a different idea of what "low volume" means than their parents did when they screamed for you to "Turn it down!" Most experts consider 80 decibels the cutoff point for hearing safety, but a survey of music headset users found that their listening volumes ranged up to 102 decibels. So here's your guideline from Dr. Turner: If you can't carry on a normal conversation while wearing a headset, it's too loud. On a scale of 1 to 10, the maximum setting should not be above 4.

Don't be a fathead. Saturated fat can block the tiny arteries feeding your ears just as it does the big arteries that feed your heart. The inadequate blood flow that results keeps your ears from recovering from noise damage as quickly as they should. So watch your diet, for your ears' sake as well as your heart's.

Balance your diet. Eating well goes beyond cutting back on fat. Zinc, calcium, magnesium, and vitamin A all have been shown to benefit the sense of hearing. These nutrients are readily available in a healthy, balanced diet.

Keep the top up. If you drive long distances with the top down on your convertible, or the windows open, or on motorcycle, you're getting blasted with perhaps as much as 90 decibels worth of wind noise, Dr. Turner estimates. While that's within the range of safety set by the Occupational Safety and Health Administration, those standards are general, and your ears may be more sensitive.

Tinnitus: Don't Answer That!

That ringing you hear isn't the phone. It's your ears. And for some people with tinnitus, the ringing seldom stops. Dr. Turner estimates that one in ten Americans between the ages of 65 and 74 has this condition.

"It's with you day and night," Dr. Turner says. "It ranges from merely an annoyance to—in about 15 percent of the cases—real interference with work and life." Tinnitus is often a sign of deterioration of hearing, Dr. Turner says, although you can have one without the other. Exactly what's creating the ringing is unclear, but one theory suggests that the inner ear's sensitive hair cells get so overwhelmed with the work of transmitting noise that they start misfiring.

"Tinnitus is a monumental problem, even more than hearing loss, because there's very little that can be done to help," Dr. Turner says. "There's no medical or surgical treatment." There aren't even any safe drugs. The few that help put you at risk of heart arrhythmia, or irregular heartbeat.

So what are your options? "The only proven thing you can do is prevent it," Dr. Turner says. Since noise is the most common cause of tinnitus, using the above guidelines for avoiding excessive noise will help your prevention effort. But if tinnitus is already ringing in your ears, try out the following tips for muffling the bells:

Turn up the white noise. White noise is a kind of sound you hear when the TV station you're watching signs off for the night. There are machines that duplicate this sound, which masks the ringing of tinnitus in about 50 percent of the cases, Dr. Turner says.

Try a hearing aid. Studies show up to two-thirds of people who've tried them report reduction or total elimination of tinnitus. Why? No one knows for sure, but it may be that amplified outside noise masks the inner noise. Or at least for people whose hearing is normal or near normal, the noise produced by the hearing aid's electronic circuitry may cancel out the tinnitus.

Add noise. A tinnitus masker looks like a hearing aid but produces either a wide or narrow band of noise. You can control how wide the spectrum is and the volume. This manufactured noise drowns out the noise of tinnitus.

It's been proven effective for up to half of the people who've tried it, but the only way to know if it will work for you is to try it yourself. Your doctor can prescribe a unit, and you should be given a month-long trial to see if it's the right one for you. Some of the people who use maskers find that they have what's called residual inhibition when they don't wear the masker—a period of time when the tinnitus is totally gone. Then it gradually returns.

Give it feedback. Biofeedback training can teach you to relax to the point that your tinnitus may become more tolerable. Studies show that the majority of tinnitus sufferers benefit from biofeedback; they sleep better and need fewer tranquilizers and antidepressants.

Pack away the cigarettes. The relationship of smoking to tinnitus is much less direct than that of noise, Dr. Turner says, but the association is there nonetheless. "We think it may constrict the blood vessels feeding the inner ear, which would harm the nerve cells," he says. "And smoking definitely aggravates existing hearing problems."

Rethink your drinks. Caffeine is a well-known blood-vessel constrictor. So use it in moderation if you have tinnitus. Limit your coffee, tea, and cola. Besides caffeinated drinks, red wine, tonic water (quinine), and grain-based spirits may also aggravate tinnitus. To find out which drinks affect you, try keeping a diary of what you drink and how it relates to tinnitus attacks.

Assess your aspirin. "Aspirin is the leading cause of hearing loss and tinnitus when it comes to medication," Dr. Turner says. "But it's strictly individual. Some people with arthritis have to take large amounts before they get any tinnitus or hearing loss, while my wife can take just one and get ringing in her ears." When you stop taking aspirin, or reduce the amount, the tinnitus usually disappears, and your hearing returns to normal. If you think aspirin may be causing your problem, Dr. Turner advises switching to ibuprofen or acetaminophen.

Check the diagnosis. Tinnitus sometimes has a medical cause, which can be an aneurysm or a narrowing in blood vessels, high triglycerides in your blood, or even excessive earwax. It's best to check with your doctor to get a proper diagnosis. Above all, don't give up hope. Up to three-fourths of people with tinnitus say it improves over time.

High-Tech Help

Some experts say that hearing aids may soon become as common as glasses, as people grow more comfortable with admitting their hearing isn't what it used to be. These people will come from the ranks of baby boomers, who grew up in the world's noisiest civilization. In fact, our rock and roll culture has dropped the average age for first-time hearing aid wearers from 60 to 50.

So if you can't hear normal conversation clearly, it's time to listen up: Have your doctor first check you out and then recommend an audiologist.

How I Did It: Hearing Life Again

As a 54-year-old teacher, Eleanor Schwarz would hear laughter from her students when she answered their questions. "I soon realized I was answering something they hadn't asked," she says. "I was having trouble hearing them."

Her hearing problem worsened, but no doctor could discover the cause. Though Schwarz got along for some years with hearing aids, her impairment reached the point where she had only 4 percent of her hearing left. She began to take sign-language instruction and felt increasingly isolated from her husband, family, and friends.

Then in walked good old American know-how, in the form of a cochlear implant. Unlike hearing aids, which magnify sound to reach the inner ear, cochlear implants have tiny wires with electrodes that are surgically inserted into the inner ear to transmit sound energy. The sounds that result aren't normal, so Schwarz had some interpretive skills to learn after she got her implant at the age of 68.

A cochlear implant is expensive and not for everybody, but it worked for Eleanor Schwarz. "It has made all the difference in the world," she says. "I stopped having to learn sign language. I can talk on the telephone now, although it's hard to understand strangers. I do still have to use lip-reading, but now I can hear people talking when they're behind me. I can hear birds, rain, water running. You don't realize what you've lost until you regain it."

The good news is that the digital revolution in music technology has worked its wonders on hearing aids. New digitally programmable aids use a computer-generated signal that you can adjust with a remote-control device like the one controlling your TV. As with the finest stereo equipment, you can add bass or treble, "warm" the tone, or filter out background noise.

Behind-the-ear aids have an earpiece molded to fit in the bowl of your outer ear and a power pack worn behind the ear. They're large and moderately powerful for moderate to profound hearing loss. Even more powerful are hearing aids that connect the earpiece to an amplifier you carry in your clothing. All that juice is best for the most profound hearing loss.

Some aids can now fit into your ear canal where other people can't see them easily. But their minute size makes them difficult to manipulate and care for. For example, their batteries are tiny and hard to change, so people with arthritis in their hands may have a particularly difficult time. In-the-ear aids aren't as expensive as digital aids but cost more than behind-the-ear and on-the body aids.

Even better than aids would be a cure, and that may be on the way. Scientists had always believed that once the ear's hair cells were destroyed, they couldn't grow back and hearing was gone forever. But recently, researchers discovered that these hair cells can regenerate in animals. "The question now is, can we regenerate them in man?" says Bill Brownell, Ph.D., a researcher at the Johns Hopkins Center for Hearing and Balance in Baltimore, whose work is defining the cutting edge of otology.

It's a big question, admittedly. But if researchers can find the genetic factors that turn off cell growth after the ear is formed in the womb, they may be able to restart the growth process and regenerate damaged cells. In a sense, scientists may one day be able to grow you a new pair of ears.

Heart Disease

How to Avoid Ticker Shock

Genetic research has provided some new answers to some old problems about heart disease. But it's also prompted a new question from people in their fifties and sixties: "Why should I bother changing my bacon-crunching lifestyle if it's the genes that are gonna get me anyway?"

The truth is that what you do or don't do with your life makes a big difference, genes or no genes. "There's no way you can avoid the genetic inheritance that predisposes you to heart attack," says Edward D. Frohlich, M.D., vice president of academic affairs with the Alton Ochsner Medical Foundation in New Orleans and chairman of the American Heart Association's council for high blood pressure research. "But you have abundant opportunities to overcome other risk factors that multiply your inherited risk."

In other words, by concentrating on what you can do rather than what you can't help, you can significantly lower your risk of heart disease. Declining death rates from heart disease show that lots of people have gotten that message. But it's still the number one killer in the United States. About one in four Americans has some form of cardiovascular disease to deal with (*cardio* refers to the heart, *vascular* to the blood vessels).

Public Enemy No. 1

To prevent heart disease, it helps to know how you get it. A good starting point is atherosclerosis, resulting from deposits of cholesterol, calcium, and scar tissue, along with cellular growth, in the coronary arteries.

This hardening of the arteries is responsible for most heart disease in America and for more than 90 percent of all heart attacks, says Virgil Brown, M.D., professor of medicine at Emory University in Atlanta and president of the American Heart Association.

The first noticeable sign of atherosclerosis is often an angina attack—a crushing, burning, or squeezing pain in the chest that radiates to the left arm, neck, jaw, or shoulder blade. The pain comes when the heart needs more blood after exertion, a large meal, emotional excitement, or exposure to cold but can't get it because the arteries are too "hardened" with other debris to allow for the free flow of blood. Angina may feel like a heart attack to its victims, but it's usually only a warning. With a real heart attack, there's enough blood blockage to actually kill part of the heart muscle.

Such serious blockage does not occur overnight. It's the long-term result of atherosclerosis. Year after year, the coronary artery narrows as those deposits grow along the arterial wall. Finally, one unhappy day, the tiny remaining tunnel gets stuffed up with a blood clot. No blood reaches a part of the heart, and that part begins to suffocate. Next thing you know, you're in the hospital . . . or the morgue. (For more on atherosclerosis, see Killer Accomplices on page 555.)

Don't think for a minute that this clogging of the arteries is normal with aging, says Dr. Brown. In cultures where risk factors are low, people live to old age without significant clogging in their arteries. As a result, they have healthier hearts. "In fact, most people in our own culture can live into their nineties without heart disease if they live right," says Dr. Brown.

The Top 10 Ways to Prevent Heart Disease

There are so many things that people in their fifties and beyond can do for their heart that we dedicated two entire sections of this book almost exclusively to lifestyle strategies you can use to cut down your risk of heart disease and cancer (see part 2, The Age Extenders Arsenal, and part 3, A Lifestyle of Longevity). But according to one poll of hundreds of top cardiologists, the most vital heart-saving measures are those listed here. Depending on what you're already doing, you can choose what to add to your own strategy.

Cut your cholesterol. There's a one-in-three chance that the amount of total cholesterol swimming around in your blood is borderline high—that is, between 200 and 239 milligrams per deciliter. Such levels hike your risk of dying from coronary heart disease (the kind of heart disease caused by clogged coronary arteries) by 70 percent. If your cholesterol level is 240 or more, as it is in one in four Americans, your death risk goes up a terrifying 200 percent. At those levels, you'd have plenty of company at the morgue: The federal

Centers for Disease Control in Atlanta estimates that high cholesterol levels alone cause more than 300,000 needless deaths each year, making it the number one contributor to fatal heart attacks in America.

According to the National Cholesterol Education Project, you should aim for a total cholesterol level of less than 200, but many doctors say you should aim even lower. "Clearly 150 would be much better, because about four billion people on this earth have a cholesterol level of 150, and they don't get cardiovascular disease," says William Castelli, M.D., epidemiologist, medical director of the Framingham Cardiovascular Institute, and former director of the landmark Framingham Heart Study in Massachusetts.

How do you lower your cholesterol level? Start with cutting down on the two things in your diet most related to high blood cholesterol: cholesterol-rich foods, and foods high in saturated fat. The two mostly fall into the category of fatty meats, dairy products, and junk foods. (For more on lowering your cholesterol level, see High Cholesterol on page 450.)

Get up and go. Experts say that inactivity is the number two source of fatal heart attacks in America. By virtue of being an American, there's a better than one-in-three chance that you're not getting the exercise you need. A sedentary lifestyle gives you a 90 percent higher chance of dying from a heart attack.

We're not talking about heavy-duty training. "The message has been confused," says Thomas Kottke, M.D., a cardiologist at the Mayo Clinic in Rochester, Minnesota. "The average person is so sedentary that any exercise other than flipping through the channels or cracking a beer is great," he says. In fact, a brisk walk 20 minutes a day would make a major impact.

How I Did It: Life Before Lifestyle

Bob Finnell was living the American dream: a high-powered executive position, more frequent flyer miles than a Canada goose, gourmet meals, 40 extra pounds of fat, a heart attack. . . .

When that attack came during a Labor Day hike in Yosemite National Park, Finnell didn't think the wooziness and weakness was a heart attack. But some weeks later he saw a picture of his heart blockage, so he began to study up on heart disease. Convinced that his high-fat, high-cholesterol diet was mostly to blame, Finnell hesitated at the bypass surgery his doctor had recommended. "I realized that if I went through with the bypass, I could very easily go back to the same old habits," he says.

Instead, he got into an experimental study on re-

Lower the pressure. The chances are one in eight that your systolic blood pressure (the first number in the reading) is between 140 and 159. If so, you have a 70 percent higher chance of developing a blocked coronary artery that can lead to a heart attack. If it's higher than 159, the odds against surviving a heart attack are raised by almost 200 percent. No wonder high blood pressure is the third-leading cause of fatal heart attacks in the United States.

The time to start controlling your blood pressure was at age 20, but the benefits of lowering your blood pressure are still there at ages 50, 60, and beyond. Control your weight, cut down on dietary sodium if you're sodium sensitive (as many as one in three people are, according to Dr. Frohlich), and reduce your alcohol

versing heart disease supervised by Dean Ornish, M.D., who was then assistant clinical professor of medicine at the University of California, San Francisco. Dr. Ornish taught Finnell a completely different lifestyle, including exercise, relaxation, and a diet that cost him about $5 a day. "That wouldn't have paid for my appetizers before," he says.

Now Finnell walks for 1 hour five or six mornings a week. He does yoga and relaxation every day. Yes, his life has been restricted in some ways (he can never return to full-time work), but expanded in others. "I read much more," he says. "I've learned languages, I travel for leisure, I spend time with friends." And he's at his army-discharge weight. The only vestige of Bob's former lifestyle is a 1,000-bottle wine cellar, which he still dips into—but only on occasion.

consumption to no more than two drinks a day. (For lots more on lowering high blood pressure, see High Blood Pressure on page 435.)

Lose that excess baggage. Clothes fitting a little tighter each year? You're not alone. More than two-thirds of Americans are overweight. Those who are 30 percent or more overweight have double the chances of dropping dead from a heart attack. But being only 10 or 20 percent above your ideal weight is no cause to rejoice: You're giving a heart attack a 50 percent better chance to kill you. Excess weight, say the experts, is the number four cause of fatal heart attacks in the nation. (For advice on losing those extra pounds, see Overweight on page 482.)

Stop smoking. If you're a smoker, you're about twice as likely to have coronary heart disease and heart attacks—and you have a 70 percent greater chance of dying from a heart attack. One study traced half the heart attacks in middle-aged women to smoking. Why? Doctors think that breathing in smoke makes your blood clot more easily. Also, smoking adds to the likelihood that you'll have high blood pressure and high cholesterol. Quit and the benefits come very quickly.

Stop smoking smokers' smoke. They call it passive smoking, but it really does an active job on your heart. Secondhand smoke kills over 35,000 Americans a year via heart disease, estimates Stanton Glantz, Ph.D., professor of medicine at the University of California, San Francisco. "Nonsmokers married to smokers have a 30 percent increase in risk of dying from heart disease over nonsmokers married to nonsmokers," she says.

Take aspirin. Aspirin is rapidly becoming a mainstay in heart attack prevention. By making blood platelets slippery instead of sticky, aspirin cuts down on clotting. A six-year study of 88,000 female nurses found that the risk of a first heart attack was 25 percent lower in the women who took one to six aspirins per week than in those who did not take aspirin, says JoAnn Manson, M.D., assistant professor of medicine at Harvard Medical School and associate physician at Brigham and Women's Hospital in Boston. But you may be able to benefit from much less. Richard Milani, M.D., a cardiologist at the Ochsner Clinic in New Orleans, says that your optimum protection can come from half a baby aspirin taken daily or from a whole one taken every other day.

Don't go blithely popping aspirin and think that will solve your problem. "Aspirin should serve only as an adjunct to controlling other risk factors, like smoking, cholesterol, diabetes, high blood pressure, and overweight," Dr. Manson cautions. "And nobody should start treating themselves regularly with aspirin without first consulting their doctor." Although aspirin is usually safe, it's potentially dangerous for people with stomach problems (especially ulcers), hemophiliacs, and those already taking blood-thinning medications. Aspirin's ability to make your stomach upset or bleed can be reduced by taking it with meals or with a full 8 ounces of water and by using coated aspirin.

Open up with omega-3. Several studies have documented the positive effects of this unique fat on opening up your arteries. It's been found to lower total cholesterol and LDL (the "bad" cholesterol) levels, reduce the blood's clotting ability, and possibly help lower blood pressure. Cold-water fish, like salmon and mackerel, have the most omega-3, but all fish have some.

The only rich nonfish source of omega-3 is flax seed. "Flax seed is about 35 percent oil, and more than half of that oil is omega-3, more than you can get from fish," says Jack Carter, Ph.D., agronomist at North Dakota State University and president of the Flax Institute of the United States. Dr. Carter gets his daily dose of omega-3 by stirring 3 heaping tablespoons of flaxseed meal into his morning orange juice. He also bakes the meal into muffins and breads, which gives them a pleasant, nutty taste. You can buy the whole seed in health food stores, but the meal must be kept in the freezer. Cold-pressed flax oil is also good for salads but it's too sensitive to heat to be good for cooking.

Live longer with love. In a *Prevention* magazine survey, 64 percent of the cardiologists polled said learning to enjoy love and friendship was "important," "very important," or "extremely important" in preventing heart disease. Robert Rosenson, M.D., co-director of Preventive Cardiology at Rush Presbyterian

Hospital–St. Luke's Medical Center in Chicago, has added a therapist to his staff to come to his patients' emotional rescue. "I have patients who are overweight and inactive and resist positive lifestyle changes," he says. "And there may be some depression or low self-esteem there that I can't do much about as a cardiologist."

Consider hormones. Postmenopausal women are more at risk for heart disease because they stop producing estrogen. Estrogen replacement seems to help keep arteries clean by keeping cholesterol levels in check. Remember, though, that while estrogen can do your heart good (and is a proven osteoporosis preventer), it can also increase your risk of breast cancer. "We're not ready yet to make a blanket recommendation that says all postmenopausal women should take estrogen," says Frank Sacks, M.D., assistant professor of medicine at Harvard Medical School. Make the decision to take estrogen only after consulting with your doctor about your particular needs, weighing the benefits for your heart and bones against your risk of breast cancer.

When There's No Other Choice

If you have heart disease, it was probably a doctor who first told you about it. Stick with a doctor. He or she will likely tell you to lose weight, exercise, and learn to relax, but you may need more. Doctors have a wide range of drugs and surgical procedures to call on to treat heart disease.

The kind of medications for heart disease vary greatly, depending on specific conditions. Many people with high blood pressure, for example, also have high cholesterol levels. The drugs given for these disorders have to be carefully balanced and stringently monitored to prevent or reduce side effects. At all times you must

Artificial Vessels for Life

They answer the phone with a breezy "Plastic lab!" but they're not perfecting beach balls. They're letting the air out of synthetic blood vessels, a research advance that can overcome one of the major stumbling blocks in heart disease treatment.

Most people have coronary bypass surgery using their own vessels, which themselves can eventually get plugged up, requiring further surgery. "The reason for the bypass in the first place is because the person has arterial disease, and it's often throughout their body," says physiologist Bruce Klitzman, Ph.D., director of Duke University's Plastic Surgery Research Laboratories. "So you're replacing a very bad vessel with one that's only a little bit bad."

Synthetic vessels have had a similar problem. The Teflon material they're made from is 70 percent air. And when blood contacts air, it clots.

So Dr. Klitzman and his team devised two methods of removing the air from synthetic vessels: soaking it out with acetone, and squeezing it out with pressure. Their success bodes well not only for coronary bypasses but also for bold new forays into artificial organs.

"What called a screeching halt to the artificial heart was clotting," Dr. Klitzman says. "The more we understand about how blood reacts to synthetic materials, the better we can design a variety of artificial organs." This means an artificial heart that won't produce stroke-causing blood clots.

communicate with your doctor, who needs your feed-back to find the drugs and dosages that work best for you.

Sometimes your heart's arteries may be so blocked with plaque that a trip to the hospital is your only recourse. Here's a look at the three common hospital procedures for heart disease.

Angioplasty is a procedure in which doctors try to reopen a clogged blood vessel. In balloon angio-plasty, they insert a tiny balloon into the artery and in-flate it. The balloon squashes the deposit against the artery wall, making more room for blood to flow. In cold-laser angioplasty, a laser beam literally vaporizes the plaque. Angioplasty is safer than bypass surgery, but there can still be serious complications. Roughly 1 in 100 angioplasty patients requires emergency bypass surgery because of such complications.

The "success" rate for both balloon and cold-laser angioplasty is about 96 percent, says James Tcheng, M.D., assistant professor of medicine at Duke University. But success is measured by whether the artery is opened up at all, not by how long the opening lasts. In 30 to 40 percent of the people receiving an angio-plasty, the arteries become blocked up again, usually within six months, says Dr. Tcheng.

Atherectomy, like cold-laser angioplasty, is a rel-atively new procedure. It opens your artery like Roto-Rooter does your plumbing, albeit with more finesse. A motorized device the size of a matchstick with a miniature drill attached to the end is slipped into the artery through a pencil-size plastic sheath. The drill shaves away the plaque on the artery wall. The shav-ings fall into a little receptacle, which is removed through the sheath.

"Atherectomy holds promise for people with

blockages of the largest coronary artery," says Jeff Brinker, M.D., associate professor of medicine at Johns Hopkins Medical Institutions in Baltimore. It can cut the reblockage rate in half, he says.

Bypass surgery is open-heart surgery. Surgeons take a blood vessel from another part of the body and use it to construct a detour around the blocked artery. Serious business, the bypass should only be done when the heart arteries have multiple blockages or after all other attempts to clear the arteries have failed. In a nonemergency bypass, the risk of a fatal complication is usually less than 1 in 50. Proceed with caution and always get a second opinion.

High Blood Pressure

Go with the Healthy Flow

Like poet Carl Sandburg's fog, high blood pressure silently steals in on little cat feet. It seems to come out of nowhere. There are no symptoms. Its cause is a mystery.

What's not a mystery is the damage high blood pressure can do. Untreated, it can lead to heart problems, stroke, and kidney disease, among other afflictions.

The only way to know if you're one of the nearly 60 million Americans with high blood pressure is to get tested. Blood pressure tests are simple, painless, and often free. (You can find blood pressure measuring machines in many department stores and malls as well as in doctors' offices.) Experts say persons over 50 should have their pressure checked at least every two years, and more often if you've been diagnosed with high blood pressure.

What the Numbers Show

Your blood pressure measurement has two numbers. The higher number (called systolic) is the pressure exerted when your heart muscle beats—that is, when the muscle contracts to squeeze blood out through the arteries. The lower number (diastolic) measures the pressure when the muscle is relaxed, allowing blood to flow back into the heart. If someone were to tell you that your blood pressure is 110/75 (said "110 over 75"), that would mean that your systolic pressure is 110 and your diastolic pressure is 75.

Blood pressure tends to rise with age, so a "normal" reading for you now may be higher than what it was decades ago. Furthermore, what's normal for one person isn't for another. In general, however, for most adults, a normal blood pressure is a diastolic (bottom number) reading of less than 85 and a systolic reading of less than 140.

A diastolic reading of 85 to 89 is considered "high normal," but one over 90 clearly qualifies as high blood pressure. On the systolic side, a reading of 140 to 159 is usually considered borderline; above 160 is high. Because of the different factors involved, even a high normal or a borderline reading should be carefully discussed with your doctor.

The Risks You Can't Control

Although doctors can't be certain what causes high blood pressure (also called hypertension), there are several risk factors closely associated with it. Some you can't control. And, unfortunately, aging is at the top of that uncontrollable list.

Perhaps more than 60 percent of Americans between the ages of 65 and 74 have high blood pressure. "If you're an adult man, you have a better than one-in-five chance of developing high blood pressure," says Edward D. Frohlich, M.D., chairman of the American Heart Association's council for high blood pressure research and vice president of academic affairs with the Alton Ochsner Medical Foundation in New Orleans.

Genetics is another uncontrollable risk. High blood pressure tends to run in families, and black families are especially susceptible. "If you're an adult black man, the odds of developing high blood pressure approach 40 percent," Dr. Frohlich says. Whatever your race, if you have a family history of high blood pressure, you should begin to have it checked early in life, he says.

Then there's gender. Men are more at risk until about age 65. But in the golden years, women catch up and then pass the men.

Blood Pressure Reducers

You can't choose your age, gender, or family, but there are many things you can do to beat hypertension. "High blood pressure is largely a disorder of lifestyle," says John Martin, Ph.D., clinical psychologist and high blood pressure researcher at San Diego State University. The three most important things you can change

How I Did It: Never Too Old

Bob Schoenberg will always remember the Thanksgiving he spent in an emergency room recovering from his second heart attack. For 30 years, Schoenberg took diuretics but his blood pressure was still borderline high and probably linked to his heart attack. If it remained high, his doctors said, he might have another heart attack. Lying on the table in the ER that Thanksgiving, the man from Fair Lawn, New Jersey, made a promise to himself: "I decided right there I was not going to die. I was going to turn it around."

Schoenberg had been an active bowler, hiker, and skier for most of his 72 years, but he describes his past diet as "typically unhealthy," consisting largely of pizza, cheeseburgers, and fried foods. To lower his blood pressure, he learned, he would have to change that diet and de-stress his life.

So over the next six to eight months he gradually stopped eating meat, most dairy products, and salt. He gave up caffeine. He took up yoga, meditation, and deep-breathing exercises. He even learned that something as simple as chewing his food more slowly could have a calming effect. "I look at things entirely differently now," he says.

Did it work? And how! Schoenberg lost 45 pounds and lowered his blood pressure enough for his doctor to take him off the diuretics. It's now 120/70, a healthy 20 points below what it was when he was on medication.

In fact, life in general has changed for the better, even in some unexpected ways. "My bowling average has jumped 13 points," Schoenberg says.

are your waistline, your physical fitness, and your level of stress, he says.

Send those pounds packing. Of all the controllable risk factors, body weight is the most closely associated with high blood pressure, Dr. Frohlich says. If you are overweight and have high blood pressure, losing weight may bring your blood pressure down to normal. Or at least you may be able to reduce your dosage of hypertension medication.

The best protection against high blood pressure is to never get overweight in the first place, says Edward Freis, M.D., chief of the Hypertension Clinic at the Veterans Administration Center in Washington, D.C. Thin people don't develop high blood pressure nearly as often as the overweight. To control your weight, watch your diet, get lots of exercise, and read Overweight on page 482 of this book.

Get moving. Get up off that BarcaLounger. Get out of that car. Get out of that office. Move your body. Walk. Run. Lift weights. Pull weeds and plant tulips. Do something physical. For the vast majority of people who have high blood pressure—and for those who want to prevent it—being active may be the ticket.

Why does exercise work? Certainly it helps to keep off those extra pounds, but there's more to it than that. "The exact mechanism is not clear, but it may well be that the amount of inactivity many of us have been accustomed to is simply unnatural from a biological point of view," says Dr. Martin. "A certain level of physical movement may be necessary to keep the body's blood-pressure-regulating mechanisms working as they should." Scientists now know, for example, that small arteries can begin to shut down through lack of physical activity and that blood-pressure-regulating hormones can be adversely affected.

Find your level. Getting active doesn't mean you have to run marathons. In one study done by Dr. Martin and colleagues at the Veterans Administration Medical Center in Jackson, Mississippi, the people exercised at levels well within their comfort zone. "That exercise consisted of either walking, jogging, or cycling or doing any combination of these activities for approximately 30 minutes, four times a week," Dr. Martin says.

And what happened? Previously sedentary subjects with mild high blood pressure didn't lose much weight or body fat, but they definitely lost points on their blood-pressure readings. In only ten weeks, they took seven points off their average systolic pressure and ten points off their average diastolic, dropping the average from 145/97 to 131/84. "The results suggest that even fairly light physical activity may be more helpful against high blood pressure than previous research has led us to think," says Dr. Martin.

Be aware, however, that other research shows conflicting results. In a study done at Duke University, researchers found no great differences in the blood pressure of exercisers and nonexercisers. Given the controversy, you'd be wise to exercise if you have high blood pressure, but exercise should not be your only action.

Calm down. Whatever your level of blood pressure, stress can only make it higher. One study at Cornell Medical College found that those who experience chronic stress on the job are three times as likely to develop high blood pressure.

There are lots of ways to reduce stress. Studies have shown that mild high blood pressure can often be successfully treated by using relaxation techniques such as yoga, biofeedback, and meditation. Exercise is also a good way to relieve stress. Another option might be to seek professional therapy. A good therapist might teach you a new and calmer way of looking at life. Or you might consider a lifestyle change, such as looking for a new, less stressful job.

Take your last puff. Doctors say that smoking doesn't cause high blood pressure, only that it can worsen the condition. In fact, studies have shown that a higher percentage of smokers have high blood pressure than do nonsmokers. Smoking is also a large risk factor for heart disease in and of itself.

Diet for a Lower Blood Pressure

The verdict's not in, but certain nutrients may have an impact on your blood pressure. There's enough evidence for the following recommendations.

Watch that sodium. Dr. Frohlich estimates that as many as one third of people with high blood pressure may be sodium sensitive and may benefit from reducing sodium intake. About 50 percent of dietary sodium comes in the salt we eat. The rest comes in the form of sodium-containing food additives and preservatives such as monosodium glutamate (MSG) and sodium benzoate. "If high blood pressure runs in your family, then you should probably start reducing sodium," says Dr. Frohlich. Start by tossing the salt and carefully reading food labels.

Load up on calcium. Several studies have shown that adding calcium to your diet can lower your blood pressure. In one study, more than half of the women and a third of the men shaved more than ten points off their systolic blood pressure by taking extra calcium. Because of the interaction between calcium and salt, a diet rich in calcium works especially well if you're salt sensitive.

(continued on page 444)

Where You'll Find the Sodium

The sodium found in salt plays a vital role in body chemistry, especially in the regulation of water balance. But too much sodium may contribute to blood pressure problems in sensitive individuals. American adults eat an average 3,000 to 7,000 milligrams of sodium a day, far above the high-health range of 1,000 to 1,500 milligrams. The foods listed here all contain substantial amounts of sodium. And keep in mind that table salt is 39 percent sodium.

Food	Portion	Sodium (mg)
Salt	1 tsp	2,300
Dried beef, chipped	2 oz	1,988
Sauerkraut, canned	1 cup	1,560
Alaska king crabmeat, cooked	1 cup	1,436
Potato salad	1 cup	1,322
Enchilada dinner, beef and cheese	8 oz	1,260
Spaghetti and meatballs, canned	1 cup	1,220
Ham, canned	3 oz	1,086
Cream of mushroom soup	1 cup	1,076
Refried beans	1 cup	1,071
Chop suey with beef and pork	1 cup	1,053

Food	Portion	Sodium (mg)
Bread stuffing, from mix	1 cup	1,008
Dill pickle	1 med.	928
Tomato juice, canned	1 cup	881
Cashew nuts, dry roasted, salted	1 cup	877
Cheese pizza	2 slices	811
Creamed corn, canned	1 cup	730
Chinook salmon, smoked	3 oz	666
Turkey hot dog	1	642
Green olives, canned	5 large	463
Beef bologna	2 slices	460
Parmesan cheese, hard	1 oz	451
Vanilla pudding, canned	½ cup	441
American cheese	1 oz	406
Carrot cake	1 slice	373
Total cereal	1 oz	352
All-Bran cereal	1 oz	320
English muffin with butter	1	310
Pickled herring	1 oz	262
Pita bread	1	215
Bagel	1	198

Add calcium to your diet by eating tofu, low-fat dairy products such as nonfat yogurt and skim milk, and certain fish such as canned sardines and salmon. Do check with your doctor, however, before you start dropping calcium pills—you may be in a small group whose blood pressure actually goes up with calcium. A family history of kidney stones may also make you a poor candidate for calcium supplementation.

Reduce the pressure with potassium. Potassium is a natural diuretic, helping your body excrete water and sodium, thus possibly lowering blood pressure. In fact, there's evidence that salt sensitivity may be caused by too little potassium in the diet, says high blood pressure researcher G. Gopal Krishna, M.D., associate professor of medicine at Temple University. Studies have shown that the lower the potassium intake, the higher the blood pressure, and the higher the ratio of potassium to salt, the lower the blood pressure.

Lucky for you, potassium is easy to come by in a normal diet. Fresh fruits and vegetables are rich sources for the 3,000 to 4,000 milligrams of potassium you should be getting each day. Do not take a potassium supplement without first checking with your doctor, though, particularly if you have a kidney disease.

Magnesium keeps calcium from making your heart beat too strongly. It may also help regulate sodium levels. Most Americans don't get enough of it in their diets (350 milligrams daily for men and 280 for women).

In fact, studies say magnesium intake has been dropping steadily over the past 100 years, and maybe it's not a coincidence that blood pressure has been rising during the same time. Research shows that people with low magnesium levels often have high blood pressure, especially if they have a family history of high blood pressure. And when people with low magnesium levels and high blood pressure are given magnesium supplements, their blood pressure drops.

This mineral is found in many foods. The richest sources are dried beans, nuts, whole grains, bananas, leafy greens, and hard water. Although magnesium is generally safe, too much may actually lower your blood pressure too far or put too much strain on badly working kidneys. Be sure to check with your doctor before taking supplements, especially if you're on high blood-pressure medication.

Try C. Vitamin C seems to be recommended for just about everything these days. Some researchers say that C may be important in regulating blood pressure as well. The relationship between the two has not been solidly proven, but "we have a suspicion that it's real," says physiologist David Trout, Ph.D., of the U.S. Department of Agriculture. Vitamin C is part of a healthy diet, and the foods it comes in—citrus fruits, green peppers, potatoes, broccoli, tomatoes, strawberries, cantaloupe, grapefruit, and spinach—are also full of other good things, including taste.

Drink less alcohol. The more alcohol you drink, the more at risk you are for high blood pressure. Alcohol abuse has been shown to be the most common cause of reversible high blood pressure. Experts say that alcohol use may increase blood pressure by washing calcium out of your system.

Switch to decaf. The conventional wisdom on caffeine has been that although it does raise blood pressure, the effect is only temporary and even then disappears once you become habituated. But now research is overturning the conventional wisdom.

(continued on page 448)

Guard Against False Readings

Your physician takes your blood pressure and it's sky high. Get it done outside that setting and it's just fine. This odd phenomenon is called "white-coat hypertension" and it's just one of the ways your blood pressure readings can be skewed.

In one study, researchers looked at a group of 292 supposedly hypertensive adults, comparing blood pressure measurements taken around the clock by a carry-along device to measurements made by a doctor. Over 20 percent of those who had high in-office measurements turned out to have normal pressure at home and at work.

The danger is that a doctor may prescribe medication based on high in-office readings. "That's why your doctor should take the average of the high and low readings over time to get a more accurate picture," says Thomas G. Pickering, M.D., of the Cardiovascular Center at the New York Hospital–Cornell University Medical Center.

The culprit in white-coat hypertension is the anxiety that comes from seeing a doctor. Research suggests that the simple presence of the physician can boost blood pressure regardless of the setting. So one way to beat white-coat hypertension is to have someone other than a doctor do the measurement. Blood pressure readings have been shown to be markedly lower when taken by a nurse or a medical technician instead of a doctor.

An at-home measuring kit would be a big plus for those concerned about their blood pressure, Dr. Pickering says. They're fairly cheap and accurate, when used properly. Ask your doctor or check with your pharmacist for more information.

Keep in mind that other factors may influence blood pressure measurements, too. No one knows why yet, but a full bladder at the time of a measurement tends to raise the numbers. Also, a person with fat arms may get an inaccurately high reading because of the narrow cuff of the measuring device. Use a wider cuff if you have plump appendages.

More variation comes with the natural peaks and valleys of circadian rhythm (your built-in biological clock). Blood pressure drops to a low point around 4:00 A.M., then tends to rise as you wake. "Our hearts beat faster, we breathe faster, and our blood pressure increases as we go about our morning activities," says William Frishman, M.D., professor of medicine and epidemiology at Albert Einstein College of Medicine in New York City.

These cyclic changes in blood pressure are mostly harmless, but they may complicate drug treatment in people with high blood pressure. That's why it's key, Dr. Frishman says, for people on blood pressure medication to make sure they take it regularly to cover those volatile morning hours.

Twenty healthy young men—all regular coffee drinkers with normal blood pressure—were given three cups of coffee a day in a study at the University of California, Los Angeles. The researchers found that even after 12 hours of overnight abstinence, the morning cup raised the men's systolic and diastolic blood pressure readings an average of six points. After their morning coffee break, their blood pressure rose more than two points (systolic) and five points (diastolic). The researchers noted that had the young men's pressure been taken 1 hour after drinking the coffee instead of only 10 minutes, the hikes in blood pressure would have been even greater. The conclusion: If you have high blood pressure, consider the caffeine risk.

When Medication May Be the Answer

Doctors disagree about medication for high blood pressure. Some say medication is the best and most responsible way to treat all high blood pressure. Others say borderline and mild high blood pressure are being overmedicated. But if your diastolic pressure is 95 or more, or your systolic pressure is 160 or more, you need medication, says Dr. Freis.

No drug gives you a license to ignore your lifestyle. On the contrary, if you're on blood pressure drugs, it's exceptionally important to watch your weight, follow a diet low in saturated fat and cholesterol, exercise, and do everything else you can to help the drugs do their job.

There are currently four main kinds of drugs doctors can give you.

Diuretics are usually the first drugs given. They work by increasing the excretion of sodium and water by the kidneys (sodium makes the body retain water), thereby reducing the volume of blood and lowering pressure in the arteries. Their success rate is in the 40 to 50 percent range. Possible side effects include higher cholesterol and triglyceride counts, weakness, and sexual dysfunction.

Beta-blockers reduce the amount of work the heart has to do. They're the drug of choice for people who have had a heart attack. A mainstay of drug treatment, they have a 40 to 50 percent success rate which climbs to 80 to 85 percent when given with a diuretic. Among possible side effects may be insomnia, fatigue, nightmares, sexual dysfunction, and depression.

ACE (angiotensin converting enzyme) inhibitors are becoming more popular because they're very effective with relatively few side effects. They prevent the production of the enzyme that constricts blood vessels. ACE inhibitors are successful in 60 to 70 percent of people with mild or moderate high blood pressure. Combining them with a diuretic raises the success rate to about 80 percent. They're especially good for people with heart failure or diabetes.

Calcium-channel blockers work by relaxing the blood vessels, thus lowering blood pressure. These medications have a success rate of about 30 to 40 percent. Side effects can include swelling of the legs, dizziness, and headaches.

With any of these drugs, your goal will be to take the minimum amount possible to keep your blood pressure in check. To accomplish this, you should work closely with your doctor.

High Cholesterol

Finding a Lifestyle with a Heart

You might think cholesterol, that waxy goo sloshing about in your bloodstream, is all bad. Actually, you couldn't live without it. Cholesterol is a vital ingredient in fat-digesting bile, in all cell membranes, and especially in brain and nerve cells. Only when it comes in surplus does the stuff wreak havoc.

You might also think that cholesterol is fat. Actually, it's more related to alcohol. And if your doctor has just told you that if cholesterol were vodka, you'd have enough in your blood to see the Russian army through the siege of Stalingrad, your heart's got a problem.

"If you could wave a magic wand and change the one thing that would have the most impact in preventing or reversing coronary artery disease, that thing would probably be your cholesterol level," says Virgil Brown, M.D., professor of medicine at Emory University in Atlanta and president of the American Heart Association. "If you look at societies where cholesterol is low, coronary artery disease is low."

The United States is not one of those societies. As you might expect in a country where heart disease ranks as the number one killer, American cholesterol levels are way too high.

How Much Is Too Much?

In a general sense, your total cholesterol level should be less than 200 milligrams per deciliter (mg/dl), according to the American Heart Association and the National Cholesterol Education Program. Push above that, especially up around 240, and your heart disease risk is getting too high, especially if you smoke, are overweight, or have high blood pressure.

But total cholesterol level doesn't give you the whole picture. That's because there are two kinds of cholesterol—low-density lipoproteins (LDL) and high-density lipoproteins (HDL). You want your LDL level to be low and your HDL level to be high, since HDL cholesterol actually carries potentially dangerous fats and alcohols out of the bloodstream.

"LDL and HDL tell a more complete story than total cholesterol," Dr. Brown says. "You should think independently about each, because the things you do to lower LDL may not be the same things you do to raise HDL." Your LDL level should ideally be under 100, says Dr. Brown. "If we all kept it at that level, coronary artery disease would probably be cut by 90 percent."

But that level may be a little impractical. And for many people—especially those with no other risk factors—it's probably not necessary. "So we tell most people that their LDL level should be below 130," says Dr. Brown. An LDL level of 130 to 159 puts you at borderline high risk, while a level of 160 or more is clearly bad news, he says. If, however, you already have heart disease, or if you have other risk factors, an LDL level of only 130 may put you at too high a risk.

Regardless of your LDL level, your level of HDL,

the good cholesterol, should be at least 35 mg/dl and ideally quite a bit higher. Those blessed with an HDL of 80 have little worry of heart disease, even with a high total cholesterol level, says William Castelli, M.D., epidemiologist, medical director of the Framingham Cardiovascular Institute, and former director of the Framingham Heart Study in Massachusetts.

Another way to look at this whole numbers business is to divide your HDL count into your total cholesterol figure. This gives you your cholesterol ratio. If the number on your calculator is 3.5 or less, you may still be in pretty good shape, even if your total cholesterol is slightly high.

You find out these numbers by blood testing. A simple finger-stick test at your local mall is fine, but for accuracy's sake, get another test within eight weeks, this time hypodermically drawn and analyzed at a laboratory certified by the federal Centers for Disease Control for testing blood lipids.

If the second measurement is within 30 points of the first, take the average of the two tests as your cholesterol level. But if the discrepancy is more than 30 points, have a third test done in another one to eight weeks. The average of the three tests is your cholesterol level.

Those in the high risk zone—240 or more—get a lipoprotein analysis, which will measure LDL and HDL, as well as levels of a fat in the blood known as triglycerides. For this test, you'll have to fast 10 to 12 hours beforehand. It's expensive, and it's debatable whether you need it if your initial cholesterol count is below 240 and you have no other risk factors, such as family history of heart disease.

Attack the Fat

So what do you do if you find out your cholesterol level is high enough to qualify as a professional bowling score? Don't run for the drugs just yet.

"The knee-jerk reaction of most doctors in this country would be to put you on cholesterol-lowering drugs," says Dr. Castelli. "But before you spend money on medication, you should talk to your doctor about investing a good six months in a solid cholesterol-lowering diet and exercise program." Even if your cholesterol level is a sky-high 300 or above (which, in most cases, would be the result of your genetic makeup), Dr. Castelli still recommends an initial drug-free attack plan, starting with reducing the fat in your diet.

The effect of dietary changes on LDL is powerful. "LDL is clearly the one that's most out of line in Americans, and it's the one that's linked most clearly to diet," says Dr. Brown. The average American gets 40 percent of calories from fat, with 13 percent of the total coming from saturated fat, which is the kind most likely to raise your cholesterol level. Americans also eat too much cholesterol directly, which comes in nearly all animal products. "The first and safest and only remedy that goes right to the heart of the problem is to lower the amount of saturated fat and cholesterol in the diet," says Dr. Brown.

After more than half a century worth of eating habits, you may dread change. But the happy truth is that most people can cut their fat intake fairly easily. Many who do find that they enjoy their food more and have the added benefit of fewer stomach problems. "So this idea that people have to eat a horrible, unpleasant diet to stay healthy is totally wrong," says Dr. Brown. "In fact, it's just the opposite."

Attitude Matters

Before jumping into your new cholesterol-lowering lifestyle, consider these few words from the experts on how your attitude can make all the difference.

Set measurable goals. Get a certain amount of exercise and make one dietary change each week. Do this and you'll feel good about your accomplishments, so you'll want to do more.

Focus on what you *can* eat. Instead of lamenting the loss of bacon and eggs, get your mouth watering over whole wheat pancakes with maple syrup. Or French toast made with egg whites and topped with jam. Or a bagel topped with jelly or low-fat cottage cheese and herbs.

Count your blessings. Think about how nice it is to eat more and not hike your cholesterol. That's exactly what happens when you follow a low-fat, high carbohydrate diet. Your food intake isn't limited, so you'll rarely feel hungry.

Enjoy the feeling. Do it because it makes you feel good, not because you're afraid of dropping dead. Fear will motivate you only for a short time, says Dean Ornish, M.D., president and director of the Preventive Medicine Research Institute in Sausalito, California, and author of *Dr. Dean Ornish's Program for Reversing Heart Disease.* He emphasizes that people who make positive lifestyle changes stay motivated because they feel so much better.

The American Heart Association suggests a diet limited to 30 percent or less fat, and many doctors say you should shoot for even less. But the kind of fat you're eating may be more important than the amount. "Vegans, people who don't eat any animal products at all, tend to get 35 percent of their calories from fat, but it's vegetable fat, and their cholesterol levels are extremely low," says Dr. Brown.

Unless you're going totally vegetarian, try to drop your fat calories to 20 percent over the next two months. You should also limit the amount of dietary cholesterol you consume. Fortunately, foods high in fat tend to be high in cholesterol, and vice versa, so you can pretty much avoid both villains at once by following these guidelines.

Cheat on the meat. Have no more than one serving of meat, fish, or poultry a day. Make it lean, and limit that serving to 3 or 4 ounces (about the size of a deck of cards). Limit red meat to two or three servings a week. Avoid cholesterol-laden organ meats, like liver.

Grab the grains. Have two servings of whole grains, breads, or starches (like pasta and potatoes) with every meal. Have even more if you can afford the calories.

Go part-time vegetarian. Have at least one totally vegetarian meal each day. Combine pasta, rice, barley, and starchy vegetables, such as potatoes, corn, and winter squash.

Switch to skim. Each day, substitute two servings of nonfat milk products (such as skim milk and nonfat yogurt) for two servings of fattier ones.

Know your oils. Each day, use no more than 2 to 4 teaspoons of added fat or oil on foods. When you do, stick with olive, canola, corn, sunflower, or safflower oil. Choose margarine with one of these oils

What about Triglycerides?

With smoking and cholesterol and blood pressure and stress, and HDL and LDL and obesity and genes, figuring out your heart disease risk is complicated enough. But there's another risk factor to throw into the picture. The evidence is far from clear, but high triglyceride levels may contribute to heart disease.

Triglycerides are the principal fat in your blood. They're necessary for energy, insulation, organ protection, cell membranes, cell metabolism—but you can have too many.

Among older women participating in the Framingham Heart Study in Massachusetts, those who had heart disease also tended to have high triglycerides. But these same women also tended to be dangerously overweight, making it hard to pin the rap for their heart disease on high triglycerides , says Virgil Brown, M.D., professor of medicine at Emory University in Atlanta and president of the American Heart Association.

Still, you should save a little of your concern for your tryclicerides level, if only because high triglycerides rarely come alone. "High triglycerides are often associated with obesity and several other important risk factors, such as a high-fat diet and sedentary lifestyle," says Dr. Brown. Medical experts generally agree that a triglyceride reading of more than 250 (milligrams per deciliter of blood) is an indication of possible trouble. When you cut down on dietary cholesterol and saturated fat, you also cut down on triglycerides, Dr. Brown says.

listed as the first ingredient. But remember that margarine is made with hydrogenated vegetable oil, which acts the same as saturated fat, so use margarine especially sparingly. Avoid shortening and lard, butter, and palm and coconut oils, all loaded with saturated fat.

Top it right. Use only low-fat condiments or toppings, like fat-free butter substitutes, nonfat salad dressings, prepared mustard, horseradish, catsup, chili sauce, relish, and salsa.

Yoke the yolks. Eat no more than one egg yolk a week. Cholesterol-free egg substitutes or two egg whites can often be substituted for one whole egg in recipes. Remember that one egg yolk has about 240 milligrams of cholesterol (while experts recommend no more than 300 milligrams for an entire day).

Fill Up on Fiber

Eating high amounts of fiber, particularly soluble fiber from sources like oat bran and beans, can help lower blood cholesterol, says James W. Anderson, M.D., professor of medicine and clinical nutrition at the Veterans Affairs Medical Center in Lexington, Kentucky. Soluble fiber works in two ways: It takes its own sweet time going through your digestive tract, so you may feel fuller and won't be inclined to eat as much as you might of other, fat-containing foods. And it may also transform in the colon into substances that interfere with the body's production of cholesterol.

Actually, there's some controversy about whether fiber itself lowers cholesterol, with some arguing that people who fill up on fiber are simply eating less fat. But however it works, it works. In one study, men asked to eat heaping amounts of fiber-rich fruits, vegetables, salads, berries, and bran lowered their total cholesterol by 5 percent in only four weeks.

To avoid digestive upsets, increase your fiber intake gradually, and be sure to drink plenty of water to avoid constipation. Here's how to make sure you get enough fiber.

Go for cereal. Eat a bowl of high-fiber cereal daily, preferably one with oat bran or psyllium. Some research suggests that rice bran may have similar cholesterol-lowering effects. Inspect cereal labels for fiber content.

Add in legumes. Slowly work up to ½ to 1 cup of legumes a day—kidney beans, chick-peas, lima beans, lentils, navy beans, or pinto beans. A cup of lentils provides about 10 grams of fiber. You'll find that legumes can provide that pleasant, full feeling you thought you could get only from meat. Combine legumes with small amounts of meat, chicken, fish, rice, or pasta, or add them to hearty salads, soups, casseroles, stir-fries with vegetables, or pita-bread sandwiches with sprouts and low-fat cottage cheese.

Feel your oats. Add oat bran to foods whenever you can. One-third cup of oat bran contains about 4 grams of fiber. Try it in low-fat muffin recipes, as a meat-loaf extender, as a thickener in soups and stews, as an ingredient in blender shakes, baked into breads and rolls, in place of bread crumbs, in pancake batter, and in casseroles.

Help other nutrients. Consider taking a multiple vitamin/mineral supplement containing iron and zinc. All that fiber you're now getting can interfere with the absorption of these and other nutrients.

Go Aerobic

As with fiber, there's some controversy about the role of exercise in combating cholesterol. A number of studies have indicated that vigorous aerobic exercise can raise levels of HDL, the good, protective kind of cholesterol. In fact, aerobic exercise may be the only thing you can do to raise your HDL level. It may also lower your LDL and total cholesterol levels.

Still, no one can pin down the link between huffing and puffing and strong blood. But when researchers from the University of Texas looked at a large group of very athletic people (who averaged 9 hours of exercise a week), they found the men had total cholesterol levels 29 mg/dl lower than the average for their age. The women had levels 17 mg/dl lower than average. Just as impressive, both the men and the women had levels of HDL that were at least 15 mg/dl higher than average.

Of course, exercise does a lot more for your heart than help battle cholesterol, like helping you stay thin and lowering blood pressure. Running, swimming, biking, cross-country skiing, and walking are excellent aerobic exercises. Walking may be the safest and easiest aerobic activity. Work up gradually to a minimum of two brisk miles a day.

Getting Tougher

After two months of following your new diet and exercise program, it's time for another blood test. Discuss the findings with your doctor.

By now you should know if the program is working for you. If your cholesterol level has dropped to within the healthy range, congratulations! But remember, the lifestyle changes are forever, or your cholesterol is going to climb right back up. "One way to stay on the straight and narrow is to have your blood tested regularly for the rest of your life," Dr. Castelli says. "I recommend every three to four months for

(continued on page 462)

How I Did It: A Wish Come True

Twenty-nine years ago, at age 25, psychologist Peter A. Wish, Ph.D., had a total cholesterol level of 330 and a family that was getting heart disease the way other families get the flu. His aunt had a heart attack at age 37. His father died from one at age 50. One uncle died at 39, another at 54.

Dr. Wish knew that longevity was not something he was going to fish out of this particular family's gene pool. But it wasn't until he developed a fatty bump on his elbow that he finally looked for help.

His family doctor told him that the fatty bump was a symptom of familial hypercholesterolemia—a $12 word that means genetically influenced high cholesterol—and prescribed medication that would lower his triglyceride (another type of dangerous fat) levels, and suggested that he eat less fat.

Of course, "eating less fat" back then meant going from hamburgers, whole milk, and cheesecake to a lean steak, 2 percent milk, and pound cake. It was a step in the right direction, but it sure didn't lower cholesterol much. So Dr. Wish looked around and, down the street from where he worked in Framingham, Massachusetts, he discovered epidemiologist William Castelli, M.D., then associate director of the Framingham Heart Study.

Dr. Castelli disclosed up front that most scientists thought he was a nut. "I'm everything the medical establishment doesn't like," Dr. Castelli reportedly told Dr. Wish. "Are you ready to be a guinea pig?" The answer was strong and sure: "Absolutely."

Over the next six weeks, Dr. Castelli put Dr. Wish on a cholesterol-lowering drug and a stringent low-fat diet that even today would raise eyebrows: No red meat. No shellfish. Lots of fruits and vegetables. Lots of whole grains. When his total cholesterol got stuck around 200, the lifestyle was radicalized even further to a more vegetarian style of eating and an exercise program consisting of $1\frac{1}{2}$ hours a day divided between a treadmill, a stair climber, and a stationary bike. Only then did the final 30 points that stood between him and longevity drop away. The bumps around his joints disappeared, and today, Peter has a total cholesterol level of 170.

Obviously, such an accomplishment demands motivation, but Dr. Wish had an advantage. As a psychologist, he understood that to make any significant lifestyle change he would have to learn a whole new way of thinking—what psychologists call a cognitive shift. Since you can't see or feel high cholesterol, that's not easy to do.

The way to overcome this handicap, Dr. Wish says, is to make the changes so gradually that your body hardly knows what's going on. Implement the changes in bite-size chunks. Set yourself a specific goal—say, a drop in total cholesterol of 50 points—then break it down into small, realistic steps and reward yourself as you accomplish each step.

"This is a lifelong process," Dr. Wish says. But it produces a long life.

the first three to four years, then every six months thereafter."

What if your cholesterol level is still too high after two months of diet and exercise? Then you need to take stronger steps. Start with psyllium, which will give you a hefty soluble fiber boost. A tablespoonful of this crushed seed (available in any pharmacy) boasts about as much fiber as an entire bowl of bran cereal. Dr. Castelli's advice is to add a daily tablespoon of psyllium to your diet for a month, then have your cholesterol rechecked. If it's still not low enough, double the dose for another month, then check your blood cholesterol again.

Psyllium is powerful stuff, as your digestion will no doubt tell you. Give yourself time to adapt to its laxative effects, and be sure to drink plenty of water, since psyllium absorbs large amounts of fluid. Don't take more than 2 tablespoons a day. Some people are allergic to psyllium; stop taking it if you experience wheezing, itching, or shortness of breath.

If you really want to do everything in your power to lower your cholesterol without medication, it may be time to go on a strict vegetarian diet. Research by Dean Ornish, M.D., president and director of the Preventive Medicine Research Institute in Sausalito, California, and author of *Dr. Dean Ornish's Program for Reversing Heart Disease*, suggests that such a diet, coupled with exercise and stress-reduction techniques (plus quitting smoking), may lower cholesterol and even reverse existing blockages in the arteries. Other research shows that this kind of very low fat diet is associated with extremely low LDLs, total cholesterol, and triglycerides (fat in the blood).

Although it can be tough to follow a strict vegetarian diet, Dr. Ornish thinks it's important that you realize you may have an alternative to drug therapy. Once you have your doctor's approval, here's what you need to do.

◆ Stop eating all meat, poultry, and fish. Let every meal feature vegetables and greens, beans, sprouts, egg whites, and grain products such as bread, cereal, rice, pasta, and tortillas. Tofu and tempeh, which are high in vegetable fat, are okay in moderation.

◆ Limit dairy products to 1 cup of skim milk or nonfat yogurt a day. Eat no cheese.

◆ Use no oil or egg yolks and only a moderate amount of sugar and salt.

◆ Eat no butter, margarine, shortening, or lard.

◆ Limit "taste enhancers" to seasonings like herbs, mustard, or salsa. Entirely lay off of the mayo and sour cream.

◆ Take a multiple vitamin/mineral supplement to ensure you're not missing any nutrients because of the dietary restrictions. Yes, switching to such a diet may be a large effort at first, but Dr. Ornish has plenty of now-healthy patients who can attest that adapting to and enjoying this new way of eating is possible for anybody.

When Diet and Exercise Aren't Enough

It's six months since you started and stuck to your war against cholesterol. But the war isn't going well. Your doctor tells you there's still too much cholesterol swimming around in your veins and you'll need medication. Even so, since you've done everything you can to avoid reliance on drugs, you have something to be proud of: You're eating better, and you're healthier.

Those achievements mean you'll likely be able to

get by with far less medication should your doctor say you need it. "We want you to be on the smallest amount of the drug that will be effective," he says. That's because they tend to have side affects, such as nausea and constipation.

Once you're on cholesterol-lowering drugs, you have to stay on them or your cholesterol will shoot right back up to where it was, says Dr. Castelli.

But there's no doubt that medication—cholestyramine, colestipol HCL, lovastatin, simvastatin, and atorvastatin are most prescribed—works. A large number of studies show that you can lower your total blood cholesterol level by 10 to 35 percent on medication.

Still, says Dr. Brown, drugs are not for everyone. In nearly all cases, he says, "the first therapy is still lifestyle change."

Memory Loss

It's Probably Nothing Serious

Your body slows down as you age, so why not your memory? Some memory loss is indeed natural as you grow older—half of all people over age 60 have memory problems—but only an unlucky few have conditions that can really do damage to their memory, like Alzheimer's disease or the after-effects of stroke.

The rest of us might have "benign senescent forgetfulness," a relatively new term that refers to the natural lapses in memory that often come with aging. Memory is just another physical process, says Frank Benson, M.D., behavioral neurologist and professor of neurology at the University of California, Los Angeles. And like all physical processes, it slows down with age.

"It happens to all of us," Dr. Benson says. "Look at the difference in the best marathon times between a well-conditioned young runner and a well-conditioned elderly runner," he says. "The older runner's times are darn near twice as long."

Still, Dr. Benson notes, your memory is better than you think it is. "A sizable number of people complain that they're forgetful, but when they're tested, they test well," he says. "Maybe not as well as most people, but good enough."

In fact, as you age, you probably lose much more time off the 100-yard dash than in your ability to remember things. "We simply don't see devastating losses in memory in older people who aren't sick," says Curt Sandman, Ph.D., neuropsychologist and co-director of the Memory Disorders Clinic at the University of California, Irvine, Medical School.

Mind Your Body

Your memory is in your brain, and your brain is in your body, living on the same blood and nutrients as the rest of you. To be at its best, it needs the rest of you to be at its best.

And there's plenty you can do to keep your

body in good enough shape to preserve and improve your memory.

Go that extra mile. A brisk, daily 20-minute walk is enough to get your blood pumping all the way up to your head to feed those hungry memory cells, Dr. Sandman says. But he found you can do more than that to help your memory. "We assigned elderly people as foster grandparents to neurologically impaired children," Dr. Sandman says. "The foster grandparents had to walk several miles a day, they had social interactions they otherwise wouldn't have had, and there were physical demands on them in caring 20 hours a week for another human being." EEGs showed the foster grandparents had higher brain activity, better memory, and better sleep, he says.

Sleep soundly. Be sure to get a good night's sleep, so that you can be alert enough the next day to learn and remember what you want to, say memory experts. Your chances of sleeping well are increased if you don't eat and drink late at night. Sleeping pills don't help much either—they knock you out rather than let you sleep, and you can really feel sluggish the next day.

Bite down on brain food. Your diet plays a big role in memory function. The B-complex vitamins are especially important, along with the right amounts of protein and carbohydrates. A balanced and varied diet of fresh foods—fruits, vegetables, dairy products, fish, poultry, and grains—is an easy way to get your brain everything it needs.

Go for the glucose. One food in particular has been shown to improve memory: a fruit drink sweetened with the simple sugar known as glucose. University of Virginia researchers found that people who drank the glucose drink just before memory tests did much better than those who drank a fruit drink sweetened with sodium saccharin. But check with your doctor before you start guzzling glucose-sweetened lemonade, because people with high blood sugar levels (like those caused by diabetes) did poorly on the memory tests. In fact, if your memory is failing, you may want to have your blood sugar checked.

Variety Is the Spice of Memory

The older you get, the less likely you are to pay attention to details, Dr. Sandman says. "What we think happens is that you pay more attention to general principles," he says. "You may ignore the details younger people concentrate on in favor of understanding how the world works. So if you're tested about details that have just happened, you may have ignored them, and you're said to have a bad memory. What really happened is that those details didn't really change the world and so you didn't pay attention to them. It's not really a loss of memory; it's a way of adapting to the world, and we call that wisdom."

But even the wisest of us can minimize memory loss. Many of the secrets of a better memory are right in the mind.

Use it. If you've never run 100 yards, you never will unless you get your rear off the couch, your feet into running shoes, and your body in gear. The same goes for memory, Dr. Benson says. "The old use-it-or-lose-it idea may be just as true for mental activity as it is for physical activity," he says. "Keeping an active mind is something you should do all your life."

Challenge it. "People who are using their memory and pushing themselves and really maintaining as much interest in what goes on around them as they did when they were kids may well get along better than those who are pretty complacent and going about doing the same things day after day and not challenging their minds," says Dr. Benson. "You've got to learn new things in order to remember them."

Spice it up. "The number one stimulus is variety," Dr. Sandman says. One of his studies challenged Alzheimer's patients and their spouses to do something different each week. Then the couples were given memory tests—not for that special event but for all the little details of their lives that week. "We found that adding spice to their lives improved their memories significantly," says Dr. Sandman.

What kind of spice? "Some of them had romantic lovers' picnics in the park, the kind of thing they hadn't done for 55 years," Dr. Sandman says. Others took short trips. "As they get older, many people tend to become tied very closely to their house," he says. "We encouraged them to take some risks, buy things they had put off buying, indulge in dining out on food they've never tried before. Those were all ordinary, simple, enjoyable things that had a jarring effect on their memories."

Update it. Reminiscing is the opposite of variety, and it hurts your ability to remember details, Dr. Sandman says. That's because it's a seductive and satisfying substitute for engagement. After all, what's a more exotic place to travel than in time? "You completely block out the rest of the world," Dr. Sandman says. "Everything going on around you is quite secondary. But it produces memory loss."

Instead, Dr. Sandman advises, "replace the satisfaction of internal trips with external trips."

Test it. If you watch any TV at all, you know that TV people don't think much of your ability to concentrate for any length of time. Prove them wrong. All you have to do is watch a program and write down ten questions. Three days later, ask yourself those questions. Do this regularly. "It's amazing what this will do for your memory," Dr. Sandman says.

He even conducted a study in which he and his patients watched the same programs at home. "Then we all made up tests about the details of the programs," he says. "They asked me questions, and I asked them questions. Even though the questions weren't the same, their ability to answer my questions improved remarkably, just because they themselves drew up questions to ask me. As a matter of fact, I could answer their questions better, too, because I had also drawn up questions to ask them."

Relax. One of the memory problems that causes the most anxiety is the ability to remember names. Well, you can relax. Really.

"Just become less anxious about remembering names," Dr. Sandman advises. "Instead, after you're introduced to someone, don't even focus on the name and the face. Instead, focus on interests, on things you have in common with the person. You build an emotional halo around the person."

Because you find out more about the person, including things you have in common that you hold dear, this person registers in your emotions. "Emotional memories never die," Dr. Sandman says. Having this emotional focus gives you something to talk about and relieves anxiety in a social situation. Result: It helps you remember the name.

Go over it. Rehearsal is a tried-and-true method of remembering. "If you want to learn and remember something, just rehearse it," Dr. Sandman says. Dr. Sandman points to a project he did with his

When Is It Alzheimer's?

Fear of Alzheimer's disease is common. It's often the first thing to pop into your mind when you start forgetting things. Yet it's not likely your memory problems are the beginning of Alzheimer's.

The fundamental difference? "People with Alzheimer's don't learn," says Frank Benson, M.D., professor of neurology at the University of California, Los Angeles. "People with slowing memories can learn." For fast relief from the fear and trepidation of Alzheimer's, take a look at this table, prepared by social worker Lisa Gwyther, assistant professor of psychiatric social work and director of Duke University's Alzheimer's Family Support Program.

Activity	Alzheimer's	Normal Memory Loss
Attending an event	Forgets the whole experience	Forgets parts of experience
Following directions	Gradually unable	Usually able
Taking notes; using reminders	Gradually unable	Usually able
Caring for self	Gradually unable	Usually able

Alzheimer's patients. "We had a group of our patients take pictures of each other and write the names on the backs," he says. "Then they went over and over the names. At the same time, they used the emotional associations—what these people do for a living, trips they'd taken, how many children they had, anything they felt they could identify with. Now these were people who were having a hard time remembering their spouses' names. After four weeks, they were remembering all the names of the people in the group."

More Words of Wisdom

Although memory problems are a normal part of aging, they can sometimes be a symptom of physical or emotional disease. There's a long list of conditions that affect memory, including Alzheimer's disease, depression, fatigue, grief, artery disease, alcoholism, and diabetes. So if you notice your memory is starting to slip, discuss it with your doctor.

Of course, you've got to be able to hear and see in order to remember. As you age, the lens of your eye yellows and impairs vision. The power of your ears to hear high-pitched sounds declines. So be sure to have your vision and hearing checked and remedied. And while you're with the doctor, ask if any medications you're taking could be making you forgetful.

If it turns out that your health is on your side, improving your memory is a simple question of exercising your body and mind.

Menopausal Problems

Smooth Changes

Imagine standing beside a roaring bonfire. Your face turns beet red and your chest and arms sizzle with a zillion hot pinpricks. In seconds, your blouse is soaked with sweat, and your hair mats to your brow. You feel uncomfortable and clammy, like you've been shrink-wrapped in plastic.

Now picture yourself standing crimson faced and sopping wet before a meeting room full of people. That's what a hot flash, the most common, uncomfortable and embarrassing symptom of menopause, is like.

A generation ago, there wasn't much a woman having a menopausal hot flash could do. As one woman put it, "with each wave of heat, I felt my body was broadcasting to the world that I was going through the change of life."

Technically, a woman reaches menopause on the date of her last period, usually around age 50, although early signs of menopause can begin four to six years before. Menstruation ceases because the ovaries no longer produce enough of the hormone estrogen to trigger the regular monthly cycle.

When estrogen output grinds to a halt, however, more than the menstrual cycle is affected. Estrogen affects many different tissues and organs throughout your body. So when the hormone flow is stopped, your entire body feels the difference—from your brain down to your bones.

"When estrogen wanes, your body reacts like it's going through a drug withdrawal," says Brian Walsh, M.D., director of the Menopause Clinic at Brigham and Women's Hospital in Boston. The more serious effects involve changes you can't even feel.

Life without Estrogen

Without estrogen to help your bones absorb calcium, you're at increased risk for osteoporosis. And people who have advanced osteoporosis—a disease that involves gradual degeneration of the bones—are more susceptible to bone fracture. Estrogen also helps keep artery-clogging blood fats in check. So a decreased estrogen level may increase your risk of heart disease and stroke.

Most women are all too well aware of other troublesome menopause symptoms. Hot flashes head the list. Three-fourths of all women going through menopause experience these internal heat waves. For many women, they're infrequent and no more intense than a blush after a bawdy joke. Others have severe, sweat-soaking flashes that come in rapid-fire succession. They interfere with daily routines, from driving to conducting meetings, and can jolt you awake again and again throughout the night. These sleep-robbing "night sweats" may be why some women feel wrung out, edgy, and muddle-headed during menopause, experts say.

"In a nutshell, a drop in estrogen makes the body's thermostat go haywire," says Dr. Walsh. "The body thinks it's too hot, so blood vessels near the skin's surface dilate, causing the pink flush. Then you sweat to cool off. This gives you the shivers."

Next to hot flashes, vaginal discomfort is the second most vexing menopausal complaint. It's easy to see why. As estrogen dwindles, the vaginal walls shrink and become thinner, drier, and inelastic. This can cause painful friction during sexual intercourse. Blood flow is reduced, so the touch sensation is altered. These symptoms can quickly squelch sexual desire.

Additionally, the vagina becomes more inviting for bacteria, possibly triggering a merry-go-round of vaginal and bladder infections.

Thinned urethral tissues may also increase the frequency of urination. And lax bladder muscles may cause unexpected dribbling when you laugh, sneeze, or cough.

A Decade of Dwindling Hormones

Fortunately, the effects of estrogen withdrawal don't hit all at once (unless you've had a total hysterectomy—in effect, a surgical menopause in which the ovaries are removed).

Normally, a woman's ovaries start gradually slowing down their output of hormones—both estrogen and progesterone—in her forties. During this winding-down phase, sometimes called the perimenopause, she may notice subtle "mini-changes." Periods become erratic, for example, or bleeding may get either scantier or, more typically, heavier. As hormones fluctuate, a woman may ride a roller coaster of changing moods.

Then the other menopausal symptoms emerge, usually hitting in full force within three years after periods stop. Some symptoms subside, others may continue for ten years or more.

But here's encouraging news: Many women are able to ride out the waves of menopause until their symptoms subside without undue strain. In fact, even among women who may suffer severe symptoms, few sink into the depths of despair.

Women are developing an upbeat, take-charge attitude about menopause, according to Cynthia Stuenkel, M.D., medical director of the Menopause Clinic at the University of California, San Diego. "They're seeking (and finding) methods that ease them through menopause and help them stay healthy in the years beyond," she says.

Many of those methods are easy-to-use home remedies, but by far, the most effective treatment is one that comes from the doctor—hormone replacement therapy (HRT).

Help from HRT

Ever since its introduction in the 1960s, hormone replacement therapy has profoundly improved the quality of life for many women going through menopause. As its name implies, HRT replaces hormones that the body no longer produces. Today, a common HRT formula consists of an estrogen pill taken daily for 21 days, followed by a progestin pill, a synthetic version of progesterone, taken for the remaining days of the month. This hormone duo closely mimics the interplay of hormones that a woman naturally experiences during her childbearing years.

Having the option of taking HRT means you don't have to suffer through debilitating symptoms until they finally subside years later.

For instance, if night sweats are so severe that you're changing sheets like they change guards at Buckingham Palace, HRT can usually eliminate them in short order, according to Lila E. Nachtigall, M.D., associate professor of obstetrics and gynecology at New York University School of Medicine in New York City and author of *Estrogen: The Facts Can Change Your Life*. Within a week or two, for many women, night sweats will be a memory. Once hot flashes are extinguished, many women sleep better, feel less edgy, and have more energy.

HRT can also help end vaginal symptoms, according to Dr. Nachtigall. Estrogen toughens up painfully thin vaginal tissues and increases lubrication. Tenderness, itchiness, and vaginal infections may vanish for as long as you take the hormones. This can lift your libido. At the Yale University School of Medicine, researchers found that sexual desire—and sexual activity—increased after three months of estrogen in 90 percent of women who reported a lack of desire.

While the research is inconclusive about HRT's effects on mood, many women find that HRT helps them feel less anxious and irritable.

HRT also helps prevent bone loss and staves off osteoporosis. Estrogen replacement is the main way to effectively stem the unrelenting loss of your bone as you get older, according to Dr. Nachtigall.

When started within a few years of the onset of menopause, estrogen can actually help women recoup lost bone. As for fractures, women who take estrogen may have fewer broken bones than those who do not take it, studies show.

"Very simply, HRT can renew your life," says Dr. Walsh. It can also save it. In a ten-year study of nurses at Harvard Medical School, women who took estrogen cut their risk of heart disease by nearly half. "It appears that estrogen raises the good lipids and decreases the bad

Hormone Replacement: A Look at the Options

A popular replacement therapy (HRT) regimen is estrogen in daily doses for 25 to 30 days, accompanied by progestin for the last 10 to 13 days. Sometimes physicians prefer to prescribe the estrogen for only three weeks, with one week off—plus the overlapping days of progestin.

The problem is that two-thirds of HRT users stop their medication because of period-like bleeding. The good news is that it's possible to sidestep bleeding and other side effects by customizing your HRT formula. Here are your choices.

Daily low-dose progestins. A low dose (2.5 milligrams) of progestin given every day produces bleeding only for about six months. There's no final word yet on how this regimen affects bones or blood fats.

The patch. A medicated adhesive is attached to your abdomen, where it releases estradiol, a pure form of estrogen thought to be less cancer causing. Estradiol bypasses the liver and is best for women who can't take HRT orally but who have severe hot flashes and vaginal problems. Early studies indicate the patch may protect the bones and heart.

Vaginal estrogen cream. It increases lubrication and relieves dryness and itching. Effects may be noticed in less than a week. You can use cream on and off and resume treatment when symptoms return. Estrogen is absorbed by the bloodstream but has fewer risks than when taken orally. You may need an occasional progestin pill.

lipids," says Dr. Walsh. "This is significant, since heart disease is the number one killer of women over age 50."

Concerns about HRT

Despite all that HRT has going for it, only one-third of the women who receive prescriptions actually take it. The major reason? "Fear of cancer," says Dr. Walsh.

That's understandable. Early versions of HRT contained more potent doses of estrogen and produced five times more endometrial cancer in the women who took it. Excess estrogen causes endometrial (uterine) tissue to grow abnormally.

Today's HRT formulas contain a safer, lower dose of estrogen coupled with progestin, a combination that prevents the buildup of uterine tissue.

But there's still one hard-to-ignore problem: Some preliminary evidence suggests that progestin may contribute to breast cancer. In a much-publicized Swedish study, for example, women using HRT had four times more breast cancer than women who were not using it.

To complicate matters, it appears that progestin reverses to a degree estrogen's heart-healthy effects: It raises the bad lipids.

Even with this uncertainty, doctors believe that if you have severe vaginal dryness or hot flashes, or if you're at high risk for heart disease or osteoporosis (you're thin, fair skinned, or have a family history of osteoporosis, or a bone density test reveals dangerously thin bones), the benefits of HRT outweigh any possible risk of breast cancer.

"Women have far greater odds of getting heart disease than breast cancer," says Dr. Walsh. Until further studies can resolve these perplexing issues, says Dr.

Walsh, women should stay up-to-date on HRT information and carefully weigh the benefits and risks with their doctor based on their own medical history and lifestyle.

At this point, HRT may be used with caution by women at risk for breast or uterine cancer or by those with uterine fibroids or liver or gallbladder disease. If you have high blood pressure, HRT may be okay with close monitoring. All HRT users should have regular breast exams and report any unexplained bleeding to their doctor.

You should, however, expect regular period-type bleeding if you take the combined HRT. Progestin's job of controlling endometrial tissue means the tissue gets sloughed off each month. While these periods may be briefer and lighter and may eventually disappear, they can still be a nuisance, especially when the one plus of menopause is not having periods.

Progestin also brings back other unwelcome PMS-like symptoms, such as breast tenderness, headaches, and moodiness. Some newer HRT regimens may minimize these side effects.

Taking Charge

"HRT is not a substitute for good prevention habits that can help you stay healthy in the postmenopausal years," says Dr. Stuenkel.

Menopause isn't about popping pills to resolve your problems. "It's about finding ways to take control, so you can make the most of your life as your body changes," says Dr. Stuenkel.

The following nonhormonal self-help techniques have made it possible for many women to take control of troublesome symptoms. You might want to try one or several of these approaches before turning to more potent medication. If you are already using HRT, these methods may boost its effectiveness.

Skip the alcohol and coffee. These beverages can make the blood vessels dilate and worsen hot flashes. So can hot and spicy food.

Try vitamin E. If your hot flashes aren't devastating, this nutrient could help you have fewer, less intense episodes, according to gynecologist Susan Lark, M.D., director of the PMS and Menopause Self-Help Center in Los Altos, California, and author of *The Menopause Self-Help Book*. The recommended dosage is 400 international units (IU) twice a day. If that doesn't do the trick, double the dose. (Check with your doctor first; Vitamin E can be blood thinning.)

Chill out. In one six-week study of menopausal women, stress was associated with an increase in the frequency, intensity, and duration of hot flashes in half of the participants. Try meditation or a soothing tub soak.

Shift your view. You may be able to lessen the intensity of a hot flash by changing how you think about it, says Dr. Lark. One woman associated the sweaty feeling of hot flashes with how she felt after playing tennis. "The hot flashes still came, but I felt less negative about them," she says.

Lubricate. Vitamin E oil rubbed in vaginal tissues can ease your discomfort, says Dr. Lark. You might also try Replens. This over-the-counter lubricant and moisturizer plumps up the vaginal lining cells with moisture and can actually return shrunken vaginal lining tissue back to normal, studies show. Another plus: Replens creates an acidic environment, which keeps bacteria at bay.

Avoid antihistamines. These drugs dry out mucous membranes in your vagina as well as in your nose.

Engage in regular sex. "Regular orgasm and tender, sensitive lovemaking can help to relax the pelvic muscles, improve blood flow, and keep natural moisture in vaginal tissues," says Dr. Lark.

Practice Kegels. These specially designed exercises improve muscle tone and blood circulation in the pelvic area, says Dr. Lark. To contract the pelvic muscle, use the same motion you would to stop a stream of urine. Do 10 contractions a day—5 fast, plus 5 held for 3 to 5 seconds. Build up to a total of 50 to 100 contractions a day.

Sip passionflower tea. This herb—along with others such as chamomile, hops, and catnip—has been found to elevate serotonin, which triggers sleep and calmness, according to Dr. Lark.

Walk it out. "Exercise helps discharge excess anxiety-causing adrenaline that many women experience around menopause because of a shift in hormones," says Dr. Lark. Regular exercise may improve your mood by raising endorphins (feel-good hormones that are known to drop during menopause).

Give it a rest. Take an afternoon or midmorning meditation breather. Sit quietly with closed eyes. Let your muscles go limp and breathe slowly.

Strong Bones and Heart

Experts now say that you need three things to build strong bones: estrogen, exercise (especially weight-bearing exercise like walking), and calcium. But even if you can't take estrogen for some reason, the other two factors may be enough to slow bone loss if you are not high risk for osteoporosis.

In a two-year Australian study, researchers found

that postmenopausal women who participated in exercise and brisk walking three times weekly and also took 1,000 milligrams of calcium daily showed a significant slowdown of bone loss.

You can also fortify your bones by avoiding the calcium bandits such as excess coffee and salt.

There are also several strategies to help protect your heart that you should incorporate into your life, whether you take HRT or not.

"Stopping smoking, eating a high-fiber, low-fat diet, getting regular aerobic exercise, and practicing stress management are all proven, nonhormonal ways to prevent heart disease," says Dr. Lark. "The sooner you start using these preventive strategies, the more likely you'll remain disease-free in the years beyond menopause."

Overweight
Take It Off and Keep It Off

O ne thing's different about excess weight in your fifties or sixties than in your twenties or thirties: You've probably spent a lot more time losing it and then gaining it back than your younger partners in pounds.

Feel frustrated? Helpless? Like you're condemned to a life of love handles or saddlebags? You're not alone.

Between 90 and 95 percent—that's right, nearly all—of people treated for being overweight fail to keep it off.

So maybe sometime around your sixtieth birthday the temptation is to throw up your hands. Why bother if you're doomed to fail?

Because you're not doomed to fail. You can, in fact, achieve a lower, healthier weight after age 50. How? By exercising and learning to eat low-fat meals, says G. Kenneth Goodrick, Ph.D., an assistant professor of medicine at Baylor College of Medicine in Houston.

A Corpulent Corpse

Not to scare you, but death could come quicker if you're overweight. Body fat increases blood pressure, lowers the level of high density lipoproteins (HDL, the "good" cholesterol) in the bloodstream, and heightens the chance of developing diabetes, according to JoAnn Manson, M.D., assistant professor of medicine at Harvard Medical School and an associate physician at Brigham and Women's Hospital in Boston. "All increase the risk of heart disease, coronary artery disease, and stroke," she says. "They're major risk factors."

To some extent, being fat is determined genetically. "But it's not destiny that you're going to be fat or have these health complications," Dr. Manson says. Genes aside, people gain weight when they consume more calories than they expend.

Truth is, society may be more of a factor than genetics. "In a Westernized, industrial environment such as the United States, it seems as if we're almost predisposed to gain weight," says Patrick M. O'Neil, Ph.D., clinical psychologist and director of the Weight Management Center at the Medical University of South Carolina in Charleston. "There's ready access to lots of high-fat food, high-calorie food, and there's usually no great deal of physical exertion required."

This is where your own personal behavior comes in, according to Dr. Goodrick. Rather than lamenting genetics and society, it's up to you to overcome inactivity and indulgent eating.

The Diet of a Lifetime

Any weight-loss expert will tell you: Crash diets and fad diets don't work. Severe calorie restriction or unnatural reliance on certain foods while avoiding all others may work initially, but not in the long run, says Dr. Goodrick. A diet that treats food as the enemy is simply not realistic.

"With food as your foe, the idea of eating becomes anxiety-provoking, and you have even less control," says Dr. Goodrick. What's more, crash diets actually set up the body to crave high-fat foods. "It's no wonder to me that 90 percent of overweight dieters relapse," Dr. Goodrick says.

Such yo-yo dieting isn't just frustrating. It's downright dangerous. "Weight cycling appears to be even more harmful than maintaining an elevated weight with no loss," Dr. Manson says. The reasons aren't clear, she says, but it appears that yo-yo dieting is associated with higher fat deposits in the abdomen and upper body. Once you've lost and then regained fat, it tends to accumulate in the torso. And upper-body fat, as opposed to fat on the hips and legs, is a strong predictor of stroke and heart disease.

In addition, Dr. Manson says, "It's extremely stressful to the system physiologically and emotionally to constantly diet and regain."

Liquid meal substitutes are appropriate only in certain situations that are carefully supervised by a physician. "They're a way to help the more overweight person lose a significant amount of weight pretty quickly," says Dr. O'Neil. Liquid meal supplements are recommended only when part of a comprehensive program to help you make long-term lifestyle changes, he says.

Otherwise, liquid nostrums are completely unrealistic, weight-loss experts say. You need to eat. And you need to exercise to maintain any lower weight you achieve. "If you're expecting the powder alone to keep the weight off, then you're barking up the wrong tree," says Dr. Manson.

Successful, permanent weight loss demands a lifelong monitoring of what you eat and what you do to burn those calories. And the only way to balance that scale is to make everlasting changes in diet and exercise. If you want to shed your excess pounds and keep them off, incorporate these principles into your lifestyle.

Cut the fat. One of the most important causes of obesity is dietary fat, which not only has more calories per forkful than either protein or carbohydrates but also may be more likely to be stored as fat in the body. Trim fat from the meats you eat, and use only low-fat dairy products, desserts, and salad dressings.

Low-fat eaters naturally eat fewer calories, Dr. Goodrick says. And eating fat may make you more lethargic. "People eating high-fat diets sleep more," he says. "They're sluggish. Their red blood cells tend to sludge together and don't transport oxygen as well."

Ease into change. Don't make abrupt alterations in food choices or calorie intake. A body drastically deprived of sustenance thinks it's starving. "We're programmed to conserve calories," Dr. Goodrick says. If you starve yourself, your metabolism slows to a crawl, and your body begins to store—as fat—whatever it does consume.

The trick, Dr. Goodrick says, is to switch to low-fat eating gradually. "If you do that, you can lose excess weight without feeling deprived," he says.

Know your nutrition. Learn about healthier food choices, so that you can eat wisely. Take the skin off chicken. Broil or bake; don't deep-fry. Drink skim milk. Eat low-fat frozen yogurt instead of ice cream. Buy tuna packed in water, not oil. Armed with such knowledge of fat facts, it's much easier to eat low fat even when you're not preparing the meals or when you're dining out.

"Alternative menu planning is easy," Dr. O'Neil says. "It has been estimated that people routinely eat only about ten different meals, and they rotate among them. And they have even less variety in their breakfasts. When you think of it that way, making long-term changes is pretty manageable."

Mind your menu math. You certainly don't have to count every calorie, Dr. O'Neil says, but you should be aware of certain nutritional rules of thumb. "A pound of body fat contains roughly 3,500 calories," he says. "To gain a pound of body fat, you need to eat 3,500 more calories than you burn. To lose a pound, you have to do the opposite."

Overall, fat should comprise no more than 20 to 30 percent of the calories you consume. Protein should make up another 15 percent, with the remainder coming from carbohydrates, preferably complex carbohydrates from grains and vegetables, Dr. Goodrick says.

Break it down. Losing weight is clearly easier when you break down the math into 100-calorie increments—the equivalent of a can of light beer or two-thirds of a regular 12-ounce soft drink. "One hundred calories a day is roughly 10 pounds a year," Dr. O'Neil says. "On a daily basis, if you eat 100 calories more than you burn, expect to gain 10 pounds in a year. Ten pounds is not that much, but 10 pounds a year for ten years is 100 pounds."

Now turn that formula on its head and consider cutting just 100 calories a day. "That seems more doable," Dr. O'Neil says. "Extrapolate it to a year or more, and you can see where you're really making a difference in weight loss."

Fitness Fights Fatness

In stripping off the weight and keeping it off, exercise is very significant, especially in the long run, Dr. O'Neil says. "It's even more critical in maintenance than in weight loss itself," he says. These exercise basics should become routine parts of your life.

Muscle up your metabolism. Your metabolic rate—how many calories you expend while at rest—is determined by the amount of lean muscle in your body. "Strength training is good," Dr. Goodrick says, "because it increases lean tissue, and you won't lose the muscle you otherwise would lose from decreasing calorie consumption."

And don't worry if you see the needle on the scale rising a pound or two after you begin a strength-training regimen. "With muscle gain, you actually have an increase in weight," Dr. Manson says, "because muscle weighs more than fat."

Take a walk. Brisk walking is a fine way to begin

How I Did It: Picturing the Future

Youth, you might be pleased to hear, offers no immunity from obesity. By the time she was 17 years old, Rachel Socas Irizarry tipped the scale at 307 pounds. "I had severe high blood pressure in the 200/100 range and an enlarged heart," she remembers. Not a promising health profile for one so young.

But she was determined to lose weight, and she started by eating salads and walking. Within eight years, she was 5 feet 11 inches tall and weighed 153 pounds as she stood before photographers and television cameras as a part-time model. And what of her rampant high blood pressure? She was able to control it completely through losing the weight, giving herself a health profile that matches her figure.

"I never thought I'd get as far as I did," she says with some degree of disbelief. "But I did."

Here's how:

Irizarry first developed a mental image of what she wanted to look like. "You need to visualize yourself and the body type you'd like," she says. "Or picture yourself doing some hobby you can't do now because of the weight. Use that as an incentive to get started. I

a new fitness lifestyle. Ease yourself into hour-long hikes three or four times a week, Dr. Goodrick says.

Prepare for the long haul. Take a walk on the mild side at first. But for maximum benefit, build up to more than a half-hour exercise session. "During the first half hour, you're just burning glycogen stores in the body," Dr. Goodrick says. "You don't

chose modeling, as it was something I always wanted to do."

She then altered her eating patterns by eliminating fat. "You have to change your eating habits, not just diet," she says. "Once you make the adjustment, it becomes a permanent part of your lifestyle. I used to always put butter and sour cream on my baked potato. Now I wouldn't even think of it. I automatically just eat it plain."

Once the pounds began to drop, weight loss became its own incentive. "All the positive feedback I received was so inspiring," she remembers. "You see the changes in the mirror, and you want to continue."

Exercise helped Irizarry lose the fat and keep it off, and her Orlando, Florida, home now resembles a small gymnasium, complete with a treadmill, stair-climbing machine, stationary bicycle, mini-trampoline, dumbbells, and stacks of work out videos. She walks the treadmill for 30 minutes five days a week and uses the other devices often.

"If I can do it, anyone can," she says. "You need to choose a goal you really desire. You have to do it for yourself. No one else."

burn excess fat until you've been exercising beyond a half hour." The psychological high sparked by the body's production of mood-elevating endorphins also doesn't kick in during exercise routines shorter than 30 minutes.

Enjoy yourself. Just as you should avoid short-term dieting binges, you should also shy away from excessively strenuous or exceedingly demanding workouts that no one realistically could maintain. Select an exercise program that you can see yourself doing for the rest of your life, Dr. O'Neil says. That's because you *will* be doing it for the rest of your life.

The New You

Once you're on a weight-loss roll, the results themselves should provide ample encouragement to stick to your new eating and exercising regimens. "You'll see it on the scale, you'll hear the compliments as people notice the change," Dr. O'Neil says. "You'll feel different."

But it's at this point that some people may let down their guard. "It's easy to make dietary and exercise changes when you're seeing the results so quickly," he says. "The real difficulty starts when the rate of weight loss slows down, and you and others don't notice as much change. The compliments wane, and you start to take your new size for granted." This is when people often think they can revert to old habits, says Dr. O'Neil. They can't. "These are eating and exercise patterns that you have to stay with forever," he says. The weight-loss pros have some suggestions for doing just that.

Take it easy. "One of the most important challenges is that obesity is a chronic problem that needs a long-term solution," Dr. O'Neil says. "Everybody wants a quick fix; it's human nature." Weight loss won't come easy, and it won't come fast. Expect to lose only about ½ to 1 pound of fat a week.

Make it easy. "You don't get extra credit for difficulty," Dr. O'Neil says. "Don't get into a sackcloth-and-ashes mind-set of severe calorie restriction and exhaustive exercise. You won't be able to continue that for long."

Plan for setbacks. "Draw a line a few pounds above your maintenance weight—3 to 5 pounds, not 30 or 50," Dr. O'Neil says. "Then plan what to do if your weight ever goes above it." You might want to consider drinking one fewer beers or colas a night or skipping that buttery bag of popcorn at the movies. Continue this recovery plan until your weight is safely below the line.

Pneumonia

Stand Up To a Killer

Richard Levine of Albuquerque eats well, sleeps well, and looks like a weight lifter—the rewards for spending thousands of hard, hot days making bricks at one of the largest adobe-brick manufacturing plants in the Southwest. But despite nearly 60 years of robust good health, Richard has two weak points: his lungs.

"The first time I had pneumonia, I was a student at Berkeley in 1968," Richard remembers. "My chest hurt like crazy, and I couldn't breathe. It was terrible. When I went to the doctor, he listened to my lungs and slapped me into bed in the hospital for a week. I just couldn't move."

Levine's second bout with pneumonia—and another week in the hospital—came ten years later. After the third time, he finally took his doctor's advice and stopped smoking. "You know, I haven't had pneumonia since," he says.

Actually, it's not cigarettes that cause pneumonia but viruses and bacteria moving into your lungs and bronchi, causing infection, inflammation, and congestion. The germs that often cause pneumonia—*Streptococcus pneumoniae*, for example—normally live harmlessly in your throat and airways. They can even dip down into your lungs without causing any trouble. It's usually when your guard is down (after years of smoking and drinking, for example) or when you've been sick with another illness that your lungs become vulnerable to these everyday bugs, says Steven W. Stogner, M.D., a fellow in the Division of Pulmonary and Critical Care Medicine at Louisiana State University School of Medicine at Shreveport.

When it's mild, pneumonia can be mistaken for a cold, Dr. Stogner says. In more serious cases, it can put you to bed for days with wracking coughs, burning fever, and teeth-chattering, bone-rattling chills. In fact, pneumonia ranks sixth among death-causing diseases, killing more than 40,000 Americans every year. This is because pneumonia often strikes people whose systems are already weakened by other underlying health problems, like heart disease, asthma, or emphysema.

Keeping the Killer At Bay

Since pneumonia tends to strike when your natural resistance isn't up to snuff, the best way to prevent it simply is to stay in tip-top shape. Of course, no one is healthy all of the time, and it's impossible to avoid entirely the multitudes of pneumonia-causing germs. But you can keep your defenses in fighting form. For starters:

Encourage productive coughs. "One of the risk factors for pneumonia is being unable to properly clear secretions from the airways," Dr. Stogner says. People who smoke or who have frequent colds or other respiratory tract infections will often harbor large amounts of mucus in their lungs and airways, he explains. Bacteria love phlegm. And the more bacteria you have in your airways, the greater your chances for getting pneumonia. In other words, those productive coughs—those that bring up phlegm—really are protective coughs.

Keep your distance. Some pneumonias are contagious while others are not, but catching a lungful of anyone else's germs is pushing your luck. If you're in the sickroom with someone with the disease, try to keep a few feet between you and whatever it is they're blowing, sneezing, or coughing. Frequently washing your hands is added insurance, Dr. Stogner says.

Snuff the cigarettes. Tobacco smoke essentially paralyzes the hairlike projections in your airways, called cilia, that help expel mucus and other secretions. If the cilia aren't working, the mucus—and hordes of bacteria—stay inside.

Treatments of Choice

If you have a stubborn cold or flu-like symptoms and congestion in the lungs that doesn't get better after a few days, you could have pneumonia, and you should promptly see your doctor, Dr. Stogner says. A course of antibiotics may be all that is needed to clear it up. If your pneumonia is caused by a virus, your doctor may prescribe a virucide such as amantadine or acyclovir.

These drugs may provide quick relief from symptoms, but the infection generally lasts longer than the symptoms. Unfortunately, many people feel so much better that they assume they're cured and quit taking the drugs. "Your doctor prescribes the exact amount of antibiotics he wants you to take," Dr. Stogner says. If you give the germs a reprieve by stopping your medication prematurely, he warns, they may very well rally and make you sicker than before.

While pneumonia can sometimes be treated at home, some sufferers need more intensive care. In the hospital, you might be given oxygen to give your inflamed lungs a little help. Or if you're having trouble cleaning the phlegm because of an ineffective cough, your doctor may insert a flexible tube into your trachea (windpipe)—a procedure called nasotracheal suction—to clear things out.

Pleurisy, an inflammation of the lining of the lung, is a common complication of pneumonia that makes coughing, even breathing, terribly painful. Your doctor might give you codeine or other drugs to ease the pain. You might even get an intracostal nerve block—an injection that dulls the nerves near the rib cage.

After you get out of the hospital, you'll still have to take things slowly for a few weeks. Your lungs have taken a terrible pounding. They need some rest. To give your healing a helping hand, Dr. Stogner recommends the following.

Fill up on fluids. Pneumonia's hot fevers will dry you out like the desert sun. You need to drink plenty of fluids—about six to eight glasses a day—to avoid dehydration.

Thin your phlegm. You already know how important it is to clear mucus from your lungs and airways. But because pneumonia often is accompanied by pleurisy, the slightest cough can be terribly painful. One possible solution to discuss with your doctor is to take over-the-counter drugs called expectorants. Essentially, these make your coughs more productive with less effort, Dr. Stogner says.

Lie on your side. By supporting, or splinting, your rib cage, this position should make coughing and breathing somewhat less painful.

Take some aspirin. Not only can aspirin help relieve your aches and pains, it will help cool your fever as well. Check with your physician about whether you should use aspirin or a substitute such as acetaminophen.

Get plenty of rest. Your lungs have been through the wringer, and they need time to recover, Dr. Stogner says. This isn't the time to overexert yourself. A gradual increase in daily activities is suggested.

A Shot of Prevention

After you've concluded the long, breathless journey into and out of pneumonia, you'll never want to get it again. But if you're in the more elderly range of 50-plus, you're at higher risk of contracting pneumonia. So are those with chronic lung disease, diabetes, or any debilitating disease.

If that's you, or if you're in close contact with anyone who has pneumonia, you should ask your doctor about a pneumonia vaccine. "For certain types of pneumonia, the vaccines are very good," Dr. Stogner says. But pneumonia is sufficiently rare in healthy persons, and easy enough to treat when it does occur, that doctors don't routinely give the vaccinations to everyone.

Because of modern antibiotics and antiviral drugs, pneumonia isn't the marauding scourge it once was. If left untreated, however, it can certainly be a very dangerous disease; people die from it every year. But most pneumonias are tamed easily with drugs. Even Richard Levine, who twice stayed in the hospital, treated his third attack at home with antibiotics. Don't panic if you think you have pneumonia, Dr. Stogner says. But don't wait to call your doctor either. Early diagnosis and treatment are of paramount importance.

Prostate Problems

Conquering Man's Greatest Fear

During a man's younger years, the prostate, a small gland at the base of his bladder, quietly churns out the semen that fuels his sex life. As he ages, however, the prostate sometimes assumes another duty: causing trouble. It can get sore, tender, and inflamed. Like a summer zucchini, it can grow large and cumbersome. Finally, it's one of the leading sites of cancer in American men.

But relatively few men are prostrate because of their prostate. Most prostate problems can be assuaged with rest, antibiotics, or surgery.

When Bigger Isn't Better

Every night, millions of older American men, with tired eyes and a brimming bladder, leave the comfort of their bed to seek relief. But to their sorrow, that relief is short-lived: No sooner do they settle back to sleep than their bladder, like an inexhaustible well, feels full again.

These uncomfortable fellows belong to what is perhaps the least exclusive club in the world: The Fraternal Order of Men with Enlarged Prostate Glands. Just about every man over 50 has an enlarged prostate, a condition doctors call benign prostatic hyperplasia. Many men with this condition feel the need to urinate often, sometimes every hour. Many will have painful urination, a diminished urinary stream, or a feeling that their bladder never is empty.

Here's what happens. As urine leaves your bladder, it first passes through a channel in the prostate gland called the prostatic urethra. An enlarging prostate gland begins to block the prostatic urethra and, consequently, the flow of urine. That's why men with enlarged prostates often have weak urinary streams. What's more, the bladder has to work extra hard to push urine through the narrowed urethra, the tube that carries urine from the bladder through the penis. Eventually the bladder gets tired and finds it more restful to stay full than to try to empty.

Many older men can hold tremendous amounts of urine because the bladder's stretch receptors have become less sensitive, says Steven R. Gambert, M.D., professor of medicine and gerontology and associate dean for academic programs at New York Medical College in Valhalla. "These men often will get an upper urinary tract disorder, which can occur if urine goes back up into the kidneys," says Dr. Gambert. "That can cause all sorts of problems including kidney failure."

Plumbing Repair

Some men can have an enlarged prostate for decades with no problems whatsoever. If the normal flow of urine gets significantly impaired, however, it may be time to open things up, says Mark S. Soloway, M.D., professor of urology and chief of urologic oncology at the University of Tennessee at Memphis and attending physician at Baptist Memorial Hospital, Memphis. Basically, you have two options: drugs or surgery.

A class of prescription drugs called alpha blockers (two examples, Minipress and Dibenzyline) can help relax the smooth muscle that surrounds the prostate, thus allowing the overgrowth to move outward from the prostatic urethra. Once the urethra is clear, urine can once again flow freely. But these drugs don't actually shrink the tissue, Dr. Soloway says. They offer temporary relief, not a cure.

Surgery, on the other hand, can cure an enlarged prostate simply by removing renegade tissue. "Many men, of course, would like to avoid an operation, but surgery is tried and true," Dr. Soloway says. In fact, approximately 350,000 surgeries for this condition are performed every year, and it's one of the most common operations performed on men 65 and older.

Surgical incisions rarely are required, Dr. Soloway says. Instead, most surgeons prefer a technique called transurethral resection of the prostate, in which prostatic tissue is removed by inserting tiny instruments into the penis, through the urethra and up into the prostate. The surgery is quite simple, Dr. Soloway says, and "about 80 percent of the people who have it are dramatically improved."

Getting the Bugs Out

Besides growth, the prostate in men over 50 can suffer from unwelcome visitors. Bacterial prostatitis—an infection in the prostate gland—occurs when bacteria from the colon get into the urethra. Once in the urethra, bacteria can take a leisurely swim upstream until they reach the prostate gland. There they make themselves at home by making you miserable. The prostate gland may get infected and painfully inflamed. Some men will need to urinate every few hours. Others will have painful urination, perhaps accompanied by fever, chills, or low back pain.

Fortunately, bacterial prostatitis is quite rare and easily treated with antibiotics, says Dr. Soloway. A few aspirin and a relaxing bath can make you feel better, but what you really need are the antibiotics, which will clear up the infection in just a few days, Dr. Soloway says.

Not so easily treated (and perhaps much more common) is nonbacterial prostatitis. It produces some of the same symptoms as its bacterial cousin, but what causes it remains a mystery. "Most men who have discomfort in the area of the prostate have a sort of nonspecific congestion, and it's unclear entirely what's going on," Dr. Soloway says.

Stephen N. Rous, M.D., author of *The Prostate Book*, suggests a very specific remedy for nonbacterial prostatitis that should be of interest to couples over 50: more sex. Because the prostate produces much of the fluid that comprises a man's ejaculate, any decrease in sexual frequency will allow semen to accumulate to potentially painful levels, Dr. Rous reasons. Some doctors, it should be noted, aren't convinced.

It's been suggested that the term nonbacterial prostatitis is incorrect because the disorder might be caused by bacteria that medical tests can't yet detect. In fact, many doctors treat bacterial and nonbacterial prostatitis exactly the same—with antibiotics. "Many men with nonbacterial prostatitis will get well, but that may be independent of the antibiotics," Dr. Soloway says.

The Cancer Trap

Are you sitting down? Good. Now read on: Doctors estimate that perhaps 30 percent of American men 50 years and older may already have prostatic cancer. Among men who live into their nineties, that number may shoot to 80 percent. In other words, if you live long enough, there's a good chance you'll get cancer of the prostate gland.

Now, those harsh facts sound scary, but they're really not as bad as they seem. Here's why.

Most of these cancers won't catch up with you. Many more men will die *with* prostate cancer than *from* prostate cancer, says Dr. Rous. This is because prostate cancer usually grows very slowly.

But cancer of the prostate is still cancer, and it can be deadly. In fact, it's the third largest cause of cancer deaths in men, Dr. Soloway says. That's why doctors advise all men over 50 to have yearly rectal examinations to screen for early signs of trouble. Catch prostate cancer in time, and you could save yourself from being a statistic.

Trim the Risk

Better yet, you may be able to prevent prostate cancer in the first place. One way to do this is at the dinner table.

Trim the fat. Researchers have found that men

Prostate Surgery: Coming Out Ahead

The same man who might run into a raging fire to rescue a kitten will buckle at the knees should his doctor mention prostate surgery. It's not merely his life that's being discussed but (gulp!) his sex life.

Guys, you can calm down, says Steven R. Gambert, M.D., professor of medicine and gerontology and associate dean for academic programs at New York Medical College in Valhalla. If you had erections before surgeons worked on your prostate, there's a good chance you'll have them afterward. If you had orgasms . . . well, you might notice some interesting changes.

Most men who have surgery for benign prostatic hyperplasia will have retrograde ejaculations, Dr. Gambert says. This means your semen, instead of coming out of the end of your penis during orgasm, will go backward into the bladder. It's painless and won't necessarily change the quality of your orgasms, but the idea does take some getting used to, he says.

More threatening to a man's sexual functioning is radical prostatectomy (removal of the entire prostate gland), a procedure sometimes required for men with advanced prostatic cancer. But there's good news here, too. "In the old days, many of the nerve fibers that control erections might have been cut, and that would lead to impotence," Dr. Gambert says. Today, however, surgeons can often spare the nerves, thus sparing erections. It may, however, take six months to a year after the surgery before a man feels like his old self again.

who skimp on high-fat foods such as eggs, meat, and cheese may substantially reduce their risks for prostate cancer. In one study, researchers in Utah investigated the diets of 358 men with cancer of the prostate. Eating high-fat foods, the researchers concluded, "was the strongest risk factor" for developing prostate cancer.

Add some fiber to your diet. Some researchers believe that foods high in dietary fiber—such as beans, dried fruit, and whole-wheat breads—can further lower prostate cancer risk. In one study, investigators examined the diets of thousands of men. Those who ate the most fiber had lower risks for prostate cancer.

Stay active. According to a Harvard study, men who stay active all their lives may have only half the risk of prostate cancer compared with those who are inactive. In the study, researchers examined the exercise habits of 17,719 men. Among men over 70 years old who were highly active, the risk for getting prostate cancer was 53 percent of the risk of inactive men. Researchers suggest that exercise, by decreasing testosterone levels, may decrease the risk for prostate cancer as well.

Stroke

Reducing the Risks

It's a fact of life: The older you get, the higher the risk you have for stroke. After you turn 55, the risk doubles every decade.

What it comes down to is that there's something your brain needs more than a large cup of coffee in the morning or a nightly dose of *Jeopardy.* It needs blood.

Without a constant flow of blood to supply your brain cells with fresh oxygen, those brain cells would quickly die. That is what happens when a blood vessel bringing blood to the brain ruptures or gets clogged. It's called a stroke, and it's America's third largest killer (heart disease and cancer hold the top spots) and a cause of serious impairment in thousands of people. The number of those stricken yearly is about a half million but it's a number that, happily, is falling every year. In fact, the number of strokes in America has declined by half in the past two decades.

Why's that? The drop is mostly the result of increased knowledge about what causes stroke and what can prevent it. If you're not already privy to this information, it's a stroke of good luck that you're reading this chapter.

The Basics of Stroke

Strokes occur in two different ways: *Ischemic* strokes are caused by blood clots that block the supply of

(continued on page 506)

How I Did It:
Can't Is a Four-Letter Word

One day in 1961, Veronica McKeen was in the shower in her home in El Paso, Texas, getting ready to go shopping. As she bathed, several small blood clots broke loose and traveled to the arteries of her brain. There they blocked the flow of blood, and Veronica collapsed. She woke up five days later in the hospital, paralyzed on her left side. She was 23.

"I was in the hospital only two weeks, including the five days I was in a coma," she says. She wasn't given any therapy, and there was no follow-up treatment. "It's hard to believe now," she says, "but that's the way things were in those days."

McKeen assumed she'd just get better, as though she were recovering from a cold, but things did not go well for the next few years. "I wasn't getting any better," she says. She wheeled herself around the house, struggled to walk, and battled her mild aphasia (problems with finding the right words). Depression and anemia set in, along with crying fits and laughing spells. Thus began six years of weekly visits to a psychiatrist, tranquilizers, even shock therapy—and she continued to deteriorate.

By 1970, McKeen had hit bottom and found there was nowhere to go but up. "I started realizing I would have to take things into my own hands," she says. "A very good friend helped. She'd say 'You can,' I'd say 'I can't,' and she'd say 'You can, and you will.'"

Will—the magic word. A horse lover, McKeen began working at the stables of a nearby racetrack, hobbling around, caring for the horses. Later she wangled herself a job at the betting window. "It helped build my self-confidence," she says. "The more I did it, the more confident I got."

After three years of confidence building, she married a man who said, "You can, you can, you can." From day one, he told her, "I don't ever want to hear you say 'I can't.'" This new, supportive husband gave her the idea for a 640-mile bicycle ride.

In April 1988, with the Organization for After-Stroke Resources as her backer, she rode from Glendora, California, to Sacramento, stopping at convalescent homes along the way to show strokers they can overcome their disability. "It was eye-opening to the people in those homes, many of whom had just given up," she says.

McKeen now has full use of her left arm; her aphasia has faded, but she still limps slightly. If a doctor tells you you'll never walk again, get another doctor, she says. "Your recovery depends on you," says McKeen. "You don't know what you can do until you try. The sooner you can help yourself, the sooner you get out of that bed or wheelchair, the sooner you can begin to re-gain your independence."

blood to areas of the brain. They account for 70 to 80 percent of all strokes. *Hemorrhagic* strokes, the more deadly of the two, are caused by blood vessels that rupture in the brain itself or on the surface of the brain.

Neither kind of stroke is actually a disease—doctors call them "events." The illness behind the event is cardiovascular disease, which is disease of the blood vessels, the heart, or both. Regardless of what we call a stroke, some people are more susceptible than others. Besides age, there are several other risk factors for stroke that you can't control.

Gender. The incidence of stroke is about 30 percent higher in men than in women.

Race. Blacks have a 60 percent greater chance of death or disability from a stroke than whites.

Diabetes. Even though diabetes can be controlled, the disease may weaken blood vessels, hiking the stroke risk for men by 40 percent and for women by 72 percent.

Heredity. If you have a family history of stroke, your own risk is higher than normal.

Prior stroke. It increases the risk of another stroke by several times.

Irregular heartbeat. A condition called atrial fibrillation can cause clots to form that may travel to the brain. It raises the risk of stroke in men by 83 percent and in women by more than 200 percent. Atrial fibrillation often results from a prior heart attack.

What You *Can* Do

Now the good part. There are lots of things you have control over that will lessen your chances of having a stroke.

Lower the pressure. Hypertension (high blood pressure) is the number one risk factor for stroke. So it should be no surprise that controlling high blood pressure has probably had more to do with the decline in death rates from stroke than has any other factor.

High blood pressure can cause and aggravate atherosclerosis—hardening and clogging of arteries that normally are open and flexible and able to adjust to temporary increases in pressure and blood flow. Controlling high blood pressure can often be achieved by eating a healthier diet and losing excess weight. Sometimes drugs can do the trick. The first step, of course, is to have your blood pressure checked. If it's high, discuss options with your doctor. (For tips on how to control high blood pressure, see High Blood Pressure on page 435.)

Avoid heart disease. Even without hypertension, heart disease more than doubles your stroke risk. The three biggies for avoiding heart disease are cigarette smoking (don't), blood cholesterol (keep it low), and blood pressure (the lower, the better). (For a heart disease prevention program, see Heart Disease on page 424.)

See red. Watch your red blood cell count. The more red cells you have, the thicker your blood, and the more likely you are to form stroke-causing clots, doctors say. If your physician determines that you have this condition, it can be treated by removing blood or by prescribing a blood "thinner" such as aspirin.

Control cholesterol. This fatlike natural blood alcohol strongly contributes to the development of atherosclerosis and heart disease. So if you can reduce your blood cholesterol, you're two steps ahead of stroke. You can keep your cholesterol under control by reducing the cholesterol and saturated fat in your diet. Start by eating more vegetables, fruits, and grains—and less meat, dairy products (unless they're

Top Sources of Potassium

Potassium is known to help control high blood pressure (the greatest risk factor for stroke) and may also have other stroke-protective effects. Your stroke prevention diet should include these foods, the best sources of potassium.

Food	Portion	Potassium (mg)
Avocado	1	1,204
Potato, baked	1 med.	844
Cantaloupe	½	825
Prunes, dried	½ cup	600
Watermelon	1 slice	560
Raisins	½ cup	545
Orange juice	1 cup	496
Broccoli, raw	1 med. stalk	490
Lima beans, large, boiled	½ cup	478
Banana	1	451

low-fat or nonfat varieties) and snack foods. (Ideas for controlling cholesterol can be found under High Cholesterol, on page 450.)

Stop smoking. Smoking tobacco hikes your risk of stroke by about 70 percent. Part of the reason is that smoking contributes to heart disease and atherosclerosis. It may also make your blood more likely to clot and your blood vessels more likely to constrict. If you

Food	Portion	Potassium (mg)
Apricots, dried	¼ cup	448
Squash, winter, baked	½ cup	445
Skim milk	1 cup	406
Sweet potato, baked	1 med.	397
Whole milk	1 cup	370
Sardines, Atlantic	1 can	365
Kidney beans, boiled	½ cup	355
Sunflower seeds, dried	⅓ cup	331
Apricots, fresh	3	313
Flounder, baked	3 oz	292
Tomato, raw	1 med.	254
Peach	1	171
Green pepper	1 large	144

don't smoke, don't start. If you do smoke, quit. Researchers from the Framingham Heart Study in Massachusetts say that after four or five clean years, quitters may find that their risk of stroke is no greater than that of someone who has never smoked.

Cut down on drinking. Let's toast water and fruit juice. Studies show that alcohol increases the risk of both types of stroke, but heavy drinkers triple their risk for the more deadly hemorrhagic stroke. If you drink, do so in moderation.

Exercise. If you lead a life of ease, sliding into the car even to go to the corner mailbox, you are increasing your risk of heart disease—and you know what that means. Exercise can help lower blood pressure, take off excess weight, control cholesterol levels, and manage diabetes (another risk factor for stroke).

Recent studies have shown that most of the health benefits of exercise come from moderate workouts. Brisk walking, for example, is an excellent exercise. You can start by hiking to the mailbox! Of course, it's a good idea to check with your doctor before starting any exercise program.

Shed excess pounds. Obesity is often a prominent partner of heart disease, diabetes, high blood pressure, and high cholesterol. Lose weight, and you lower your risk of stroke.

Control diabetes. Statistics show that diabetes increases stroke risk in men by 40 percent and in women by 72 percent. Keeping diabetes under control won't remove the risk altogether, but it boosts the odds in your favor. (For more information on controlling diabetes, see Diabetes on page 398.)

TIA: A Warning Sign

A transient ischemic attack—or TIA—is a not-to-be-ignored warning of an impending ischemic stroke. This "mini-stroke" mimics what a real stroke would do to you: weakness; numbness in the face, arm, hand, or leg; loss of the ability to speak clearly or to understand what others are saying to you; dimness or loss of vision in one eye; dizziness or loss of balance. But the symptoms rapidly disappear—in 90 percent of the cases, they fade in less than 6 hours. The importance of the TIA is that 20 to 40 percent of people who have them go on to have a full-blown stroke. Their risk is ten times greater than that of those who haven't had a TIA. If you think you've had a TIA, see a doctor immediately.

"The greatest risk of stroke is in the first week after a TIA happens," says Harold P. Adams, M.D., director of the Cerebrovascular Diseases Division at the University of Iowa. But just because you haven't had a TIA doesn't mean you're safe: Only 10 percent of strokes are preceded by a TIA.

The Road Back from a Stroke

Seven out of ten people who have a stroke live through it, although the going can be rough. Survivors may be affected in a large number of ways, from speech problems to difficulty chewing and swallowing. Of the people who survive a stroke, about two-thirds will need some form of rehabilitation, says Michael Reding, M.D., associate professor of neurology at Cornell University Medical College and director of the Stroke Rehabilitation Unit at Burke Rehabilitation Center in New York City.

Through rehabilitation, the brain can develop new pathways that circumvent damaged connections and switches. "Some cells are dead, some that were just outside the damaged area aren't dead but are not functioning," Dr. Reding says. "In the three months after a stroke, these cells will start to recover." As recovery progresses, these still-living cells may take over some of the functions the dead cells used to perform. They'll need practice.

"The whole philosophy of rehab is that if you

511

Speaking in Tongues

Sometimes a stroke can help scientists learn how the brain works. Take the Baltimore man who had a stroke in small arteries deep in his brain. "The area that was damaged was very small but very important," says his doctor, neurologist Dean Tippett, M.D., of the University of Maryland School of Medicine in Baltimore. Important enough to shed light on how the brain produces language.

The man was born and bred in the United States, and spoke no foreign languages. But after a couple of days of slurred speech, he began speaking with a strong accent. "He was pretty clear, and everyone who heard him said he sounded Scandinavian or Nordic," Dr. Tippett says. He added vowel sounds as he spoke, saying things like "How are you today-ah?" When making a statement, his voice would rise in pitch at the end of a sentence, making it sound like a question.

There have been 15 similar cases reported since 1901, Dr. Tippett says, "and each helps us learn the discrete areas responsible for very specific language functions"—like the ability to form contractions.

The Baltimore stroke victim actually stopped forming contractions (for example, saying "do not" instead of "don't"), as if he didn't know the language he was speaking. "He had to struggle with the English language, as if he were a foreigner," Dr. Tippett says. "Rather than something being added to his speech, something was actually taken away."

have trouble with something, you keep working at it," Dr. Reding says. "If you have trouble walking, you keep trying to walk. The same goes for dressing or talking. The way you learned to read and write and figure things out in the first place was practice, practice, practice. You have to relearn the basics. That's how the brain learns to adapt to its environment."

Rehab also puts the patient through exercises to keep joints mobile and muscles, tendons, and ligaments limber. Exercise provides feedback to the cells that are taking on new roles, Dr. Reding says. Recognize that after a stroke, the patient is likely to get tired even thinking about exercise. That's something he needs to work through, says Dr. Reding.

Attitude Is Everything

"People come out of rehab in all stages," says Frank Shirbroun, Ph.D., executive director of the Organization for After-Stroke Resources (OASR) in Upland, California. "Most recover many of their skills in the first six months after a stroke, and then a plateau forces them to realize that some of the effects of their stroke are permanent. That's often when depression, hopelessness, and decline set in."

If you're in that boat, know that you can bail out.

Be with your compadres. "Spend time with other survivors and their families," Dr. Shirbroun says. "They can inspire you and ignite your will to get on with life." Hospital social workers, senior centers, stroke survivors' organizations, Alzheimer's and Parkinson's groups, and YM/YWCAs are all sources of support group information.

Prove that doctor wrong. "People often don't know what they can do until they try," Dr. Shirbroun says. "You don't have to accept the doctor's verdict that you'll never walk again. It may be physically impossible, but then again, it may not. That's the unknown part of stroke. People can recover far more than many think if they have the will and the access to help. How much a stroke patient can do is very individualized."

The staff at OASR, composed mostly of volunteers, works at convincing stroke survivors and their families that they can get back into society, Dr. Shirbroun says. "Our activities are always in a public facility, like a community center or a school," he says. That means they're not shut away in homes and hospitals.

Inspiration is another factor. "We try to keep successful survivors in front of our people," says Dr. Shirbroun. "Many of these success stories were once in wheelchairs."

Sing out. About one-fourth of stroke survivors have problems talking. "But often people who can't or won't talk, whether from physical inability or lack of will, can sing," Dr. Shirbroun says.

Play games. "In one of our games aimed at regaining the ability to talk, each person has to say one word that has to do with summer," Dr. Shirbroun says. "One man who had never said one word since his stroke started saying 'bikini' over and over again. He didn't even realize he could say it. Another woman, after her stroke, could only say 'Magic Johnson.' Now she's giving inspirational speeches to other stroke survivors."

Work out. "Even if you're in a wheelchair or relying on a quad-cane, you can exercise," Dr. Shirbroun says. "We have range-of-motion exercises for people in wheelchairs. Because of aquatic exercise, one man was able to get out of his chair, then walk with a quad-cane and finally walk without a cane."

The Glutamate Connection

Hospital emergency rooms, intensive care units, and probably even ambulances of the near future are going to have new weapons to prevent stroke-caused brain damage. These weapons will target a brain chemical that makes brain cells virtually work themselves into a fatal frenzy in the hours and days following a stroke.

That brain chemical is glutamate. Glutamate normally plays an essential role in making a brain cell fire off messages to neighboring cells, says Stephen Heinemann, Ph.D., professor of neuroscience at the Salk Institute for Biological Studies in San Diego. "It does this by transmitting calcium into brain cells. But after a stroke—when there's a drop in blood supply or oxygen to the cells—glutamate builds up and keeps pumping calcium into the cells," Dr. Heinemann says. "The cells become overstimulated, firing again and again until they die."

So researchers have theorized that if they can block the buildup of glutamate, they can prevent too much calcium from setting off this brain-damaging reaction. No glutamate, no calcium, no cell damage. Cell damage is what often causes severe disabilities in victims of stroke.

When can you expect hospital emergency rooms to have glutamate-blocking drugs to prevent stroke-caused brain damage? "We will be lucky if they are available by the year 2000, but I hope they will be," Dr. Heinemann says.

The OASR even organizes after-stroke athletic games—bowling, basketball, shuffleboard, even card games—played by people who thought they could never again hold and deal a deck of cards, let alone bowl over pins.

See the cup half full, not half empty. All stroke patients fear having another stroke. Depending on your risk factors (gender, blood pressure, heart disease, diabetes), your chances of having another stroke range from 15 to 40 percent. But turn those numbers upside down. "The odds are obviously in your favor," says Dr. Reding. "There's a 60 to 85 percent chance you won't have another stroke." And thanks to recent advances in medical knowledge, those odds are getting better all the time.

Get organized. If you can't find a group, start one. You might be the impetus for saving yourself and others in the same boat from decline. "Too many stroke survivors just plop in front of a TV for the rest of their lives," says Dr. Shirbroun. "And that's a tragedy, because there's a lot of good living still to be done."

Varicose Veins

Folding Up That Road Map

Do your legs start aching in the afternoon? Do you always wear long pants, even at the beach? Do you stare at your legs and wonder, "Where's Route 66?"

Welcome to the world of varicose veins, that tortuous topography of swollen blood vessels that twist and turn like interstate highways on a road map. Caused by structural weaknesses inside, varicose veins are proof that gravity exists.

An Uphill Battle

Basically a varicose vein is a blood vessel that doesn't quite have the oomph to push its cargo—blood—back into circulation. Here's what happens: When blood exits your heart through the arteries, it shoots right along, assisted both by gravity and by the heart's pumping action. The return trip through the veins, however, is more arduous. Not only do your veins exert less pressure, but much of the journey, particularly from the feet and legs, is uphill.

To help the blood move upward, your veins are lined with tiny one-way valves. The valves open to let blood through, then snap shut as it passes. This system allows the blood to move in stages, its weight supported by the valves. Sometimes, however, the valves fail. Or in some cases, they're congenitally absent.

When this happens, the rising column of blood comes crashing down.

"Instead of carrying blood away from the skin and muscles and to the heart, the vein now is carrying blood in a reverse flow," explains Mitchel P. Goldman, M.D., assistant clinical professor of dermatology at the University of California, San Diego, and author of a textbook on the treatment of varicose veins. Since the blood has trouble going upward, it tends to pool at the bottom of the vein. When this happens, the vein becomes distended—in other words, varicose.

Varicose veins are extremely common, affecting one in five adults, Dr. Goldman says. Women are five times more vulnerable than men, and the veins often crop up during and after pregnancy. Varicose veins rarely are a serious problem, although they can make the legs achy and tired, and the impaired circulation, if left untreated, can cause ulcers to develop on the lower legs. And, of course, they don't look so good.

Keep That Blood Moving

Your heart's a real powerhouse, pumping approximately 1½ gallons of blood every minute. But varicose veins don't get enough of that action. For your blood to keep moving, it needs some extra help. With a few simple tricks, you can relieve some of the ache from varicose veins, and in some cases help prevent them from forming. For example:

Walk your dogs. Unlike arteries, veins depend on your muscles to move blood along. Every time you stand up or take a walk or flex your toes, the muscles in your legs squeeze the veins, actually squirting the blood upward. The more you move your legs, the more pressure you exert on your veins—and the less blood you have just sitting there. Every now and then, shift your weight from foot to foot. Wiggle your toes. Move your feet, heel to toe, to get a really good stretch.

Flatten those heels. "When you wear high heels, you do not activate your calf muscles properly, which allows blood to collect in the veins," Dr. Goldman says. Flat heels can give your muscles (and your veins) the help they need. Of course, flats are a bit more comfortable, too.

Prop them up. Since your blood, like Isaac Newton's apple, has a powerful tendency to go downhill, it naturally gravitates to your legs—and your varicose veins. You can reverse the flow simply by raising your legs above the level of your heart. During the day, put your feet up now and then to let the blood drain out.

Keep your weight down. This can help in two ways. First, when you're overweight, you have more blood, and this puts additional strain on your veins. Second, leaner people have more muscle, and muscle, remember, helps move the blood along. In other words, too much cushion means not enough pushin'.

Feast on fiber. "If you're straining to have a bowel movement, you're going to put a lot of pressure on the pelvic veins, which impedes the blood flow back to your heart," Dr. Goldman says. Try to eat several helpings of fruits, vegetables, and whole grains a day. This will help the stools pass more easily and will take some of the pressure off your veins.

Stay out of hot water. In fact, you should avoid all high temperatures, whether from saunas, hot tubs, or sunbaked beaches. Heat dilates your veins, which in turn lowers the pressure that pushes the blood uphill, Dr. Goldman says.

Loosen up. Those tightfitting pants, girdles, and

panty hose that flatter your figure can flatten the veins between your heart and your legs, Dr. Goldman says. Do your bloodstream a favor and stick to looser, more comfortable clothes.

Wrap them up. While tight clothes can make your varicose veins worse, graduated compression stockings, which apply prescribed amounts of pressure, can help prevent them. For stockings to work, however, they should be fitted to your legs by a doctor, Dr. Goldman says.

Going a Step Further

Most people with varicose veins don't need medical treatment, Dr. Goldman says. But when your legs really are hurting, or you're so self-conscious that you refuse to wear shorts in July, then it might be time to consider more serious measures.

If the idea of surgery scares you stiff, think how Galen's patients must have felt. Galen, a Greek physician who practiced medicine some 1,800 years ago, suggested that varicose veins be removed . . . with hooks! Today's techniques are more sophisticated, thank goodness, and the treatment—with a scalpel or, in many cases, with injections—often is the best bet for varicose veins, Dr. Goldman says.

When you have surgery, the problem veins simply are removed. "The legs have thousands and thousands of veins, and most of them are connected to each other," Dr. Goldman explains. "By eliminating the useless veins, you're going to improve the circulation to the others." Once removed, varicose veins don't come back. However, other veins may eventually become varicose, he adds.

With surgery, of course, there always are risks—

from bleeding, infection, and other complications. There's also the risk of scarring, which in some cases can be as unsightly as the veins are. To avoid these risks, many doctors now are removing varicose veins with a procedure called sclerotherapy, an injection therapy, Dr. Goldman says. With injection therapy, the doctor injects an irritating solution into the vein, which then collapses and eventually disappears.

With smaller veins, one injection may be enough; larger veins may require two, three, or even four injections, Dr. Goldman says. After each treatment, the legs are wrapped with graduated compression stockings to prevent the collapsed veins from opening up again. Should a vein reopen, another injection will close it again.

Most varicose veins are "100 percent" curable, according to Dr. Goldman. "Particularly for smaller veins, I can't see the treatments getting much better than they are now," he says.

Vision Problems

Keeping the World In Sight

There ought to be a law against what aging can do to your eyes. Getting older seems to be a major player in three of the four leading causes of blindness—glaucoma, macular degeneration, and cataracts (the fourth is diabetes). If eyes are truly the window of the soul, how is your soul supposed to see out with the blinds drawn? Why should you have to play peekaboo with the beauty of life?

Odds are you don't. The human eye is an intricately complex and delicate organ. Its components are tiny and fragile. Yet thanks to remarkable advances in ophthalmology in the past 20 years—from sunglasses to eye-drops to laser surgery—the risks of blindness are relatively slight. And for many older people, the new treatments can also curb some of the vision problems that used to be a matter of course.

Cataracts

Right behind your iris and pupil is the lens, a transparent, elastic material that focuses the light entering the eye. Tiny muscles can narrow or thicken the lens as needed. A cataract is a clouding of that lens, blocking the passage of light through it.

Getting older is a major cause of clouded lenses. By age 65, half of all Americans have some degree of cataract formation. For those over 75, the percentage jumps to 70. The most common symptom is fuzzy, blurry, or double vision that gets worse in the evening. No matter how many new eyeglass prescriptions you get, they may not help.

On the brighter side, there's only a 15 percent chance that cataracts will interfere with your normal activities. And even if cataracts do cause you trouble, surgery can help most of the time. There are also ways to stop trouble before it starts.

Shun the sun. No one really knows what causes most cataracts. But researchers do know that fishermen on the Chesapeake Bay had much greater chances of developing cataracts than miners in West Virginia. "There is evidence that ultraviolet and blue light increases the risk of developing at least one type of cataract over your lifetime," says Walter Stark, M.D., professor of ophthalmology at Johns Hopkins University and director of the Corneal and Cataract Service of the Wilmer Eye Institute at the Johns Hopkins Hospital in Baltimore. That's why protecting your eyes from the sun is your best insurance against cataracts.

Wear shades and a hat. If you do go outdoors, the American Academy of Ophthalmology (AAO) recommends that you wear sunglasses that block ultraviolet light. Studies show that regular use of sunglasses can reduce the risk of cataracts and slow their growth if you're developing them. Look for the designation Z80.3 on the sunglasses: It indicates that they filter out 95 percent of the harmful rays. A broad-brimmed hat can also help, according to the AAO.

Get a daily dose of C and E. Another theory on cataracts says that they're caused, at least in part, by the oxidation of the lens by so-called free radicals. The body's own defenses against oxidation decrease with age. Vitamins C and E, and the minerals zinc and selenium, are known antioxidants and are believed to help the body neutralize free radicals, thus helping to prevent cataracts from forming.

You can get lots of those antioxidants naturally, by eating plenty of fruits and vegetables. You can also take supplements, but not all doctors recommend them. "I don't routinely prescribe them, but I don't object either," says Michael Klein, M.D., associate professor of ophthalmology at Oregon Health Sciences University in Portland. If you decide to take supplements, Dr. Klein stresses that you consult your doctor. Vitamins and minerals can be toxic in high dosages.

Cataract Surgery: A New Lens on Life

Cataract surgery is so common (about 1.2 million operations are performed each year in the United States) that it tends to get trivialized, Dr. Stark says. "But it's major surgery," he points out. It virtually always involves the implantation of a synthetic lens to replace your old, cloudy one.

But do you really need this surgery? Maybe not. "A cataract is not a malignancy," he says. "It will not hurt the eye. There's no harm in putting off surgery. It does not have to be removed unless the reduced vision interferes with your life. If you can still see well enough to do everything you want to do, then you do not need surgery."

Cataract surgery also may not be enough to restore your vision, even though it's successful 95 percent of the time. "You may have a moderate cataract but severe macular degeneration, and cataract surgery will not help you," Dr. Stark says. "On the other hand, you may have a severe cataract and severe macular degeneration, and cataract surgery may help restore some of your vision."

You can usually have cataract surgery as an outpatient. You'll go to the hospital, where the surgeon will make a small slit in the eye and slide out the lens. Then the new synthetic lens will be inserted and the incisions will be closed. The operation to remove the lens takes only 45 to 60 minutes, but preoperative and postoperative procedures boost the total time to about 10 hours, Dr. Stark says. You can go home the same day.

Recovery is usually swift, he says. "You can do pretty much what you want to do the day after, using

Vision Aids and Attitude

If you have any vision left at all, says Lorraine Marchi, executive director of the National Association for Visually Handicapped, you can read if you want to. "It's a re-education of the brain," Marchi says. "The more you use your reduced vision, the better the brain interprets what it sees."

What you need is motivation. "The motivation comes from being able to understand what the problem is," Marchi says. "We have a 97 percent success rate with our people, because we explain everything to them."

The other part of the equation is vision aids, which help those with glaucoma, macular degeneration, and other eye diseases. They include simple things like:

Telescopic lenses. They can be built right into a pair of glasses. One type looks like a tiny camera viewfinder perched on top of your glasses.

Closed-circuit television. It lets you read print enlarged up to 60 times on a TV screen.

Field enhancer. This is a special prism that increases the peripheral vision of someone with glaucoma.

Adjustable lamps and high-intensity light bulbs. These increase the amount of light in a room.

Large-print publications. There are many books and magazines that come in large-print editions. There are even large-print telephone dials, calculators, and needle threaders.

common sense," he says. "The main thing is not to get hit or bumped in the eye. You can go back to work as soon as you want, but you should avoid strenuous activity or contact sports for a few weeks."

In about 30 to 40 percent of the cases, another operation is needed within five years, Dr. Stark says. And this is where lasers come in. In the first operation, he says, the doctor puts the new lens in the old lens capsule. "Over time, the capsule itself becomes hazy," he says. In effect, it's formed its own version of a cataract. The doctor can use a special laser to fire light through the lens and into the capsule, punching a tiny hole in the capsule and clearing up your vision.

Glaucoma

They call glaucoma "the sneak thief of sight" because it doesn't affect your central vision at first, says Cynthia Bradford, M.D., assistant professor of ophthalmology at the University of Oklahoma Health Sciences Center in Oklahoma City. "It creeps in from the side," she says. "If you first learn you have glaucoma by noticing you can't see as far as you once could, you already have very significant damage. When you lose this peripheral vision, it can't be restored. Your vision can be 20/20 straight ahead, but only straight ahead—it's tunnel vision, like peeking through a straw."

A normal eye is filled with fluid, and that fluid drains through tissues between the iris and cornea (the clear membrane covering the iris). In the most common form of glaucoma, the drains get backed up (no one knows why) and the fluid either flows out more slowly or stops flowing completely. The fluid buildup increases pressure throughout the eye, damaging the tiny blood vessels that feed the retina and optic nerve. Without nutrients, the cells of the optic nerve begin to die, and your vision begins to die, too.

Glaucoma is a leading cause of blindness in America. About one of every seven legally blind Americans has lost his or her vision to this progressive eye disease, and nearly a million have become visually impaired. Heredity plays a significant role in glaucoma: Your risk is far greater than normal if others in your family have had the disease. If you are African-American or have diabetes, anemia, or atherosclerosis, your risk is also considerably higher.

There's no cure for glaucoma; it can only be controlled. But controlling it can save your sight. "It's very amenable to treatment," Dr. Bradford says.

The key to successful control is early diagnosis. "By the time the doctor can see any damage, the actual damage to the optic nerve is significant," Dr. Bradford says. "It's like not weighing yourself until you've gained 200 pounds." Once you've lost some vision, you can lose your remaining vision even faster, she says.

Thankfully, an ophthalmologist doesn't actually have to see damage to detect glaucoma. There are seven or eight different tests that reveal pressure, vision loss, and nerve damage, Dr. Bradford says. "You put all the tests together and decide whether there's enough suspicion for glaucoma damage to put the person in treatment."

One crucial test is measuring the pressure inside your eye. Just because your fluid pressure is high doesn't mean you have eye damage, Dr. Bradford says. "Some people can have higher than normal pressure yet never have glaucoma damage," she says. "Others get damage at lower pressures."

The key to early diagnosis is a yearly eye exam if you're over 40 years old, Dr. Bradford says. "If everybody in your family gets glaucoma at age 20, you should be checked earlier," she says. "I've had people come in nearly blind from glaucoma at age 40, and they say, 'Yes, Dad went blind from glaucoma at 42.'"

Getting the Drop on Glaucoma

Medication in the form of eyedrops is the first line of glaucoma treatment, Dr. Bradford says. A class of drugs called beta-blockers is often the first medication prescribed. In eyedrop form, they're known by such brand names as Optic, Betagan, and Betoptic.

The main problem with medication is side effects, sometimes so severe that people refuse or "forget" to take it, Dr. Bradford says. Glaucoma patients are supposed to drop the medication in their eyes up to four times a day to keep the pressure steady. But in one study, one-fourth of the patients missed an entire day of medication each month, and 30 percent used their entire daily dosage in a short period instead of spreading it throughout the day.

"Any medication can have side effects, and even physicians forget potential side effects from eyedrops," Dr. Bradford says. "Most people don't have any trouble at all, but older people can get a dramatic slowing of the heart rate, so they need their pulse checked before they're put on the drops. In fact, some patients' heart rates drop so much it can put them at risk for heart failure." Other side effects can include hallucinations, male impotence, and exacerbation of asthma.

Other antiglaucoma drugs also have side effects. "So you still have to be careful," Dr. Bradford says. "I tell my patients to let me know if they're having problems and to let other physicians know they're on the eyedrops." Also be sure to ask your doctor or pharmacist *exactly* how you should take the drops—how much you should take and how often. It's not a guessing game.

One antiglaucoma drug, pilocarpine, now comes in a wafer form, so you don't have to remember to use drops and can't take it improperly. The contact lens-size wafer, called Ocusert, slips under either your upper or your lower eyelid and works steadily for a week. The main disadvantages are that it's more expensive, you may have trouble adjusting to the feeling of something under your lid, and it can fall out, especially when you're sleeping.

"It's very frightening to be told you have glaucoma," Dr. Bradford says. "But it's like being told you have high blood pressure. If you take the drops and have follow-up exams, you should do fine and keep your vision. You're not going to go blind."

Glaucoma Surgery: Turning On the Faucet

With the side effects that come with medication, it's no wonder that many people with glaucoma ask for surgery. In fact, British ophthalmologists favor surgery over medication, Dr. Bradford says. In America, laser surgery (called laser trabeculoplasty, or LTP) is the second choice if medication fails. The surgeon focuses the laser light on the eye and makes about 50 tiny burns in the drainage area, where the cornea and iris meet. "It doesn't punch a hole in the area," Dr. Bradford says. "It just shrinks one area with scar tissue. That pulls open other areas, and the fluid can drain out." It's an outpatient procedure with little pain.

If more conventional surgery fails to control your glaucoma, your doctor may decide to give you some high-tech plumbing called the Molteno implant. It's a small plastic plate that's attached to a ¾-inch-long silicone drainage tube. The surgeon sews the plate onto the white of your eye and inserts one end of the tube into your eyeball and the other end behind the eye. The excess fluid will drain out to the back of your eyeball, where your body will absorb it.

This little faucet can be installed in a 40-minute hospital operation. You'll use antibiotic-steroid eyedrops for about six weeks after the surgery. Your eye should lose the redness and regain its normal vision in about two weeks.

"There are certain people for whom other methods to control glaucoma have failed," Dr. Bradford says. "That's when the Molteno implant might be used. There are risks with it, too. Any time you put a prosthetic piece in the body, you risk infection or failure of the piece. Certainly there are people who have had their vision saved by the Molteno implant."

Macular Degeneration

Approximately 10 in 100 people over the age of 60 will have some vision loss from macular degeneration, according to Dr. Klein. In fact, it's official name is age-related macular degeneration.

"If you live long enough, you're going to have some macular degeneration," Dr. Klein says. "But it doesn't necessarily have to influence your sight to a significant degree," he says.

Indeed, there's only a 4 in 100,000 chance you'll go blind from macular degeneration. Still, it's second only to glaucoma as a cause of legal blindness in America, and it's the number one cause of new cases of blindness in people over 65.

The macula is the central area of the retina, which

lines the back of the eye. It's responsible for sharp central vision, necessary for reading, driving, and recognizing faces and fine details. With increasing age, this tissue can break down and lead to vision loss. The major symptoms are a blurring of central vision, development of a blind spot, and distortion of straight lines into wavy lines. The degeneration usually affects both eyes to some degree, but only one eye might suffer significant vision loss.

Macular degeneration is usually classified into two general types—dry and wet. The dry type is the most common, accounting for 80 to 90 percent of the cases, Dr. Klein says. Its symptoms evolve so slowly that you may not notice them, except to become aware that "Hmm, I can't see as well as I used to." It's usually not enough loss to become legally blind, but it can interfere with driving and reading, he says.

"One theory suggests that it's caused by exposure to light over a lifetime, especially the shorter wavelengths like blue and ultraviolet," Dr. Klein says. "The retina has to react to this light, and the tissues lose their ability to handle the waste products this reaction produces. Free radicals accumulate and destroy the tissues."

The wet, or exudative, form is less common and much more serious. It comes on quickly and progresses rapidly—usually over a matter of weeks. New blood vessels start growing beneath the macula (again, no one knows why, although the body might be trying to repair the macula). These blood vessels bleed and leak and form scar tissue.

"The wet form is responsible for approximately 90 percent of legal blindness caused by macular degeneration," Dr. Klein says. "And it's the one form that is sometimes treatable by lasers."

Early diagnosis is important to be able to treat it with lasers. If you're at risk, you need at least annual eye checkups, Dr. Klein says. Often the first sign is a distortion or blurring of vision in one eye when you read or look at objects with straight lines.

Having the dry type doesn't protect you from getting the wet type, Dr. Klein cautions. "If you have the dry type, you have to be aware of precipitous changes," he says, "especially a rapid development of blurriness or developing a central blind spot over a period of days or weeks." These symptoms could herald the onset of the wet type. If this happens, see a doctor immediately.

Delaying Degeneration

There's no known cause for macular degeneration and no known way to prevent it, Dr. Klein says, although the likelihood you'll develop it is higher if your family has a history of it. What's more, there are no effective medical treatments for the more common dry type, which may get worse with time.

One hope comes from a theory that oxidation and free radicals play a part in the disease. "If somehow we can help the eye get rid of those waste products, maybe we can help macular degeneration," says Dr. Klein. That's why some doctors prescribe supplements of antioxidants like vitamins C and E and beta-carotene. Other often-recommended supplements are the trace minerals zinc and selenium, which are important in the retina's metabolism.

There is some evidence that at least zinc can be of some benefit. A study at the Louisiana State Eye Center found that patients who took 100 to 200 milligrams of zinc twice a day had less vision loss and less deterioration of their retinas than patients who took a placebo. The researchers, however, warned that the study was small—only 151 people—and that excess zinc can have dangerous side effects. Large amounts of vitamin E can also have side effects. For these reasons, self-treatment with nutritional therapy is not recommended.

Detached Retina

No one can describe a detached retina in quite the same way as ophthalmologist Wayne Fung, M.D., consultant to the Retina Clinic at the California Pacific Medical Center in San Francisco. Imagine a basketball, Dr. Fung suggests, inflated with gelatin. Now imagine that gelatin melting, from the center outward. Imagine that the only firm part of the gelatin left is an outer shell; the rest has turned to liquid. Now imagine that outer shell finally collapsing inward.

That's about what happens to your eyes as you age. The basketball is your eyeball. The gelatin is the vitreous humor, a gel that fills the eyeball and that's as firm at birth as an ice-cold batch of gelatin. "By the time you reach 30 or 40 years old, the vitreous humor begins to melt like gelatin sitting on the kitchen counter," says Dr. Fung. As it melts, "floaters" appear—tiny, unmelted pieces of the gel that appear as little spots or strings in your vision.

Finally, the solid outer layer of the gel caves in—and there's no more gelatin in contact with your retina. You feel nothing. There are no symptoms. "It happens safely in 9,999 of 10,000 people," Dr. Fung says. But if you're that 1 in 10,000, you get a detached retina.

The retina is the crux of your vision. It's literally an extension of the brain that lines the inner surface of the

(continued on page 536)

Coming: Blindness Prevention Techniques

We asked vision experts to look into the future for insight as to what's possible for the prevention of blindness. Here's what they had to say.

Glaucoma. Researchers are studying the use of computers for early diagnosis of glaucoma, says ophthalmologist Cynthia Bradford, M.D., assistant professor of ophthalmology at the University of Oklahoma Health Sciences Center in Oklahoma City. "You take a picture of the optic nerve and have the computer analyze it," she says. "Then you repeat the process six months later and see if the computer can be more sensitive in picking up any changes in the optic nerve." She also thinks lasers will become even more popular, allowing people who don't respond to medication to get surgery sooner.

Cataracts. "The instruments used in cataract surgery will get smaller and smaller," Dr. Bradford says. "And eventually the solid lens implant will give way to a substance that's injected through a little hole. It will be able to focus just like your natural lens. There are a lot of bugs to be worked out still, but it could be wonderful, and people will line up for that one."

Macular degeneration. Ophthalmologist Wayne Fung, M.D., consultant to the Retina Clinic at the California Pacific Medical Center in San Francisco, is working on using a natural immune system chemical called interferon alpha-2a as a treatment for the wet (and more serious) form of macular degeneration. In this disease, the eye for some reason goes overboard in producing masses of tiny blood vessels, which bleed and form scar tissue under the retina. Dr. Fung believes that the distressed macular cells are telling the body to make the abnormal blood vessels. He also thinks that this type of interferon can nullify the messages the distressed cells are sending. Another possibility is that interferon "turns off" the cells that are sending the distress signal. Injections of this type of interferon can reverse or at least slow down this abnormal growth of blood vessels and can clear up the bleeding, Dr. Fung says.

Other advances could come in the form of chemicals that can be applied directly to the retina to loosen the scars of macular degeneration, Dr. Fung says, "without dissolving the retina." The scars could then be peeled off, smoothing out the retina and restoring sight.

Eye transplants? Not much chance of eye transplants anytime in the near future, says Dr. Fung. "We can't transplant nerve tissue, and the retina and optic nerve are extensions of the brain," he says. "It's the same reason we can't transplant spinal cords." Some neurologists are now trying to grow retinas in test tubes using natural body substances called nerve growth factors (NGF). "In macular degeneration, the outermost colored layer of the retina gives out," Dr. Fung says. "Researchers are trying to apply NGF to this layer to see if it can be regenerated."

Another, so far unlikely, development is a visual aid like a miniature camera inside a glass eye. The miniaturization is attainable, Dr. Fung says, "but there's no way to transfer the image to the brain." Again, nerve tissue is involved, and man has not been able to duplicate it.

eyeball and transmits visual signals to the brain's vision centers. What happens is that the collapsing gel, rather than peeling cleanly away from the retina, instead pulls a chunk of the retina with it, leaving a hole. "The now-liquefied gel flows through the hole and collects beneath the retina like water behind wallpaper," Dr. Fung says.

As the fluid accumulates beneath the retina, it detaches the retina from the wall of the eye. It's painless, but you do get visual symptoms. "You may notice a gray or dark curtain coming in from the top, bottom, or side of one eye, depending on where the hole is," Dr. Fung says. "When the hole first forms, you may see a shower of hundreds of black dots and a lot of strings." These aren't floaters. "Blood from the torn retina is bleeding into the eye," he says. "Some people have described it as black ink being dropped into clear water or hundreds of blackbirds flushing out of a tree."

If you see these symptoms, get to an ophthalmologist immediately; your vision is in danger.

Surgery for Detached Retina

Treatment for a detached retina keys on the hole or holes. "We can't patch the retina, because we have no good glues that the human body will tolerate," Dr. Fung says. Surgeons can't take the eye out for repairs, either. "I tell my patients that if I could do that, I'd take your eye home tonight, and after dinner, I'd take it down to the shop and fix it, and you could pick it up in the morning," Dr. Fung says.

In a surgical procedure called the scleral buckle, the surgeon first finds the hole. In cryosurgery, the wall of the eyeball is frozen at the place where it adjoins the hole in the retina. Or a laser can be used to burn the area from inside the eye. Either method makes the body's immune system inflame the area, sealing up the hole with a scab, "using the body's own glue," Dr. Fung says. Then tiny, sterile sponges are sewn in that force the outer wall inward to meet the retina.

The success rate of a scleral buckle is about 90 percent, and you're usually out of the hospital the following day. You'll have some pain for a few days, but you should be able to return to work in about a week.

A newer technique is the pneumatic retinopexy. The hole in the retina has to be in the upper half of the eyeball for this method to work. That's because the surgeon injects an expandable gas into the eyeball, and as the gas expands inside the eye, the gas bubble naturally moves up. The surgeon then has you sit up and positions your head so that the expanding gas blocks the hole. Sometimes a laser will be used to reinforce the seal. The body absorbs the fluid that has built up beneath the retina, and the retina gradually settles back into place.

The entire procedure can be done right in the doctor's office in 30 to 60 minutes. You do have to be careful for the next few days, holding your head in the position the surgeon suggests in order to keep the gas bubble over the hole.

"You don't have to walk on eggshells, but the hole does have to be in the upper part of the eye, because we can't expect someone to stand on their head for 8 hours a day," Dr. Fung says. Again, the success rate is about 90 percent.

PART 5

Answers for a Longer Life

Screenings
and Self-Exams

How Important Are They?

Let's rephrase that question. What's the most important thing in your life? Your spouse? Your grandchildren? That little sports car you just bought, knowing that passing 50 doesn't mean slowing down?

Screenings and self-exams are at least as important as those things because they protect you from cancer, heart disease, and stroke. That in turn makes it possible for you to enjoy your marriage, your family, and all the other good things in your life.

But it's clearly not practical to walk into your doctor's office and ask for every test in the book. Besides, some of them just aren't worth taking. In the Medical Testing chapter on page 55, you got a quick read about the important medical tests for adults over 50. Now it's time for a closer look at what they're all about and why you need them.

Blood Pressure Screening

"Testing for high blood pressure is at the top of the list of needed tests," says Timothy A. McAfee, M.D., associate director of preventive care at the Group Health

Cooperative of Puget Sound in Seattle, the nation's oldest and largest consumer-governed HMO. High blood pressure damages artery walls and dramatically increases your risk of heart disease and stroke (see High Blood Pressure on page 435).

It's easy enough to get a reading on the machine at the drugstore or even to take your own at home, but this test also is part of just about any visit to your doctor's office. Your doctor will place an inflatable cuff on your upper arm. When the cuff tightens, the doctor will get a reading of how forcefully your blood is being pumped by your heart. According to the American Heart Association, acceptable blood pressure falls within a range rather than a set number. While a "normal" reading is around 120/80 millimeters of mercury (mmHg), for most adults, a reading less than 140/90 is good news. Talk to your doctor about what is a good blood pressure for you to aim for.

Blood pressure goes up and down over the course of the day, so a random reading may not be accurate. Here's how to get the best reading, says Lawrence LaPalio, M.D., medical director of geriatrics at Columbia La Grange Memorial Hospital in La Grange, Illinois.

Control consumption. Avoid stimulants that speed your heart rate, such as coffee or alcohol. A drink the night before can interfere.

Get comfortable. Five minutes before the test, sit in a comfortable, relaxed position with your arm at heart-height. Rest quietly.

Take the average. Ask your doctor to take several readings and average them. Get a reading before you head for home—you may be more relaxed. Or average the readings taken over several office visits.

Beware of the white coat. For some people, just being in the doctor's office causes nerves to surge and blood pressure to rise. And there could be more to it than that. "If your blood pressure rises due to stress in the doctor's office, it may also rise in response to everyday events," says Dr. LaPalio. "If it goes up every time you drive in traffic or go to a new place, it should be treated."

Get the full picture. For high blood pressure, you need treatment immediately, says Dr. LaPalio. But if you fall in the mild to moderate range, get the true picture by monitoring your own blood pressure for a month or so. Dr. LaPalio recommends that you measure your blood pressure at different times of the day, and when you're in different moods (stressed, relaxed, happy, depressed, active). Write down the readings, the time, and other relevant factors—what you ate and drank, if you exercised, if you took medications, and what you were doing when you took the measurement.

Breast Examination and Mammography

Since the risk of breast cancer increases with age, women over 50 need all the parts to get the whole picture. Tumors that distort the breast's structure or have absorbed calcium often show up on the mammogram you take yearly. Further physical examinations by your doctor (who feels for any lumps in the breast), as well as your monthly self-exam, can pick up what the mammogram misses. While this trio may not find all cancers, their use provides earlier diagnosis and saves lives.

A mammogram consists of compressing the breast between two plates (which may be a little uncomfortable) so a low-dose x-ray can record two or three images of the tissues. There is some controversy over whether screenings are needed after age 60 (because few studies have been done of that population), but "from an individual's point of view, it makes sense to continue to get mammograms," Dr. McAfee says.

What can screening do? A 20-year study of breast cancer published by the American Cancer Society showed that screening results in a survival rate of 86 percent in women diagnosed with breast cancer. Here are some suggestions for getting the best results from your examination, from Joseph Aisner, M.D., director of clinical sciences at the Cancer Institute of New Jersey in New Brunswick.

Check for quality. Make sure that the facility you go to for a mammogram is accredited by the American College of Radiology. That tells you the machinery is adequate and the staff is trained.

Make one trip. Use a facility that develops the pictures on the spot. That way, if there's a problem with the film, the technician can reshoot. You don't have to return for a second test.

Tune your technique. Ask your doctor or nurse to show you exactly how to perform a self-exam. Or ask for a referral to a class, especially one where you can learn by using a "phantom," a silicone model in which several tumorlike BBs have been implanted. You can learn what to feel for in your own breasts.

Get Yourself Covered

Many health insurance programs cover preventive care such as health screenings. So check your policy or call your agent.

If you're 65 or older (or have a disability), you probably use Medicare. Although regulations may change in the future, this program routinely covers only a few screening tests. It doesn't cover checkups. "But if you visit the doctor because something's wrong—if you have a symptom—Medicare will cover the visit," states an official of the Health Care Administration in Baltimore. "It covers tests your doctor decides that you need."

Medicare does cover two key tests for women.

Mammograms. If you're at low risk, the program picks up the tab for one mammogram every three years. High-risk women can get one every 11 months if they're age 64 or younger, and one every 23 months at age 65 or over.

Cervical screening. Medicare covers one Pap test every three years, unless your doctor considers you to be at risk. In that case, there are no restrictions on how often you can have this test performed.

Some states get grants from the Centers for Disease Control and Prevention to provide screenings for breast and cervical cancer. That means free mammograms and Pap tests, says Joseph Aisner, M.D., director of clinical sciences at the Cancer Institute of New Jersey in New Brunswick. So ask your doctor or call the American Cancer Society or an area hospital to check on the availability of low-cost or free mammograms and Pap tests.

Cervical Screening

"Pap tests have reduced death from cervical cancer by more than 95 percent in the past 35 to 40 years," notes Dr. Aisner. A lot of women stop getting their yearly Pap tests as they get older, but they shouldn't, he says.

It's a relatively painless process in which your doctor inserts a speculum into the vagina, opens it to reveal the cervix, and takes a small sample of cells from the vagina and the cervix. The cells are examined for cancer.

Unless you've had a full or partial hysterectomy, your doctor should get samples both from the vagina and from the endocervix, which is the cervix at its opening, says Dr. Aisner. A vaginal Pap test isn't always enough because the most common site for cancer is at the opening to the cervix. However, in post-menopausal women it may not be possible to obtain an endocervical sample, he says.

Cholesterol Testing

You'll need to donate just a very small sample of blood for a lab test to determine your levels of each of LDL cholesterol (which you want low) and HDL cholesterol, which you want high. Inexpensive home test kits give you the total cholesterol but not the level of important HDL cholesterol. Still, these tests may provide a starting point for you and your doctor to determine your risk, says Dr. LaPalio. If your doctor thinks that you're at risk for heart disease, more expensive cholesterol testing for HDL and total cholesterol will probably be covered by Medicare or other insurance.

From Dr. LaPalio, here are three suggestions for making your readings more accurate:

Get Your Levels in Line

Here's a scorecard to help track your progress in controlling your cholesterol levels. To lower your risk of heart disease, you generally want higher levels of the beneficial HDL cholesterol and lower readings for total cholesterol and the harmful LDL cholesterol. The key point to remember is: the lower your LDL level, the lower the risk. Here's a rundown of what the cholesterol readings indicate when you get a blood test, according to the American Heart Association.

Total Cholesterol (mg/dl)	Evaluation
Less than 200	Desirable
200 to 239	Borderline high
240 and over	High

LDL Cholesterol (mg/dl)	Evaluation
Less than 130	Desirable
130 to 159	Borderline high
160 or more	High

HDL Cholesterol (mg/dl)	Evaluation
50 to 60	Desirable for an average woman
40 to 50	Desirable for an average man
Less than 35	Low

Take a seat. Sit down for between 5 and 15 minutes before your test. Standing up or lying down can affect the readings.

Keep it low-key. Don't do strenuous exercise the day before your test. It will temporarily elevate HDL levels.

Test dry. Keep away from alcohol for 48 hours before your test, because it artificially raises HDL levels.

Colon and Rectal Screening

Colon cancer, the third leading cause of cancer death in the United States for men and women, starts out as a benign polyp. That's why the early detection that comes with screening can make such a big difference. "Screening decreases colon cancer mortality," says James E. Allison, M.D., clinical professor of medicine and assistant director of the internal medicine program at the University of California, San Francisco. "It can have the same life-extending benefits as breast cancer screening."

Here's a review of the more common ways doctors test for colon and rectal cancer.

The fecal occult-blood test. There are several ways to get this done. One involves the doctor taking a smear sample as part of your physical examination. Another test can be done at home using a kit from your doctor. You just wipe a stool sample on pieces of cardboard that are then analyzed by a laboratory.

Chemicals used in the testing react to some foods, says Dr. Allison, so to get an accurate reading, change your diet a few days before the test. Stay away from red meat, turnips, horseradish, broccoli, radishes, cauliflower, cantaloupes, and other melons. But do eat lots of other fresh vegetables and fruits, because they'll help stimulate bleeding from lesions, increasing the chances that they'll show up on the test.

Test results may also be skewed by vitamin C supplements (which will give false negatives), and aspirin and other nonsteroidal anti-inflammatory drugs (which will give false positives). Avoid medication that can cause gastrointestinal bleeding. If your hemorrhoids are flaring up, wait until they quiet down, suggests Dr. Allison.

And any fecal testing for colon cancer is prone to false positives because it's simply looking for blood in the feces, which can be caused by hemorrhoids, diverticulosis, or a host of other noncancerous conditions. And no fecal occult-blood test picks up nonbleeding cancerous lesions.

Still, this is a test worth taking because it's very inexpensive (under $20 for the lab work). Even if you have to pay for it, a positive reading means that the more expensive tests that give you maximum protection will probably be covered by Medicare and other insurance.

Flexible sigmoidoscopy. Okay, now we're into the stuff you don't want to read about, even though the usual schedule for women and men over 50 calls for a sigmoidoscopy only about once every five years. In this procedure, a thin, hollow, lighted tube is inserted into the rectum and lower colon. There, it picks up precancerous polyps and removes them before they turn dangerous. The device also spots cancerous lesions.

The downside is that sigmoidoscopy views only one-third of the length of the large intestine's left side. That's where many cancers develop, notes Dr. McAfee, but not all.

Colonoscopy. "I think colonoscopy is probably the best screening examination," says Dr. McAfee. That's because the thin tube travels the entire length of your large intestine, allowing your doctor to find and snip off any polyps, as well as identify any cancerous formations. Sure, it's more uncomfortable (and more expensive) than the other tests, but since colon cancer takes so long to develop, "you're home free for 5 to 10 years, maybe longer," after the test, notes Dr. McAfee.

Diabetes Screening

Talk about easy! Testing for diabetes only requires one drop of blood. So if you're overweight, get thirsty often, urinate more frequently than you used to, or just don't feel well, ask your doctor to test levels of sugar in your blood, advises Dr. McAfee.

Electrocardiogram

The electrocardiogram that you get at least once every decade of your life (especially if you already have heart disease or risk factors for heart disease, such as smoking, diabetes, or hypertension) gives a printout of your heart's activity. That lets you know whether your heart is working efficiently.

Lung Cancer Screening

This one's not on your screening calendar, and for good reason. "We don't recommend chest x-rays or any screening for lung cancer anymore," says Dr. McAfee. Studies show that by the time you can see a lesion on an x-ray, it's already spread too far. Also, doctors worry that clean x-rays lull smokers into a false sense of security.

Oral Cancer Screening

"I've never seen oral cancer in a patient who didn't smoke or drink," says Dr. McAfee. All the same, he notes, there's no reason not to make this part of your visit. Your doctor will simply perform a visual check of the inner workings of your mouth to look for suspicious-looking growths or lesions.

Ovarian Cancer Screening

Your doctor may recommend an ultrasound examination if you have a close relative who was diagnosed with ovarian cancer at a young age, says Dr. McAfee. Since your family history puts you at extra risk, your insurance will probably foot the bill. In this test a probe is inserted into the vagina, transmitting images of the uterus and ovaries to a monitor. Your doctor will look for changes in the cells lining the ovaries.

Prostate Cancer Screening

Eighty percent of prostate cancer cases are diagnosed after age 65, and 40,000 men die from it every year. Testing is a simple two-part affair: Your doctor will perform a rectal exam to check the prostate. And a blood test, called the PSA (prostate-specific antigen) test, will measure levels of a protein produced by the prostate.

But you should know that many doctors don't agree with the once-a-year PSA screenings recommended for men over 50. Since the disease develops slowly, most men never experience any symptoms, and only 1 in 380 diagnosed with prostate cancer die of it. Biopsied tumors that look dangerous under the microscope sometimes turn out to be slow-growing. On the other hand, points out Gerald W. Chodak,

M.D., director of the Prostate and Urology Center at the University of Chicago Hospitals, tumors that look easy-going can suddenly shift into high gear.

Dr. Chodak suggests considering these factors when deciding whether to follow the once-a-year recommendation for PSA testing for prostate cancer. Get tested if:

♦ You want to minimize your risk of cancer and increase your chances of living as long as possible, regardless of side effects from prostate surgery or radiation, which can include impotence and incontinence.

♦ You expect to live for another 10 to 15 years.

♦ You and loved ones can handle the psychological burden of watching and waiting—one option for some slow-growing tumors.

Just say no if:

♦ You're more interested in the quality than the length of your life.

♦ You want to minimize your risk of complications from treatment to eradicate the tumor.

♦ You only want to take tests that have been proven effective. Prostate screenings miss 20 to 30 percent of cancers.

Skin Cancer Screening

This one you do yourself. Examine your body—from the top of your scalp to the bottom of your feet. If anything looks suspicious, consult your doctor. And remember, you're at extra risk for skin cancer if you spend a lot of time indoors and then go out and get "burned and blasted" by the sun, says Perry Robins, M.D., president of the Skin Cancer Foundation in New York City. "It's the sudden shock or intense exposure to sun that increases your risk."

Also at risk are those who had bad sunburns as children or who sunburn easily or who have a family history of the disease. If you're in the high-risk group, ask your doctor to supplement your own monthly checks with a yearly skin check for you, says Dr. Robins. A doctor will be able to get a better look at hard-to-see places.

What are you looking for? The Skin Cancer Foundation has developed a self-exam guide called "The ABCDs of Moles and Melanomas."

A is for asymmetry. An irregular shape is a sign of trouble.

B is for border. Beware of irregular, scalloped, or notched borders.

C is for color. Different shades of brown or black signal a problem.

D is for diameter. Anything larger than the size of a pencil eraser may indicate a melanoma.

Also, count your moles. You're at risk if your total exceeds 100. And check for changes by keeping a record. Use two line drawings of the human body, one of the back view and one of the front to make a chart (or ask your doctor for illustrations you can use). On the drawings make marks that correspond to the location of moles on your body. Draw a line from the mark to the margin and write down the size, color, and shape of each mole, along with the date of the examination. Use the chart to keep track of changes when you do your next self-examination.

Stroke Screening

Since many people experience symptoms before a stroke, there are things you and your doctor can look for. In fact, your body does some screening for you. As many as 40 percent of strokes are preceded by transient ischemic attacks, or mini-strokes. Symptoms, which may last just a few minutes, include blurred vision, numbness, or weakness on one side of the body, slurred speech, inability to talk, or difficulty in thinking. All these symptoms shout out that your brain isn't getting the blood supply it needs, says Dr. McAfee.

Your doctor can also use a stethoscope to listen to the carotid arteries on either side of the neck that carry blood to the brain. A soft, whooshing sound (called a bruit and pronounced *BRU-ee*) may indicate blockage in the arteries, says Dr. LaPalio. If your doctor hears the sound, an ultrasound test is usually called for, using sound waves to provide a picture of the inside of the arteries.

Okay so far. But here's the problem: The surgery used to clear the blockage can also *cause* a stroke. And the jury is out on just how effective such surgery is. "So far, one good study has shown that screening in certain select populations and then operating on the carotid artery does lower the stroke rate," says Dr. McAfee. "But we need to know more."

Killer
Accomplices

Other Maladies That Contribute to Cancer, Heart Disease, and Stroke

By now you've surely got the message: Cancer, heart attack, and stroke are the big—but beatable—health threats to anybody on the wiser side of 50. And if you read part 4 of this book, Defeating Disease, you're also familiar with a number of other medical conditions that people over 50 can cure, control, or prevent.

A lot of those conditions are of special importance because they lead to or encourage heart disease. Topping that list are high cholesterol, high blood pressure, diabetes, overweight, and depression. You'd probably prefer to hear that the list ends there, but the truth is that there are some more pesky problems that can help cancer, heart attacks, and stroke do their dirty work.

Here, then, is the rest of the story—a rundown of the remaining culprits that help pave the way for the high-profile diseases. The good news is that if you control them, you can outflank the big three.

Atherosclerosis

Atherosclerosis is just the fancy name for hardening of the arteries. And that's what happens—they get stiff and narrow. Low-density lipoprotein (LDL) cholesterol starts the process, attaching to artery walls and even attracting other cells to the site. The walls thicken and stiffen. Tiny shards of bone actually form within the walls, which become inflamed. The body tries to repair the damage but ends up making plaque, the stuff that can break loose and form a clot—and increase your risk of a heart attack or stroke.

The destructive process picks up speed if you already have high blood pressure, diabetes, or high cholesterol levels. But you can fight the effects, says John Cantwell, M.D., director of preventive medicine and cardiac rehabilitation at Georgia Baptist Hospital in Atlanta.

Get hormonal protection. Until menopause, estrogen provides women with protection from hardening of the arteries. Hormone replacement therapy will help restore the benefits.

Slow it down with exercise. Exercise slows the progress of atherosclerosis. It doesn't matter whether you go to an exercise class, take walks, or just work in the house or garden. Strive for 30 minutes or more of vigorous exercise just about every day, says Dr. Cantwell.

Get control. If you can control your high blood pressure and cholesterol, you will help put the brakes on atherosclerosis, says Dr. Cantwell, who notes that just being 20 percent overweight can trigger insulin resistance or diabetes, key contributors to hardening of the arteries.

Adjust your diet. If you cut cholesterol and animal fats, you will also cut your risk, advises Frank

Don't Get X'd Out

Even it's name sounds scary. *Syndrome X*, a cluster of medical conditions that dramatically increase your risk of heart disease and stroke, is composed of (among other things) high blood pressure, high triglyceride levels, low high-density lipoprotein (HDL) cholesterol levels, and premature coronary heart disease. Researchers see indications of this syndrome even in children, but it usually doesn't become a major problem until much later in life.

"All the components of Syndrome X are related to insulin resistance," says Gerald Reaven, M.D., the researcher at Stanford University who coined the term and has pioneered the research into Syndrome X. When insulin can't get into the cells, the body gets the message and mistakenly thinks it needs to make more.

High blood levels of insulin lead to high levels of triglycerides, fats in the blood. This high triglyceride level is related to a low HDL cholesterol level—that is, the level of good cholesterol in the blood.

"You can make a big improvement with lifestyle changes, such as eating a healthy, low-fat diet and doing some aerobic exercise," says Dr. Reaven.

Barry, M.D., a family practice physician in Colorado Springs and author of *Make the Change for a Healthy Heart*. You increase the effects of insulin resistance and diabetes (both of which speed up hardening of the arteries) if you consume a lot of polyunsaturated oils, such as corn, safflower, and sunflower oils. Monounsaturated fats, such as olive and canola oils, provide a healthy alternative.

Take vitamin E. Vitamin E spurs insulin activity and can prevent LDL cholesterol from being oxidized in the body, notes Dr. Barry. One study designed to find out how much vitamin E is necessary for this protection found that 400 international units of vitamin E is the minimum needed to prevent damage. It also found that 800 to 1,200 international units of vitamin E provided more protection. But talk with your doctor first, especially if you are already taking anticoagulant drugs, says Dr. Barry.

Think small. Large meals send insulin and blood sugar up steeply, giving your system more problems to deal with, especially if your cells aren't taking in insulin and sugar as effectively as they used to. Smaller, more frequent meals will take off some of the pressure, says Dr. Barry.

Atrial Fibrillation

With atrial fibrillation, your heart loses its sense of rhythm—and your risk of stroke shoots up, because blood tends to pool and be more likely to congeal. According to the American Heart Association, this disorder is responsible for 75,000 strokes a year.

Symptoms of atrial fibrillation are subtle, including palpitations and shortness of breath. Often, you don't know that you have it until a routine physical picks up the irregular beat or an electrocardiogram maps it out.

Atrial fibrillation usually goes along with other heart problems. You're at risk if you have had a stroke, heart attack, high blood pressure, congestive heart failure, hyperthyroidism, heart valve or rheumatic heart disease, or if you have abused alcohol.

Your doctor will probably prescribe an anticoagulant, followed by a regimen of drugs to help your heart keep its steady beat.

Barrett's Esophagus

It seems pretty innocent at first—little benign tumors on your esophagus, the pipe that moves food from mouth to stomach. The growths frequently start out as irritations caused by digestive juices that spurt upward from the stomach. Symptoms include heartburn and difficulty in swallowing.

But, as in the case of many cancers, harmless little lumps can turn malignant. Doctors once thought that this condition also increased your risk for colon cancer. But a study performed in five French hospitals suggests that is not the case.

Chronic Infections

When your body's cells are damaged, repaired, then damaged again on a frequent basis, you're setting the stage for cancer, says Dr. Cantwell. Pay attention to skin sores, especially if they are exposed to the sun. Scar tissue, too, is more at risk.

"We know that chronic ulcerative colitis, an inflammatory disease of the colon, seems to be associated with increased risk of cancer," says Dr. Cantwell. "It is very likely that all of the body's tissues react the same way to chronic irritation."

Colds and Respiratory Infections

In an English study of 96 older men and women, researchers found that the increased risk of winter colds may make the blood more likely to clot in the arteries that supply the heart. That may be caused by increased levels of fibrinogen and factor VIIc, substances in the blood that lead to increased clotting.

Fibrinogen actually provides the scaffolding around which clots form, and it is linked to higher rates of heart disease. An Israeli study, for instance, followed more than 3,000 male heart patients for three years. The 111 men who died during the study all had higher levels of fibrinogen than did the survivors.

One theory is that respiratory infections trigger the body's infection-fighting mechanisms, which also increase blood clotting. But the increase in winter strokes and heart attacks could also be due to seasonal variations in high blood pressure, weight gain, and lack of activity when the temperature drops.

One common bacterium, *Chlamydia pneumoniae*, may be tied to higher rates of heart disease. This bacterium causes upper and lower respiratory tract infections. It increases the concentration of fibrinogen and sialic acid in the blood, which is also associated with higher rates of heart disease. Furthermore, research shows that people with the high levels of fibrinogen may have twice the amount of the harmful LDL cholesterol. Their levels of protective high-density lipoprotein (HDL) cholesterol are lower than normal, too.

Still, experts aren't willing to put too much emphasis on colds and bacterial infections as risk factors for heart disease, cancer, and stroke. "It's much less significant than other factors, such as high blood pressure, cholesterol, and diabetes," says Dr. Cantwell.

All the same, you can make changes in your lifestyle to keep fibrinogen levels down: Lose weight and eat a diet low in saturated fat. Include vegetables, fruit, and fish in your diet, says Dr. Cantwell.

Insulin Resistance

Insulin resistance often leads to diabetes—and that's not all. "Insulin resistance and the abnormalities associated with it accelerate atherosclerosis, which leads to heart disease and stroke," says Gerald Reaven, M.D., a researcher at Stanford University. He estimates that insulin resistance affects 25 percent of all Americans.

If you have insulin resistance, your system doesn't respond to the insulin you make. That's a problem because insulin is the substance that makes it possible for sugar to get into your cells and provide important nourishment. So your pancreas gets the signal to work overtime to produce extra supplies of insulin because the insulin it makes is insufficient to do the job. Over time, it may not be able to sustain the extra insulin production, and you end up with not enough insulin. That's when insulin resistance turns into diabetes.

But insulin resistance alone leads to its own share of problems. Several studies show that insulin resistance and high blood levels of insulin appear in as many as half of the patients with high blood pressure. And it changes the size of your LDL cholesterol, which is a risk factor in coronary heart disease. In this instance the LDL cholesterol particles become smaller and denser and more easily oxidized, allowing them to grab on to artery walls and narrow them.

There is much you can do to help your body use sugar and insulin more efficiently, reversing insulin resistance and preventing or minimizing diabetes.

Get active. People who exercise can enhance their body's insulin, decreasing insulin resistance, says

Dr. Reaven. The American Heart Association recommends that people get 30 to 60 minutes of aerobic exercise three or four times a week.

Lose weight. Being overweight is not the only risk factor in insulin resistance, but it's an important

Prescription for Prevention

Cancer, heart disease, and stroke don't arrive out of the blue. Lots of little problems pave the way for these major maladies. So all the little things you can do to assure your general health play important protective roles.

Do:

■ Keep cholesterol, blood sugar, blood pressure, and body weight within normal limits.

■ Exercise regularly to prevent the circulatory slowdowns that lead to heart disease and stroke.

■ Take vitamin E at 400 international units daily to activate your insulin reserves and protect your cells from damage.

■ Eat small meals to help your system take in insulin and sugar more efficiently.

Don't:

■ Smoke.

■ Let winter weather make you inactive.

■ Be a hot reactor.

■ Get low on potassium. You risk getting high blood pressure.

one. If you're overweight and subsequently lose weight, your body will improve its sensitivity to insulin, and you will become less insulin-resistant, says Dr. Reaven.

Check your inheritance. There is a genetic component to insulin resistance and diabetes. Your risk of developing insulin resistance or diabetes is higher if you are of non-European ancestry. If that fits your family's description, be particularly careful to lower your risk, advises Dr. Reaven.

Put out the cigarettes. Another good reason to quit now: Smoking increases insulin resistance, says Dr. Reaven.

Hepatitis

This highly infectious disease comes in several forms. Two kinds, hepatitis B and C, are linked to liver cancer. You get type C through blood transfusion or sharing contaminated needles. Type B can get into your system through blood transfusion, sexual contact, or sharing contaminated needles or instruments.

Stomach Ailments

Results from one study suggest that stomach cancer may be tied to a type of common bacteria, *Helicobacter pylori*. The little organisms produce chronic upset that may eventually allow cancerous cells to take over. In an American study, doctors found that half of the people who visited their family doctors for stomach complaints had these bacteria to blame. Antibodies that your body produces to fight the bacterial infection may actually stimulate cancer cells in the stomach. The infection can be treated with antibiotics.

Are You Hot?

The standard tests that doctors use to tell whether you're an easily stressed "hot reactor" (and at greater risk for disease) are pretty simple, so take your pick, says Frank Barry, M.D., a family practice physician in Colorado Springs and author of *Make the Change for a Healthy Heart*. For the first two tests, you'll want to take a blood pressure reading twice—once before the test and once during the test for comparison.

Test 1: Chill out. Put your hand into a cold bucket of water for 1 minute and have someone measure your blood pressure right after you take it out. If it goes up into the high range in response to physical stress, you're a hot reactor.

Test 2: Do some math. This one's a little more cerebral. Start with the number 100 and mentally subtract 7, then continue to subtract 7s until you get to 2. In the midst of your figuring, have your blood pressure taken. "There's no exercise, no threat to your life, but a lot of people still feel mental stress and their blood pressures shoot up," says Dr. Barry.

Test 3: Talk to yourself. You can also test yourself without the shock of cold water or math. Ask yourself: Are you working toward your own true goals or someone else's? If you're busy trying to keep up with the Joneses, "you're still in the rat race, even if you have retired. You're much more likely to feel the effects of stress regardless of whether you're a hot reactor," says Dr. Barry.

Stress

In the film *West Side Story*, members of the Jets, a New York street gang, urge each other to "stay cool." Researchers who study stress say the same thing: Stress can make you vulnerable to heart disease, cancer, and stroke.

Feeling stressed or overwhelmed raises your blood pressure and can even trigger heart arrhythmias. "We know that stress can contribute to increased cholesterol and hypertension," says Robert Carney, Ph.D., professor of medical psychology at Washington University School of Medicine in St. Louis.

People who react strongly to stress are called "hot reactors" by cardiologists and psychologists. Their stress triggers an extra release in the flight-or-fight hormones that gave your Stone Age ancestors an edge over saber-toothed tigers. The hormones tell your heart to pump faster, which increases your blood pressure.

Stress also releases free fatty acids into your system, giving your body the energy boost it needs. But unless you're really going to wrestle a prehistoric feline, your body doesn't have a use for these compounds. They turn into dangerous, artery-clogging cholesterol.

Chronic stress may also decrease your body's immune response, leaving you more vulnerable to a cancer. Researchers at the National Institute of Mental Health in Bethesda, Maryland, found that stress activates hormones that allow viruses and cancerous cells to get to work.

How do you lower stress? It depends on what motivates you. "Some people, in their heart of hearts, decide that it's easier to take a pill to reduce high blood pressure," Dr. Barry says. "Others prefer to make lifestyle changes."

Whatever your approach, you'll feel less stress if you feel in control of your life, notes Dr. Barry. Get that control by establishing goals, writing them down, and working toward them, giving less attention to little things that aren't really important to you. Ask yourself, "What do I want to accomplish in life?" Here are techniques that many people find effective in relieving stress.

Relax and enjoy. Believe it or not, relaxation and enjoyment take some effort—or at least some calculation. "A lot of people realize that if they sit in a chair all day, they will make their health worse, but in the years of work, they have forgotten how to enjoy themselves," says Dr. Barry. "If you enjoy life and develop a sense of playfulness and humor, you'll be less prone to stress, anxiety disorders, and depression."

Heed changes. Stress goes up with major life changes, such as the first few months after retirement. "Your routine changes immediately, but your mind and body are still tuned to the habits that may have taken 65 years to form," says Dr. Barry. Often, just acknowledging the stress helps to bring it down.

Remember that less is more. Many older people feel the stress of a fixed income. "Take advantage of the burgeoning simplicity movement," says Dr. Barry. When you sit down and think about what makes you happy and what makes you worry, you may find that you don't need the second car, the cabin in the mountains, or the new furniture. You may find that what makes you happy are family and friends, and fewer material things. Letting go of what's not important helps cut costs and stop stress.

Get on with life. Especially when you retire, you may be tempted to live vicariously through your children and grandchildren. That always produces stress because it doesn't work. Instead, live your own life. Do volunteer work to establish a larger circle of friends and responsibilities. Take courses at your local college.

Change your inner environment. Biofeedback or meditation will relax you mentally and lower stress, says Dr. Barry. Try reducing the psychological stress that raises your blood pressure by repeating a sound, word, phrase, or muscle activity while you passively disregard other thoughts.

Say good-bye to beepers. A lot of people feel as though they are always on call, says Dr. Barry, thanks to pagers, cellular phones, and the like. Take a break from technology, perhaps spending a restful day with the phone unplugged. Get *unbusy*. Allow yourself time to do nothing.

Thyroid Imbalance

In a study of 2,000 men and women age 60 and over, researchers found that thyroid imbalance can interfere with the rhythm of your heart's beat. Those with slightly overactive thyroids were most at risk, a condition called subclinical hyperthyroidism. If you have it, your thyroid releases a low level of thyrotropin, a pituitary hormone that controls the production of the thyroid hormone. Your doctor can prescribe medication to regulate hormone production.

Index

Underscored page references indicate boxed text and tables.

F

579

M

MACARONI AND CHEESE,
LOW-FAT, 131
MACULAR DEGENERATION,
524, 530–33,
<u>534–35</u>
MAGNESIUM
for blood pressure control,
444–45
for hearing loss, 418
recommended amount of,
<u>79</u>, 83
MAMMOGRAPHY, 543, 544,
<u>545</u>
MANGOES, 227–28
MAO INHIBITORS, FOR
DEPRESSION, 397
MARGARINE, WATER
CONTENT OF, 125
MARINADE, YOGURT AS,
132
MARRIAGE, <u>37</u>
for extending life span,
14–15
MASSAGE, FOR BACK PAIN,
379
MAYONNAISE
alternatives to, 122
in restaurant food, 136
MEATS, 130–31, 455
buying, 127
deli, low-fat, 127–28
iron in, 363–64, 365
lean cuts of, <u>194</u>
trimming fat from, 295
"A MEDICAL ADVANCE TO
EASE QUITTING,"
<u>353</u>
MEDICAL HISTORY, FAMILY,
18–19, <u>22</u>, 57

MEDICARE, SCREENING
TESTS COVERED BY,
<u>545</u>
MEDICATIONS. *SEE ALSO
SPECIFIC
MEDICATIONS*
exercise and, 313, 322–23
MEDITATION, 72
for menopausal problems,
481
for smoking cessation,
354, 356
in yoga, 75
MEDITERRANEAN DIET,
<u>110–11</u>
MEMORY LOSS, 464–65,
471
preventing, with
alcohol, 31
diet, 466
exercise, 466
Ginkgo biloba, 50
glucose, 466–67
mental stimulation,
467–71
sleep, 466
vitamin E, 81
MENOPAUSE, 472–74, 478,
481–82
hormone replacement
therapy (HRT) for,
475–76, <u>477</u>, 478
self-help for, 479–82
MENTAL FUNCTIONING,
EXERCISE FOR
IMPROVING, 313
METAMUCIL, 48, 155
MICROWAVING, AS LOW-
FAT COOKING
METHOD, <u>114–15</u>,
130